MEDICAL HISTORIES OF CONFEDERATE GENERALS

Medical Histories of Confederate Generals

BY JACK D. WELSH, M.D.

The Kent State University Press
Kent, Ohio, and London, England

© 1995 by The Kent State University Press, Kent, Ohio 44242
All rights reserved
Library of Congress Catalog Card Number 94-8673
ISBN 0-87338-505-5
ISBN 0-87338-649-3 (pbk.)
Manufactured in the United States of America

06 05 04 03 02 01 00 99   5 4 3 2

LIBRARY OF CONGRESS CATALOGING-IN-PUBLICATION DATA
Welsh, Jack D., 1928–
    Medical histories of Confederate generals / by Jack D. Welsh.
    p. cm.
    Includes bibliographical references (p.).
    ISBN 0-87338-505-5 (cloth : alk. paper)   ∞
    1. United States—History—Civil War, 1861–1865—Medical care. 2. Generals—
Medical care—Confederate States of America. 3. Confederate States of America.
Army. 4. United States—History—Civil War, 1861–1865—Medical care—
Bibliography.
5. Medicine, Military—Confederate States of America. I. Title.
E625.W45 1995   94-8673
973.7'75—dc20   CIP

British Library Cataloging-in-Publication data are available.

Dedicated to

ROBERT MONTGOMERY BIRD, M.D.
February 1, 1915–December 30, 1976

Friend, Mentor, Teacher,
Physician, Virginian

Contents

Acknowledgments

IN THE LIMITED space allowed, I cannot adequately express my deep thanks to the literally hundreds of individuals who have contributed to this project over the years. Many searched local, family, archival, and newspaper records during lunch hours, weekends, and evenings. Appreciation should be expressed also to all those who made a stranger feel welcome, who answered my inquiries and helped me make the transition from one research world based on observations, experiments, and statistics, to one with even more uncertainties. Dr. Richard J. Sommers, Archivist-Historian, Department of the Army, U.S. Army Military History Institute, Carlisle Barracks, Pennsylvania, consistently shared his broad knowledge, understanding, and patience. Michael P. Musick of the National Archives was always able to find just what I needed or to provide that extra source of information. Dr. LeRoy H. Fischer, Oppenheim Professor of History, Emeritus, Oklahoma State University, provided encouragement over the years. Madel Morgan, Director, Archives and Library Division, State of Mississippi Department of Archives and History, and Richard A. Shrader, Reference Archivist, Southern Historical Collection, The University of North Carolina at Chapel Hill, stand out as individuals who displayed professionalism and wonderful understanding.

Two who made unique contributions were Dennis E. Todd of Cayce, South Carolina, and E. M. Clark, Jr., of West Columbia, South Carolina, who shared information on the generals' burial sites. One or both have visited over half of these sites and verified the information. Without these data it would not have been possible to determine the cause of death in many cases.

Typing from my illegible notes and collating the information over the years were Debby Ann Frazier, Annis Dick, Glenda Dickson, Margaret M. Thompson, and Kristi Wasson. Mrs. Thompson was particularly helpful when I needed her to put it all together.

The dean of the University of Oklahoma College of Medicine, the provost, and the Board of Regents are to be commended for their enlightened view in allowing a six-month sabbatical for research in an area away from the "cutting edge" of modern medicine. Col. David A. Peura, M.D. (Ret.), and his wonderful wife, Kristin, provided a place to stay during my visits to Washington, D.C. Dr. John T.

Hubbell, Director of The Kent State University Press, made the call expressing an interest in the manuscript and made it possible to reach this point. Linda Cuckovich, Assistant Editor, not only took care of the multitude of editing details but tried to understand why I did all of this in the first place. She also became interested in the lives of the generals. Thanks also go to Diana Gordy, who supervised the design of this volume, and to Julia Morton and Flo Cunningham, both of whom offered valuable suggestions in the early stages.

The one who put up with the most during this period has been my secretary, Sylvia B. Mason, who had to contend with house officers, patients, and the medical academic world and still try to locate death certificates and shift her thinking to the mid-1800s.

Introduction

EZRA J. WARNER stated in his preface to his book *Generals in Gray* that his "interest was aroused" by reading Douglas Southall Freeman's *Lee's Lieutenants*. The idea to research medical-related material for this book was also stimulated by reading this three-volume study. Freeman's books, dealing with the command structure of the Army of Northern Virginia, frequently mention the absence of various offices because of wounds or illness, and the influence of the resulting changes in command on the military events. In pursuing my interest in the Civil War, it soon became apparent how little was recorded about these medical occurrences, and how difficult it was to find specific details. It was not clear why some men who had sustained a "severe" wound reappeared on the field in a few days or weeks, whereas others who had received a "slight" wound might not reappear. The types of wounds and how they were cared for were usually not mentioned. What specifically were the medical illnesses and how were they treated? Historians writing about the period often did not mention that a particular officer on the field was sick or had an unhealed wound. In other instances, medical events or interpretations have been reiterated without verification. As a physician, my interest was spurred by the paucity of information and inconsistencies. Consequently, I set out to compile a reference source on the medical histories (wounds, illness, accidents, and causes of death) of the 425 men described in Warner's *Generals in Gray*. This population was chosen originally on the basis of well-defined criteria, and it included Confederate officers of most interest to students of the period.

Because this work represents a collection of medical histories, to include just the events that occurred during the Civil War would provide an incomplete story and be poor medical practice. Therefore, I attempted to find out as much as possible about all medical incidents in the life of each individual. To the reader, some events by themselves may appear inconsequential or extraneous, but they are recounted because they reflect the health of the individual and are a part of his medical history. In addition, a minimum of nonmedical information concerning civilian and military careers is included to further flesh out each man's medical story. Even if medical facts were not available, I include the individual in order to document that a search of all the usual sources has been made.

There are three things the avid Civil War student will not find in this study. First, no attempt has been made to analyze the effects of the individual's medical problems on a battle or on the war. I believe this approach is better left to the military historian with more knowledge, insight, and interpretative skills in the area. Second, there is an absence of heroics and glory. Once an officer became a patient, there was little glamour in a broken arm, a suppurating wound, a shaking chill, or a recently amputated limb. Third, the events are usually not detailed as regards their location on the battlefield or the opposing units involved because these data are of little medical importance and can be found elsewhere. What is presented, when known, are factors that may have contributed to the wound, injury, or illness, and the outcome. Information on the immediate care, logistics of transportation, timing of operations, and remedies used and recommended by the physicians are included when available. Regrettably, these details are few in number. The fact that many men went into battle sick or continued on the field after being wounded is mentioned—not to show individual bravery, but more to reflect a prevalent attitude toward illness or injuries. The order issued for the general officers participating in the charge on July 3 at Gettysburg not to ride their horses illustrates this point. Among those whose physical condition prevented them from obeying the order and who did ride in on horseback were Eppa Hunton, James L. Kemper, and Richard Brooke Garnett; Hunter and Kemper were wounded, and Garnett was killed.

To the professional historian of the period, what I encountered would not be a surprise. The information found was usually fragmentary, providing just the name of a battle or simply where the individual was when he was injured or became ill—without additional details, or, in some instances, without even a date. Unfortunately, many of the original Confederate medical records that might have been helpful were destroyed when Richmond was burned at the end of the war. Many times only a lone reference to an event, lacking detail or confirmation, was all that could be found. Inclusion or noninclusion of an event in some cases was somewhat arbitrary and depended on the source and supporting data. As a consequence, a number of possible wounds are not included because of insufficient information. Although other incidents mentioned might be considered apocryphal, there were no data found to suggest that they did not happen, and they seemed consistent with other sources.

Many individuals and their commanding officers did not mention otherwise well-confirmed wounds in their official reports. In other instances, wounds, illness, or injuries were treated in camp, and reports were not made. Postwar memoirs and unofficial writings are the only sources of information regarding these events. Gilbert M. Sorrell's postwar writings detailing his multiple wounds, none of which are mentioned in the *Official Records*, provide just one of many such examples. As would be expected, I found that letters home were some of the best sources of information. However, once wounded or ill, many men traveled home or were joined by their family, and thus the letters ceased.

In other cases, there was too much information, all conflicting! Two or more dates for an event, and even varying reports on the physical location of a wound, were found. One examining physician would report a wound had occurred to the right leg, and the next would record the left. Unfortunately, physicians' handwriting then was only slightly better than it is today. Compounding the problems of trying to better identify the various medical diseases is the paucity of descriptions of the patients' symptoms. Even in the instance of a well-studied outbreak, such as that of the "National Hotel disease," which afflicted John Adams and was even discussed before the prestigious New York Academy of Science, a specific diagnosis cannot be made in retrospect. Also, sometimes two or more diagnoses were recorded by physicians who saw the patient at different times. This type of reporting was not inconsistent with a concept held by some physicians that there could be transformation during the course of the illness, for example, from malarial into typhoid fever. Symptom patterns and physical findings such as fever were used to help formulate a diagnosis, but the conclusions were not supported by laboratory or radiographic documentation. Although much was made of the various fevers, thermometers were not available to the majority of military physicians. When an apparently specific diagnosis was recorded, it must be taken into account that many medical terms used in the mid-1800s did not have the same meaning as they do today because there was not yet recognition that pathogenic microorganisms caused disease. For this reason, and as some terms may not be familiar to all readers, I have included a medical glossary. Only the present definition is given, when it has not changed over the years, but mid-1800s usage is also presented when the meaning has changed or reflects different medical concepts.

Common soldiers had rarely left their rural homes, and when crowded together, they were decimated by "childhood" diseases. Few of the general officers were afflicted by such infections during the Civil War. One of the prewar events that might have provided prior exposure to these future Confederate generals was attendance at West Point, where 146 graduated and another ten attended for varying periods. One graduated from the U.S. Naval Academy. At least 250 others went to some institution of higher learning and were exposed to other students. Forty-eight had military service in Florida, and 148 were in the Mexican War or were among the occupation troops. Thirty-one of these men served in both areas. Equally important as a source of prior exposure to disease was service on the western frontier.

The years before the Civil War were a violent time, with duels, murders, and terrible public health conditions. Some of the future Confederate generals went into the Civil War with their health already impaired from the ravages of disease or old wounds. One or more antebellum medical events were found for only a fourth of the individuals, which certainly represents underreporting, considering the times. Accidents or illnesses during the period before the Civil War were particularly difficult to identify, whereas wounds were usually better documented. Nineteen of the future generals had fought in one or more duels or street fights.

Twelve were wounded, and at least four had some residual impairment for the rest of their lives. Albert Pike and John S. Roane had a duel with each other without either being injured. Patrick R. Cleburne and Thomas C. Hindman were wounded in the same street fight. Seventeen had a recorded accident, including two who had accidently shot themselves. Wade Hampton and Ben McCulloch bore scars from fighting bears with a knife! Twenty-nine were wounded in Mexico, and two of these, James G. Martin and William W. Loring, had each lost an arm. Sixteen were wounded by the Seminoles or Plains Indians, six by arrows. One had been wounded in the Texas War for Independence. Pre–Civil War medical illnesses were found for only sixty-nine and included the usual infectious diseases of the period, such as malaria, typhoid, tuberculosis, cholera, yellow fever, and diarrhea. It was not only under combat conditions that exposure to infectious and contagious diseases occurred, because many parts of the country were noted for the "sickly" state of the population. Robert E. Lee had malaria while working in Baltimore harbor, and William N. Pendleton contracted a fever and paralysis of his limbs while traveling across New Jersey before the war.

In some instances I found verifiable evidence that the prewar medical problems continued to impair the men's health during the war. Albert S. Johnston's nerve damage from his dueling wound may have prevented him from realizing he was fatally wounded at Shiloh. Sterling Price's chronic diarrhea, contracted while he was in Mexico, persisted throughout his life and contributed to his death. Pierre G. T. Beauregard's bad throat, which had started when he was a child, was a source of almost continuous difficulty during the war.

In the sequence section I have compiled an overview by dates and geographical locations of the wounds, accidents, and deaths that occurred during the Civil War. Illnesses were excluded from this section because of the difficulty in determining a date of onset. For many wounds, two or three different dates were recorded, and for some I have selected, using the available data, a specific date as a "best bet." In a few instances, when the date of a wound or accident mentioned in the narrative was not found, the event was not listed. The time the individual was away from duty following an illness or injury was sought as an index of severity. Because unit records were usually not available, such information was obtained from *Official Records* or other sources that dealt with their combat or assignment to command. As a consequence, most of the recorded times away represent a longer period than actually occurred.

One or more nonfatal medical events occurring during the Civil War were found for 352 of the group, including seventy-three who subsequently died from other causes. Accidents, usually associated with horses, were identified for forty-one individuals, and were often severe and resulted in time away from duty. Two hundred and forty-one received wounds on one or more different occasions from shells, grapeshot, canister, or minié balls. Saber wounds were documented for seven. At least two received nonfatal wounds from "friendly" Confederate fire. Very often all that was recorded was that an individual had been wounded; there was no information regarding anatomical location, severity, treatment, or outcome. Because the available data were usually incomplete, it is impossible to gain meaningful insight into the surgeon's thinking or decision making. This is particularly true for head or body wounds. Sixty-eight individuals had eighty-one recorded fractures or joint wounds. Two had a fractured jaw and had surgical treatment, which in the case of James P. Anderson was quite sophisticated. Otherwise, little information is available on the management of fractures, except for those of the extremities. Treatment usually consisted of a splint or some form of immobilization and watchful waiting. Bone fragments were frequently allowed to work themselves out of open fractures. Surgery in some instances was performed to remove such fragments or foreign material, or in other cases was for amputation or removal of a segment of bone. Twenty-four individuals had twenty-five amputations, Francis R. T. Nichols having lost both an arm and a leg, and eleven had excision or resection of bones. Amputation was recommended for eight others, but no type of operation was performed, usually because the officer refused all surgical procedures. Six had an amputation of an arm or finger. In four instances a fracture was recorded, and the reason for the surgery in the remainder is unknown. Two died and four returned to some type of duty. Eighteen had an amputation of the lower extremity, one because of uncontrolled bleeding and the rest usually for shattered bones or a severe joint injury. Four died and seven returned to duty. The remainder did not return or their procedures occurred at the end of the war. There was recorded evidence that at least five of the officers used an artificial leg. Robert C. Tyler was on crutches because of an amputated leg when he was killed, and M. C. Butler later participated in the Spanish-American War on his wooden leg. Eleven had an excision or a resection of bone, seven of the upper, and four of the lower, extremity. Most were performed after amputation had been considered, and half were primary procedures. However, in the case of William Hugh Young, resection was delayed for about three months and was probably performed because of infection. There was no mortality, and eight were able to return to duty.

I found a recorded illness during the Civil War for 230 of the men. This number also is doubtless an underestimation, as illnesses were rarely mentioned in the *Official Records* or the men were treated by unit surgeons in camp and the event never documented. Details were few and exact diagnoses are difficult to establish in retrospect. Most of the identified illnesses were infections of the respiratory or gastrointestinal tracts, one of the "miasma" diseases, or were simply listed as "fever." Acute and chronic rheumatism were common complaints.

The sick or wounded Confederate officer usually spent little time in the hospital. He remained in his quarters when possible, went to a private residence, or returned to his home for convalescence. When he was unable to join his family, his family frequently came to him and provided care. Recovery was often delayed due to complications caused by what we know now were bacterial infections. These secondary infections could be more devastating than the original injury, and they accounted for the major suffering and time away from the field. This could explain why what appeared initially to be a "slight" wound proved later to be quite debilitating.

Ninety-six of the generals died during the war: fifteen died from disease, natural causes, or accidents; two died in duels; one was assassinated; and one committed suicide. The remaining seventy-seven were killed in action, died from their wounds, or died from complications associated with their wounds. Six of these died after an amputation, half of which were secondary procedures. Four bled to death on the field, and two bled to death later. Tourniquets were not available on the field for most of the officers, and their use was even discouraged by some Confederate surgeons. Albert S. Johnston did have a tourniquet with him at the time of his fatal wound, and had it been used early enough, his surgeon thought, his life might have been saved. Two died accidentally from Confederate fire, and it has been suggested that a third, James Dearing, was similarly killed.

After the war, some of the former generals attained high positions and their lives were well documented, but the majority held modest jobs or went off into relative oblivion. Data I was able to retrieve on the 329 survivors' postwar health were scanty, and such medical data were found for just over a third of these men. Their medical conditions on the whole were not unusual or unexpected. For a few it was documented that wartime illness or wounds plagued them for the rest of their lives, and it can only be guessed how many others suffered from residual problems. Some information was located on the cause of death for 206 individuals, with death certificates or burial records accounting for 145 of these. Infections, strokes (paralysis), heart disease, and renal disease were frequent causes of death, with a low incidence of recorded cancer. As a group, they were obviously a hardy lot, more than half of the 329 survivors being seventy years of age or more at the time of death. The last to die, Felix H. Robertson, expired in Waco, Texas, on April 20, 1928.

Because initially there was little compiled medical information on what had happened to the 425 men, this study also allowed an almost "prospective" study, something much respected by medical scientists. The incidents presented occurred throughout the whole theater of the war; therefore, as patients, the general officers were treated by various physicians with different educational backgrounds. The care received by Stonewall Jackson or Richard S. Ewell was no doubt different in degree than that given to the common soldier, but it still reflected the same medical concepts. Considered as a whole, these data present a different perspective of the actual Confederate medical system than impersonal statistics or the details of unusual happenings.

Because I had developed a physician-patient interest in all of these generals, it was very difficult to stop searching for more information. During my medical career I have taken care of veterans of five wars, and these veterans of the Civil War, in a sense, bring the total to six. Like most patients' medical histories, those presented here are incomplete, with important and intriguing loose ends, and probably some half-truths. It is hoped that this book will stimulate others to help complete these medical histories.

Abbreviations

ADAH	Alabama Department of Archives and History, Montgomery, Ala.
AGO, LR	Adjutant General's Office, Letters Received, National Archives, Washington, D.C.
BU	Baylor University, Waco, Tex.
CMH	*Confederate Military History*
CR	Confederate Records, Record Group 109, Chap. 6, National Archives, Washington, D.C.
CSR	Compiled Service Records, National Archives, Washington, D.C.
CV	*Confederate Veteran*
CWM	College of William and Mary, Williamsburg, Va.
CWTI	*Civil War Times Illustrated*
CWTI Coll.	*Civil War Times Illustrated* Collection, USAMHI, Carlisle Barracks, Pa.
DU	Duke University, Durham, N.C.
FC	Filson Club, Louisville, Ky.
LH	Lloyd House, Alexandria, Va.
LSU	Louisiana State University, Baton Rouge, La.
MC	Museum of the Confederacy, Richmond, Va.
MDAH	Mississippi Department of Archives and History, Jackson, Miss.

MHS	Missouri Historical Society, St. Louis, Mo.
MSHW	*Medical and Surgical History of the War of the Rebellion.*
MSU	Murray State University, Murray, Ky.
NA	National Archives, Washington, D.C.
NAD	Death certificate not available for time of death.
NCSA	North Carolina State Archives, Raleigh, N.C.
OR	*War of the Rebellion: A Compilation of the Official Records of the Union and Confederate Armies.* (All references are to Series 1 unless otherwise specified.)
RLB	Robert L. Brake Collection, USAMHI.
RNA	Death certificate requested and not available.
SCL	South Caroliniana Library, University of South Carolina, Columbia, S.C.
SHC	Southern Historical Collection, Library of the University of North Carolina, Chapel Hill, N.C.
SHSP	*Southern Historical Society Papers.*
TSLA	Tennessee State Library and Archives, Nashville, Tenn.
TXSL	Texas State Library, Austin, Tex.
UG	University of Georgia, Athens, Ga.
UTA	University of Texas at Austin, Austin, Tex.
UV	University of Virginia, Charlottesville, Va.
USAMHI	U.S. Army Military History Institute, Carlisle Barracks, Pa.
USMA	U.S. Military Academy.
VSL	Virginia State Library, Richmond, Va.
WLU	Washington and Lee University, Lexington, Va.

A

DANIEL WEISIGER ADAMS • *Born May 1, 1821,* in Frankfort, Kentucky. In a duel in 1843, Adams killed a writer who had been critical of his father. The man had thrown him to the ground and was on top of him when Adams pulled a derringer from his pocket and shot him in the head. Adams later became a practicing lawyer and eventually entered Confederate service as a lieutenant colonel of the 1st Louisiana Regulars. On April 6, 1862, while at Shiloh, a rifle ball hit him in the head. The projectile penetrated the skull above the left eye and came out just behind the left ear, resulting in the loss of the eye. Taken from the field in a helpless condition, Adams was thrown into a wagon with the other wounded soldiers. Progress was almost impossible because the muddy road had been torn up by the wagons and artillery. Because Adams was senseless and covered with mud, the driver thought he was dead and threw his body along the road to lighten the load. Men of the 10th Mississippi noticed signs of life and attended to him. He had nearly regained both his physical and mental capacities by the middle of May and was promoted to brigadier general on May 23. He was ordered to report for duty on August 13, 1862, and participated in the Battle of Perryville on October 8. In command of the Louisiana Brigade at Murfreesborough on December 31, 1862, he received a slight wound of the left arm from a piece of shell. Not able to go back to the field the next day, he turned over his command. In May 1863, he felt well and wanted to return to duty. Participating in a charge at Chickamauga on September 20, 1863, Adams was wounded in the left arm again. He remained in command until he became so exhausted that he was left on the field and captured by Federal troops. He was taken to the hospital at Murfreesborough without having received any medical aid. A ball had fractured the middle third of the left humerus and produced considerable tumefaction and pain. He was administered chloroform on September 23 so that doctors could determine the extent of the injury and whether amputation was required. The ball was embedded among the bone fragments, all of which were removed, together with the pointed end of the upper fragment. The specimens consisted of six pieces of bone, which represented two inches in length, and a battered conical ball. Although shortening of the limb would result, conservative treatment was selected, because any deformity was considered tolerable if the functions of the hand could be preserved. About four weeks after the operation, the arm was put up in splints of coaptation, and Adams was sent through the Confederate line under a flag of truce at the solicitation of Gen. Braxton Bragg. He went to La Grange, Georgia, to recuperate; after his recovery he was given command of the cavalry brigade in northern Alabama and

Mississippi. He was assigned to command of the District of Central Alabama in September 1864. On February 6, 1865, he was told to report to Gen. E. K. Smith, commander of the Trans-Mississippi Department, for assignment to an appropriate post duty or to any administrative department. Following his parole at the end of the war, he again took up the practice of law in New Orleans. Adams had complained of not feeling well for a few days before his death. On June 13, 1872, he was writing a legal brief at his office when his head suddenly fell forward. A physician was called immediately; he prescribed some medicine, which revived Adams rapidly. The physician left after telling Adams to go home and to continue to take the medicine. Within a short time, Adams said he felt very sick. He expired within a few minutes, before the doctor could be found again. He was buried in Jackson, Mississippi, in an unmarked grave in Greenwood Cemetery.[1]

DEATH CERTIFICATE: NAD

1. Combined Service Record, National Archives (hereafter cited as CSR); U.S. War Department, *The War of the Rebellion: A Compilation of the Official Records of the Union and Confederate Armies*, vol. 10, pt. 1:537, pt. 2:533; vol. 16, pt. 1:1122, pt. 2:756; vol. 20, pt. 1:670, 792–94; vol. 30, pt. 1:200, 379, pt. 2:222; vol. 39, pt. 2:869; vol. 48, pt. 1:1368 (hereafter cited as *OR;* unless otherwise indicated, all references are to Series 1); John Francis Hamtramck Claiborne Papers, Library of the University of North Carolina, Southern Historical Collection (hereafter cited as SHC); St. John Richardson Liddell, *Liddell's Record*, ed. Nathaniel C. Hughes, 82; *Medical and Surgical History of the War of the Rebellion*, vol. 2, pt. 2:669, Case no. 1615, incorrectly identified as Wirth Adams (hereafter cited as *MSHW*); *Southern Historical Society Papers* 10:20 (hereafter cited as *SHSP*); Glenn Tucker, *Chickamauga: Bloody Battle of the West*, 236; *Confederate Veteran Magazine* 3:278 (hereafter cited as *CV*); Gen. Clement A. Evans, ed., *Confederate Military History* 10:291, La. (hereafter cited as *CMH*); *New Orleans Daily Picayune*, June 14, 1872.

JOHN ADAMS • *Born July 1, 1825*, in Nashville, Tennessee. He graduated from USMA in 1846. Served in the Mexican War. He arrived at Fort Leavenworth in August 1846 but because of a severe attack of fever was advised not to continue his travels. He reported at Santa Fe on October 10 and was temporarily attached to Company G at Albuquerque, remaining at that post sick for the balance of the year. In November 1850 he was ordered to go to Las Vegas; though on the sick list, he had no choice but to go. In March 1851, Adams's arm was injured when one of his company's wagons fell into the Arkansas River. He applied for a twenty-day leave of absence but was refused. Although he was able to ride a horse by June, it took almost four months for his injury to heal. While in Baltimore on general recruiting duties in March 1857, he had an attack of "National Hotel disease," which he acquired in Washington, D.C. Profuse watery diarrhea, nausea, and thirst characterized this disease, which tended to relapse over a number of weeks or months. Adams was to be transferred to the Pacific, but the surgeon did not think he could tolerate it, as it would be hazardous for him to pass the Isthmus of Panama or contiguous regions. Adams's initial request for a leave was not granted. It was not until August that he received a leave, but not enough time was allowed for him to recover completely. After he resigned from the United States Army in May 1861, he received a captaincy of cavalry in the regular Confederate Army and was commissioned brigadier general to rank from December 1862. On

November 30, 1864, early in the Battle of Franklin, Adams was wounded severely in the right arm near the shoulder but would not leave the field. Later, on horseback, he attempted to jump the Federal breastworks and was mortally wounded. There are two reports as to what happened. In the first, he fell, hit by nine bullets fired by the Federal color guard, and his horse, which was also hit, fell on top of him. When they could, the Federal troops lifted the horse, while others dragged the general from under it. Adams was conscious, realized his condition, and asked for water. One of the Federal soldiers gave him his canteen, and another brought cotton for a pillow. Adams died shortly afterward. According to the other report, made by a member of the 15th Mississippi who knew Adams, after he was wounded he crawled back toward the Confederate lines and died thirty or forty yards from the Federal works. The next morning his body was recovered, placed in an ambulance, and taken to the residence of Col. John McGavock. He was buried at Pulaski, Tennessee, in Maplewood Cemetery.[1]

1. CSR; *OR*, vol. 45, pt. 1:353, 425; Rita Grace Adams, "Brigadier-General John Adams" (diss.), 30–31, 55, 59–60, 86–88; Adjutant General's Office, Letters Received, 125a/201a, May 24, 1857; ibid., 201.A/125.A, July 1857; James Wynne, "On the Disease Affecting the Inmates of the National Hotel," *American Medical Monthly* 8:347–58; *CMH* 8:285; *CV* 1:208, 264.

WILLIAM WIRT ADAMS • *Born March 22, 1819*, at Frankfort, Kentucky. After service in 1839 with the army of the Republic of Texas, he was a planter, banker, and legislator in Mississippi. He raised the 1st Mississippi Cavalry and was its colonel until his promotion to brigadier general in September 1863. Returning to Mississippi after the war, he held various positions, including postmaster of Jackson. He was killed May 1, 1888, in a street encounter by a newspaper editor from Jackson with whom he had argued. Adams was buried in the Greenwood Cemetery in Jackson.
DEATH CERTIFICATE: NAD

EDWARD PORTER ALEXANDER • *Born May 26, 1835*, in Washington, Georgia. He graduated from USMA in 1857. He left the old army in May 1861 and was appointed a Confederate captain. In mid-May 1862, Alexander had measles and remained in bed for two weeks. On May 30, when he learned that an attack was planned, he left his bed and, although still weak, rejoined the army. At Gettysburg on July 2, 1863, a spent ball ripped through his pants and bounced off of his leg. Alexander's next wound occurred in the Petersburg trenches on June 30, five months after his appointment as brigidier general. He had been walking down a path in full view of the Federal lines when a minié ball ricocheted from the hard ground in front of him and hit him under the left armpit. He walked back with help, and although the wound bled freely, he was able to ride his horse to the camp. The ball, which had just missed the artery and the shoulder joint, was removed under chloroform anesthesia. Alexander's health was already poor as he had been having fever and chills for a week. He was jaundiced and his gums were bleeding. He went home on a leave of absence as a result of his wound. On July 26, 1864, his doctor said that Alexander was suffering from intermittent fever and pain from the unhealed wound and was incapacitated. He also thought that it was not advisable for Alexander to travel to Augusta to appear before the medical examining board. The jaundice slowly disappeared, and Alexander returned to duty in mid-August, although he continued to have chills and fever. In the fall of 1864, besides having occasional aches from his wound, he was still taking medication for the recurring fever and chills that were probably due to malaria. A bout of dysentery during this period was treated by his own concoction of chloroform, brandy, peppermint, and laudanum. He was paroled at Appomattox Court-House. After the war, he held a number of governmental posts and was also a professor of engineering, a businessman, and an author. He had an unspecified illness in 1900. In September 1902, Alexander had a cerebral vascular accident and a convulsion. His convalescence was complicated by aphasia and dizziness. Throughout the remainder of his life he continued to have similar attacks. After a severe stroke in January 1910, he was diagnosed with arteriosclerosis by doctors at Johns Hopkins Hospital. He went into a coma on April 27 and died the next day in Savannah, Georgia. Alexander was buried in the City Cemetery (Magnolia Cemetery) at Augusta.[1]

DEATH CERTIFICATE: Cause of death, cerebral apoplexy, duration of about a week.

1. CSR; *OR*, vol. 40, pt. 1:759; vol. 46, pt. 1:1279; Maury Klein, *Edward Porter Alexander*, 41, 79, 124–27, 213, 221, 224, 227–29; Douglas S. Freeman, *R. E. Lee: A Biography* 3:464.

HENRY WATKINS ALLEN • *Born April 29, 1820*, in Prince Edward County, Virginia. During a duel of July 6, 1844, a pistol ball passed through Allen's upper thighs. A further description of this wound was provided in Latin: "In abdominis partibus inferioribus vulneratus fuit Allen; ictu transcidente et lacerante prorsus membra vitalia." Apparently, the ball, after passing through the soft tissue of his thigh, went across his lower abdomen and injured a vital part. It was stated that there was no conclusive evidence that his manhood was affected. His health was poor in January 1851, and he tried the waters of Cooper's Well near Jackson. In 1859, while visiting London, he almost died from an attack of "Roman fever"; although he lay in a hotel room without friends or medical care, he recovered sufficiently to return home. Poor health in 1860 prevented him from seeking the office of speaker of the Louisiana State legislature. Enlisting as a private in the Confederate Army, he was soon elected lieutenant colonel of the 4th Louisiana Infantry. On April 6, 1862, at the Battle of Shiloh, Allen was shot through both cheeks. Although blood streamed from his mouth, he continued in battle, stopping the bleeding by first placing a handful of cotton lint in the wound and then tying a handkerchief around his face. The next day, because of blood loss and intense pain, he relinquished his command and went to the hospital. After his wound was dressed, he started to lie down when a general retreat took place; he mounted his horse and tried to rally the troops. In May 1862, with his face only partially healed, Allen proceeded to Vicksburg with a detachment. On August 5, 1862, during the battle at Baton Rouge, he was severely wounded when a canister shot fired from a Federal cannon located within fifty yards hit him in both legs. The loss of blood and extreme pain rendered him almost senseless, and he was carried off the field to a private home outside of Baton Rouge. The left leg had only flesh wounds, but the bones of the right leg were shattered; although amputation was recommended, he refused. He remained at a private home for about four months, and by the end of the year he could move around on crutches. Allen left there early in December but by Christmas was again confined to bed in great agony and with little hope of recovery. In early June 1863, while escaping from a hotel fire in Jackson, Mississippi, he was injured. Later in the month he was at Bladon's Springs, Alabama, apparently for his health. Appointed brigadier general in August 1863, he was nominated for governor of Louisiana the same month and conducted his campaign and business on crutches. Allen left for exile in Mexico in June 1865 but could only travel by carriage. In Mexico he became editor of the *Mexican Times.* In October 1865, his leg wound reopened; although amputation was again considered, it was not performed. Prior to his death on April 22, 1866, in Mexico City, he had dyspepsia, increasing pain, and weakness. His physician stated that the breaking down of his whole system culminated in severe inflammation of the stomach, which in turn led to his death.[1] He was buried in Baton Rouge, Louisiana, on the grounds of the old state capitol.

DEATH CERTIFICATE: NAD

1. *OR,* vol. 10, pt. 1:489–90; vol. 15:78, 100, 103, 106; Vincent H. Cassidy and Amos E. Simpson, *Henry Watkins Allen of Louisiana,* 20, 23, 50, 61–62, 72, 77, 79, 81, 86–89, 92, 96–97, 134, 143–44, 158; *Southern History of the War,* 297; Robert U. Johnson and Clarence C. Buel, eds., *Battles and Leaders of the Civil War* 1:605.

WILLIAM WIRT ALLEN • *Born September 11, 1835,* in New York City. Leaving his life as a planter, Allen went into Confederate service as a first lieutenant and was soon promoted to major and then to colonel of the 1st Alabama Cavalry. During April and early May 1862, he suffered intensely with irregularity of his bowels. He had experienced similar attacks of dysentery during prior summers and had great difficulty obtaining relief. His condition improved, so he participated in Wheeler's operations in September 1862. On October 8, 1862, at the Battle of Perryville, he received a slight wound and was off duty for a few days. On December 31, 1862, he was disabled by a gunshot wound at the Battle of Murfreesborough. Some type of surgery was performed soon afterward, yet the injury deprived him almost entirely of the use of his right hand. On February 18, 1864, he made an application to retire. Appointed brigadier general to rank from February 1864, he was back in the field in April. During the Savannah campaign at Waynesboro on November 28, Allen was again slightly wounded. By late December he was on the picket lines, and in February 1865 he fought at Aiken, South Carolina. He was paroled at Greensboro on April 26, 1865. Although he returned to the life of a planter, he also took up railroading and held state and federal positions. At the time of his death, November 24, 1894, in Sheffield, Alabama, he had heart disease. He was buried in the Elmwood Cemetery in Birmingham.[1]

DEATH CERTIFICATE: NAD

1. CSR; *OR*, vol. 16, pt. 1:897–99; vol. 20, pt. 1:959–60; vol. 32, pt. 1:692; vol. 44:411, 988; vol. 47, pt. 1:1066, pt. 2:1147; *CV* 2:324.

GEORGE BURGWYN ANDERSON • *Born April 12, 1831,* near Hillsboro, North Carolina. He graduated from USMA in 1852. Like most West Point graduates of his time, he served on the frontier until he resigned in April 1861 and joined the Confederacy. Initially made colonel of the 4th North Carolina, he was promoted brigadier general to rank from June 1862. At Malvern Hill on July 1, 1862, Anderson was wounded in the hand and carried from the field. He was back in time to participate at Sharpsburg on September 17, 1862, where a minié ball struck him near the ankle joint. He was taken with difficulty to an improvised hospital in the rear. After examination, the wound was considered to be severe but not life-threatening. He was transported into Virginia and then on to Raleigh, where he arrived during the latter part of September. The wound became infected, and he suffered intensely because of the pain. His foot was finally amputated, but he died on October 16, 1862, soon after the surgery. He was buried in Raleigh at the Oakwood Cemetery.[1]

1. CSR; *OR*, vol. 11, pt. 2:557, 622; vol. 19, pt. 1:150, 1024; *SHSP* 14:393, 395; John B. Gordon, *Reminiscences of the Civil War,* 90.

GEORGE THOMAS ANDERSON • *Born February 3, 1824,* at Covington, Georgia. During the Mexican War, Anderson served as a lieutenant of the Georgia Cavalry. He received a commission into regular army service in 1855, from which he resigned in 1858. He was elected colonel of the 11th Georgia Infantry in July 1861 and was promoted to brigadier general in November 1862. At Gettysburg, in the fighting at the Little Round Top on the afternoon of July 2, 1863, Anderson was wounded in the flesh of the thigh and had to leave the field. On July 21, he was given a sixty-day medical furlough, and by September he had recovered sufficiently to join James Longstreet. Following the war he held various jobs in Atlanta and Anniston, Alabama, including chief of police. Anderson was very ill in March 1901 but appeared to be improving by the end of the month. On the first of April he took a sudden turn for the worse, becoming irrational and then unconscious.[1] He died April 4, 1901, at Anniston and was buried there in the Edgemont Cemetery. At his request, he was buried in the coat he had worn when he surrendered at Appomattox. Cause of death: Chronic nephritis and cystitis.[2]

1. CSR; *OR*, vol. 27, pt. 2:359, 397; *CMH* 6:391; *Anniston (Ala.) Evening Star,* Mar. 15, 27, Apr. 1–4, 1901.
2. Burial permits 1894–1903, Edgemont Cemetery, Anniston, Ala.

JAMES PATTON ANDERSON • *Born February 16, 1822,* in Franklin County, Tennessee. Anderson was a practicing physician when he raised and became lieutenant colonel of the 1st Battalion Mississippi Rifles in the Mexican War. In 1849, following the war, he had fever and ague. He served a term in the Mississippi legislature; however, in 1851 his health was so bad that he was unable to make a complete canvass of his county and thus was defeated for reelection. Despite continuing fever and ague, he resumed the practice of law, at which he was fairly successful. By 1853 his health had so deteriorated from both the effects of his sedentary habits and the agues from the miasmatic climate that he was advised to go to a dry, colder location. He was appointed United States marshal for the Territory of Washington and arrived in Olympia on July 4, 1853. His health improved after two months on the trail taking a census of the inhabitants. He later moved to Florida to manage a plantation. A member of the Florida secession convention at the start of the war, he was appointed colonel of the 1st Florida Infantry and was commissioned brigadier general in February 1862. During the retreat from Corinth, he commanded the division until it reached Clear Creek near Baldwin, where he became ill with fever. Later, after rejoining the division at Tupelo, he took part in the skirmish at Monterey, Tennessee, on April 29, 1862. Although a jaw wound finally compelled him to leave the field at the Battle of Jonesborough on August 31, 1864, Anderson had ridden fearlessly along the lines with his staff, recounted Federal general John A. Logan, doing all that a commander could do to make the assault a success. A minié ball had entered Anderson's cheek one-half inch from the angle of the jaw, producing a comminuted fracture of the middle portion of the body of the inferior maxilla. The ball also carried away the three back teeth of the lower jaw and one from the upper jaw. It then passed into the tongue near the root and came out of the top of the tongue near the tip, knocked out the right eye tooth of the upper jaw, and then passed out of his mouth. The fracture of the lower jaw reached clear around on the right side but left the teeth still attached to the dental alveoli; they projected forward some three quarters of an inch. The blow was scarcely felt when he was struck, and it was not until he found that he was bleeding profusely that he became concerned. He rode to the rear and was examined by a surgeon, who sent him back two miles in an ambulance. There a more experienced surgeon removed about an inch and a half of the fractured jawbone after ligating the lingual artery. The remaining fracture was bound up in a bandage that reached over his head, and he was laid down to sleep. Over the next two hours he continued to have serious bleeding. His tongue was so mangled and swollen that the surgeon had great difficulty locating the severed artery to ligate it. In the meantime, it had become dark outside, and they were in the woods with only a tallow candle for light. Anderson speculated the ligation of the bleeding artery was more from good fortune than skillful surgery. When he reached private quarters in Macon on September 3, the hemorrhaging had stopped and the wound was in good condition. By September 5, the swelling had somewhat subsided and there was no further bleeding. A wax impression of the upper teeth and each fragment of the lower jaw was made, and on September 10 an interdental splint was applied, which forced the teeth into place. The whole was secured by means of a mental chin compress and an occipital frontal bandage. The next day the teeth were well adjusted in the splint and in good position, enabling Anderson to take liquids through a small opening in front. The fragments were still in position by the twentieth and remained in place when the splint was removed. By November 1 the bones were perfectly united, and there was no deformity. He was able to use the teeth, and speech was only slightly impaired. Against the advice of his physician, he returned to the army on April 1, 1865, and was assigned to the command of William B. Taliaferro's division. He was required to live on wines, custards, broths, teas, and soups, all of which were hard to secure in the army. For five weeks such items were his only diet, and he could not speak a word. By December his teeth were firmly attached; although he could talk, the teeth were poor incisors. He could masticate any soft food, such as potatoes, hash, and light battercakes, but his tongue was bound down and did not allow full movement. After the Confederate surrender, he spent the first summer in Tennessee with relatives and friends, his health impaired from past wounds. Later he ran a farm newspaper in Memphis for a while and was state tax collector. He died at his residence in Memphis on September 20, 1872, and was buried in the Elmwood Cemetery. His wife attributed his death to effects of his old wounds.[1] Cause of death: Pneumonia.[2]

1. *OR*, vol. 10, pt. 1:507, 800; vol. 38, pt. 3:88, 109, 696, 775; James Patton Anderson Autobiography, SHC; Paul E. Steiner, *Physician-Generals in the Civil War*, 15–17; *CV* 3:36; *CMH* 11:195, Fla.; *SHSP* 24:57–72; *Memphis Daily Appeal*, Sept. 21, 1872; E. N. Covey, "The Interdental Splint," *Richmond Medical Journal* 1:88–91; Sister from Patton, Dec. 7, 1864, Civil War Papers Generals (Civil War Misc. Collection, James Patton Anderson), U.S. Army Military History Institute (hereafter cited as USAMHI).

2. Burial records, Elmwood Cemetery, Memphis, Tenn.

JOSEPH REID ANDERSON • *Born February 16, 1813,* in Botetourt County, Virginia. Graduated from USMA in 1836. He resigned his army commission within a year of graduation and took up engineering. His superintendency of the Richmond Tredegar Iron Works in 1841 was the beginning of his long association with that company. Commissioned brigadier general in September 1861, he saw little field service. He commanded a brigade in the Seven Days' battles and on June 30, 1862, received a blow on the forehead from a spent ball at Frayser's Farm. On July 19, 1862, he resigned to operate the Tredegar Works for the Ordnance Department.[1] After the ironworks were returned to their private owners in 1867, Anderson again took over its operation until his death. He died at the Isles of Shoals, New Hampshire, on September 7, 1892, and was buried in the Hollywood Cemetery, Richmond, Virginia. Cause of death: Cerebral atrophy.[2]

1. CSR; *OR*, vol. 11, pt. 2:880; *CMH* 6:575.
2. Burial Register, Hollywood Cemetery, Richmond, Va.

RICHARD HERON ANDERSON • *Born October 7, 1821,* in Sumter County, South Carolina. Graduated from USMA in 1842. While with the army in Mexico, Anderson and a small group of officers climbed Mt. Popocatapetl, where he suffered temporary snow blindness. Resigning his commission from the U.S. Army in March 1861, Anderson was commissioned a major in the Regular Confederate

Army. In July, he was promoted to brigadier general. A musket ball broke his left arm on the night of October 8–9, 1861, at Santa Rosa Island, Florida. The arm was set, and he convalesced in Pensacola. Although disabled for several weeks, he took part in the action at Fort Pickens on November 22. In February 1862, he was ordered to report to Gen. J. E. Johnston and was assigned to a brigade. At Sharpsburg on September 17, 1862, he was wounded in the thigh and fell from his horse. He returned December 11 and was able to take part in the Fredericksburg battle. He was unable to make a good living after the war and was serving as state phosphate agent when he died. His death was sudden, without any preceding illness, on June 26, 1879, at Beaufort, South Carolina. He was buried there at St. Helena's Episcopal Church.[1]

DEATH CERTIFICATE: NAD

1. *OR*, vol. 6:458–59, 494; vol. 19, pt. 1:150, 840; vol. 21:608; Joseph Cantey Elliott, *Lieutenant General Richard Heron Anderson: Lee's Noble Soldier*, 22–23, 33–34, 59–61, 144.

ROBERT HOUSTOUN ANDERSON • *Born October 1, 1835*, in Savannah, Georgia. He graduated from USMA in 1857. Resigning from the United States Army, he was made a lieutenant of artillery in the Confederate Army in September 1861 and a colonel of the 5th Georgia Cavalry in January 1863. He was absent in Savannah during June and July due to illness. On September 9, 1863, he was ordered to report for assignment to command of outposts on Sullivan's Island. In July 1864 he was appointed brigadier general. Wounded while putting his brigade into position at Newnan, Georgia, on July 30, 1864, he returned in mid-November. Anderson was wounded again while he and Joseph Wheeler were skirmishing with the enemy near Fayetteville, North Carolina, on March 11, 1865.[1] From two years after the war until his death on February 8, 1888, he was chief of police in Savannah. Anderson was buried there at the Bonaventure Cemetery.

DEATH CERTIFICATE: Cause of death, pneumonia congestion.

1. CSR; *OR*, vol. 28, pt. 2:354; vol. 38, pt. 3:956, 961; vol. 44:406–11; vol. 47, pt. 1:1130.

SAMUEL READ ANDERSON • *Born February 17, 1804*, in Bedford County, Virginia. Anderson fought in the Mexican War as lieutenant colonel of the 1st Tennessee Infantry. After serving as postmaster of Nashville, Anderson was appointed major general of state troops in 1861 by the governor of Tennessee. Within a few months he was made a brigadier general in the Confederate Army. Soon after being involved in an engagement near Eltham's Landing in May 1862, he resigned because of ill health. His health had improved by the following month, and in November 1864 he was reappointed to the rank of brigadier general and placed in charge of the Bureau of Conscription for the state of Tennessee until the bureau was abolished. For the remainder of his life he conducted business in Nashville. He died January 2, 1883, at his home in Nashville and was buried in the Old City Cemetery.[1]

DEATH CERTIFICATE: Cause of death, general disability.

1. CSR; *OR*, vol. 11, pt. 1:629–31; Ezra J. Warner, *Generals in Gray*, 10; *Memphis Daily Appeal*, Jan. 4, 1883.

JAMES JAY ARCHER • *Born December 19, 1817,* at Bel Air, Maryland. Served in the Mexican War. His law practice was interrupted twice by service in the regular army, first in Mexico and then again when he reentered the army in 1855. Following the Mexican War he was wounded during a duel with Captain Andrew Porter, who was supposedly the best shot in the U.S. Army. Archer entered Confederate service as colonel of the 5th Texas in 1861 and was promoted to brigadier general in June 1862. On the morning following the capture of Harpers Ferry in September 1862, Archer was too ill for duty. On the seventeenth, sick with fever, he was taken to the battlefield at Sharpsburg in an ambulance and resumed command as his troops formed for battle. The next morning, exhausted, he relinquished his command and left the field until the twentieth. On July 1, 1863, outside of Gettysburg, again sick with fever, Archer was wounded and was captured along with part of his command. He was among the officers taken to Hilton Head to be exposed to the fire of Confederate guns. After his exchange, Archer was assigned to command in August 1864. He died October 24, 1864, in Richmond, supposedly due to impaired health resulting from his wound and imprisonment. He was buried there in the Hollywood Cemetery.[1] Burial records, no information.

1. CSR; *OR*, vol. 19, pt. 1:1000–1001; vol. 21:656; vol. 27, pt. 2:638, 646, 650; vol. 35, pt. 2:147–48; vol. 42, pt. 2:1189, 1274; *SHSP* 8:195–96; James I. Robertson, Jr., *General A. P. Hill: The Story of a Confederate Warrior,* 144; *CMH* 2:171, Md.; *CV* 7:364, 8:65.

LEWIS ADDISON ARMISTEAD • *Born February 18, 1817,* in New Bern, North Carolina. Served in the Florida and Mexican wars. He was dismissed from USMA in 1836 and appointed to the regular army in 1839. He was wounded September 13, 1847, at Chapultepec, Mexico. In May 1861 he resigned to accept the rank of colonel of the 57th Virginia Infantry and in April 1862 received his brigadier general stars. He was wounded at Sharpsburg early on the morning of September 17, 1862, and had to turn over his command. Armistead was expected back within a few days; although it is not certain when he returned, it is known that he took part in the operations in early December. Months later, against the advice of surgeons and friends, he rose from his sick bed to participate in the Battle of Gettysburg. On the third day of the battle, July 3, 1863, he put his black felt hat on the point of his sword and led an assault on the center of the Federal line. Just after scaling the stone wall, he was hit in the chest and arm. With difficulty, he remained on his feet until he reached the Federal artillery, where he fell mortally wounded with his hand on a cannon. One Confederate soldier, who was firing from near his body, thought that Armistead was already dead because he did not move or groan. When the Confederate line retreated, Armistead was taken prisoner and carried to the Eleventh Corps hospital on the George Spangler farm. Armistead, with three wounds to the breast and left arm, died in the Federal field hospital on July 5. He was buried at Baltimore, Maryland, in St. Paul's Churchyard.[1]

1. *OR*, vol. 27, pt. 1:74, 428, 440, pt. 2:1000; vol. 51, pt. 1:174; C. B. Easley to Howard Townsend, July 24, 1913, in D. B. Easley Letters, Charles W. Squires Papers, *Civil War Times Illustrated* Collection

(hereafter cited as *CWTI* Coll.), USAMHI; Frederick Tilberg, "Military Life of Lewis A. Armistead," typescript, Gen. Lewis A. Armistead Misc., North Carolina State Archives, Raleigh (hereafter cited as NCSA); Francis B. Heitman, *Historical Register and Dictionary of the United States Army* 2:13; *SHSP* 10:428–29, 37:148–50, 190–91; *CV* 5:469, 19:371.

FRANK CRAWFORD ARMSTRONG • *Born November 22, 1835,* at the Choctaw Agency, Indian Territory. Following graduation from Holy Cross Academy in Massachusetts, he was commissioned into the regular United States Army and participated in the First Battle of Manassas in a Federal uniform. In August 1861 he resigned and joined the Confederacy. After staff duties he became colonel of the 3rd Louisiana Infantry and later assumed command of cavalry forces. He was promoted brigadier general to rank from January 1863. On September 30, 1863, five miles from Charleston, he was too ill to start an expedition across the mountains and wanted to be relieved from duty with his brigade. He stated that if he was not permitted to wait, he was going to forward a surgeon's certificate. In March 1864 he reported to the headquarters at Canton, Mississippi, and was assigned to the command of a brigade.[1] After the Confederate surrender, he held a number of positions, including U.S. Indian inspector and assistant commissioner of Indian Affairs. He died September 8, 1909, at Bar Harbor, Maine, and was buried in the Rock Creek Cemetery, Georgetown, Washington, D.C.

DEATH CERTIFICATE: Cause of death, myocarditis.

1. *OR*, vol. 30, pt. 4:719; vol. 52, pt. 2:650.

TURNER ASHBY • *Born October 23, 1828,* in Fauquier County, Virginia. A farmer at the start of the war, he collected a group of men who were later incorporated into the 7th Virginia Cavalry. Rising rapidly from captain, he was made a brigadier general in May 1862. On June 26, 1861, while on Kelly's Island in the Potomac River, Ashby received a slight leg wound while trying to find his mortally wounded brother. Nearly a year later, on April 17, 1862, he tried to burn a bridge over the north fork of the Shenandoah near Rude's Hill before the Federal cavalry could cross. The cavalry arrived too soon and began firing; a bullet went through Ashby's boot, grazed his leg, and mortally wounded his horse. A letter written by Stonewall Jackson from the headquarters of the Valley District, Staunton, Virginia, on May 5, 1862, reported that Ashby had been sick. An episode of fever and dysentery confined him to the camp for several days. In mid-May, Ashby was back forming a covering force for Jackson's march. He was killed on June 6, 1862, while fighting a rear-guard action four miles south of Harrisonburg, Virginia. He was attacking Federal troops when his horse was shot. As he rushed forward on foot, he was hit by a ball, which entered his right side just above the hip, passed diagonally upward, and came out under his left arm. The path suggested it had been fired by one of the Federal troops who was lying down behind a fence. Ashby was buried in the Stonewall Cemetery, Winchester, Virginia.[1]

1. CSR; *OR*, vol. 12, pt. 1:426, 782, 789, pt. 3:880; Henry Kyd Douglas, *I Rode with Stonewall*, 50; Millard K. Bushong, *General Turner Ashby and Stonewall's Valley Campaign*, 39, 102, 112; *SHSP* 10:105.

B

ALPHEUS BAKER • *Born May 28, 1828,* in the Abbeville District of South Carolina. An attorney and member of the Alabama state constitutional convention in 1861, Baker enlisted as a private in 1861 and was later elected captain of the 1st Alabama Infantry. During September and October of 1861, he was listed on the company muster roll at Pensacola as being sick. On March 13, 1862, he was placed in command of the steamer *DeSoto* for the evacuation of Fort Bankhead. At Champion Hill on May 16, 1863, in the Vicksburg campaign, Baker was wounded in the foot. One of the bones of his instep was broken; however, he got back in the saddle and remained on the field until exhausted. On May 21, 1863, he requested thirty days' leave on a surgeon's certificate because of his wound. Baker was listed as in command on November 20, 1863. Promoted to brigadier general in March 1864, he was slightly wounded at the Battle of Ezra Church near Atlanta on July 28, 1864.[1] He returned to his law practice after the war. Baker died October 2, 1891, at Louisville, Kentucky, and was buried there in the Cave Hill Cemetery.

DEATH CERTIFICATE: Cause of death, pyelitis.

1. CSR; *OR,* vol. 8, 169; vol. 24, pt. 2:77, 86; vol. 31, pt. 3:725; *CMH* 12:386, Ala.

LAURENCE SIMMONS BAKER • *Born May 15, 1830,* in Gates County, North Carolina. Graduated from USMA in 1851. Until his resignation in May 1861, he served in the regular army, mainly on the frontier. He entered Confederate service as a lieutenant colonel of the 1st North Carolina Cavalry and received his brigadier stars in July 1863. At Brandy Station on August 1, 1863, the bones of his right arm were fractured. Admitted that day to the receiving hospital at Gordonsville, Virginia, he was transferred to a hospital in Richmond the following day, where a primary excision of three inches of the shaft of the humerus was performed on the day of admission. A second operation was performed, but the reasons for it and its type were not described. He left on a furlough in October, which was extended into 1864. Because of the wound, he was unable to continue his active field service. When Wade Hampton became chief of the cavalry in the spring of 1864, he wanted Baker to accept division command. However, Baker's disability prevented him from taking the field. He was ordered to report for assignment to duty in the Second District on June 8, 1864. On December 30, 1864, Braxton Bragg ordered Baker, who was still disabled for the field by his wounds, to proceed to Richmond and to report to President Davis. He was assigned by the War Department to command of the Second Military District of South Carolina. By January, his partial disability necessitated assignment of an efficient second in command to help with his duties. In spite of his physical condition, he took part in the Battle of Bentonville in March 1865.[1] At the end of hostilities, he became a farmer for a while and finally was railroad station agent at Suffolk, Virginia. He died April 10, 1907, in Suffolk and was buried there in Cedar Hill Cemetery.

DEATH CERTIFICATE: RNA

1. CSR; *OR*, vol. 27, pt. 2:312, 324; vol. 36, pt. 3:887; vol. 42, pt. 3:1356; vol. 46, pt. 2:1037; Register Book, Receiving Hospital, Gordonsville, Va., June 1, 1863–May 5, 1864, Eleanor S. Brockenbrough Library, MC; *MSHW*, vol. 2, pt. 2:676, case no. 14; Confederate Records, RG 109, chap. 6, file 178, pp. 50, 586, 588 (hereafter cited as CR, followed by file number:page[s]); ibid. 181:35; Walter Clark, ed., *Histories of the Several Regiments and Battalions from North Carolina* 3:186; *CMH* 4:291.

WILLIAM EDWIN BALDWIN • *Born July 28, 1827*, in Statesburg, South Carolina. While running a business in Columbus, South Carolina, he became a member of a local militia company, which elected him captain in 1861. Soon he was made colonel of the 14th Mississippi Infantry and was promoted to brigadier general in September 1862. On the evening of May 22, 1863, during the siege of Vicksburg, Baldwin was wounded. He relinquished his command until June 13, 1863, when he returned to duty. He was captured at the surrender of Vicksburg but was later exchanged. He died on February 19, 1864, near Dog River Factory, Alabama, as the result of an accident. Baldwin had been horseback riding with friends when his horse stumbled. Baldwin was thrown off, and his neck was broken in the fall. It was suggested that there had been too much whiskey drinking among the whole group. He was buried in the Friendship Cemetery at Columbus, Mississippi.[1]

1. CSR; *OR*, vol. 24, pt. 2:398, 402; Claudius W. Sears Diaries, MDAH.

WILLIAM BARKSDALE • *Born August 21, 1821*, in Smyrna, Tennessee. Served in the Mexican War. Although he studied law, he became editor of a newspaper in Columbus, Mississippi. He was elected to Congress from Mississippi in 1852. At Vicksburg on July 1, 1853, Barksdale had an argument with Reuben Davis and was wounded ten or eleven times with a pocketknife. The wounds were superficial; however, his doctor ordered him to bed. Following an appointment as quartermaster general of Mississippi, he entered Confederate service as a colonel of the 13th Mississippi and became a brigadier in August 1862. He appeared on a list of casualties from Ransom's division in the First Battle of Fredericksburg on December 13, 1862, but details are lacking. There was no report by Barksdale on the battle, and Gen. Lafayette McLaws said that Barksdale had been on a leave of absence and therefore did not make a report. After the battle, Barksdale visited Jefferson Davis in Richmond. He was on the field April 30, 1863, at Marye's Hill and took part in the subsequent battles. On July 2, 1863, at Gettysburg, he was mortally wounded. Federal general Joseph B. Carr had directed his men to bring down an officer on a white horse, who they believed to be Barksdale. Barksdale was first hit by a rifle ball above the left knee but continued in command. Next his left foot was struck near the arch by a cannonball. Continuing in spite of the pain and blood loss, he was finally knocked senseless from his horse by a ball in the left breast. Left for dead on the field, he was captured and carried unconscious to the rear on a litter. He was laid in front of the field hospital on the Jacob Hummelbaugh farm and was examined by a surgeon, who considered his wounds mortal and told him so. One Federal officer thought the chest wound was too large to have been produced by a ball. He stated that with inspiration, copious amounts of blood were forced with a sputtering noise from the wound. Barksdale, alternately burning with fever and asking for water, died the next day.[1] He was buried in Greenwood Cemetery, Jackson, Mississippi.

1. CSR; *OR*, vol. 21:583, 626; vol. 25, pt. 1:839; vol. 27, pt. 1:74, 260, 436; James Willette McKee, Jr., "William Barksdale: The Intrepid Mississippian" (diss.), 46–49, 216, 290–91; David Parker to Mr. Barksdale, Mar. 22, 1882, and E. C. Barksdale to Gentlemen, Mar. 30, 1865, William Barksdale subject file, MDAH; Thomas D. Marbaker, *History of the Eleventh New Jersey Volunteers*, 98; Gen. William Barksdale subject file, RLB Collection, USAMHI; Gregory A. Coco, *Vast Sea of Misery*, 64–65.

RUFUS BARRINGER · *Born December 2, 1821,* in Cabarrus County, North Carolina. Practicing law at the start of the Civil War, Barringer became a captain in the 1st North Carolina Cavalry. At Brandy Station on June 9, 1863, a minié ball entered his right cheek. The ball passed into his mouth, fractured the superior maxilla, and dislocated the teeth of the upper jaw, producing permanent injury. Surgery was performed the same day. Barringer was hospitalized in Salisbury, North Carolina, and was absent on medical leave during July and August of 1863. The chief surgeon of the division headquarters at Asheville, North Carolina, examined him August 13, 1863, and found that he still suffered from the effects of his wound. He was slightly wounded on October 14, 1863, while at Bristoe Station but continued on duty. His rise through the ranks by comparison to many other officers was slow, and he was not appointed brigadier general until June 1, 1864. On June 4 he was assigned to the command of James B. Gordon's cavalry brigade. After the Civil War he became a Republican and was involved in politics. He was not in vigorous health the last few years of his life. In the spring of 1894 his health began to fail, and during the summer he spent a month or so in sanitariums in the North. However, when he returned home in the fall, it was obvious there was little that could be done for him. Realizing he was to die, he spent the last few months of his life setting his house in order.[1] He died near Charlotte, North Carolina, on February 3, 1895, and was buried there in the Elmwood Cemetery. Cause of death: Cancer of stomach.[2]

1. CSR; *OR*, vol. 29, pt. 1:462; vol. 36, pt. 3:873; Clark, *Histories of Several Regiments* 1:424, 427, 3:609; *Charlotte (S.C.) Observer*, Feb. 5, 1895.
2. Burial records, Municipal Cemeteries, Cemeteries Division, Charlotte, N.C.

JOHN DECATUR BARRY · *Born June 21, 1839,* at Wilmington, North Carolina. A recent graduate from the University of North Carolina, he enlisted as a private at the start of the war and was made captain of his company in April 1862. Barry was wounded at Frayser's Farm on June 30, 1862. He participated in military operations in September 1862. On July 27, 1864, at Deep Bottom, Virginia, he was wounded in the right hand by a sharpshooter. The second and third fingers were amputated the same day. He was appointed brigadier general to rank from August 3, 1864, but the appointment was soon canceled. The wound had not healed by November, and he was on extended furlough through December 1864. Because of his disability, he was assigned to departmental duty in North Carolina in February 1865 but returned to command in March during the evacuation of Petersburg. In poor health, he died soon after the war on March 24, 1867, at Wilmington and was buried in Oakdale Cemetery.[1]

DEATH CERTIFICATE: NAD

1. CSR; *OR*, vol. 11, pt. 2:892; vol. 19, pt. 1:986; Clark, *Histories of Several Regiments* 2:56, 63; *Wilmington (N.C.) Daily Journal*, Mar. 26, 1867.

SETH MAXWELL BARTON • *Born September 8, 1829*, in Fredericksburg, Virginia. Graduated from USMA in 1849. He served almost entirely on the western frontier until he left the U.S. Army and was appointed lieutenant colonel of the 3rd Arkansas Infantry in June 1861. Confirmed as brigadier general to rank from March 1862, he was captured at Vicksburg. Barton had a stormy career and was finally assigned to the defenses of Richmond in the fall of 1864. Little is known about his postwar activities. Barton died at Washington, D.C., on April 11, 1900, and was interred at Fredericksburg, Virginia, in the City Cemetery (Confederate Cemetery).

DEATH CERTIFICATE: Cause of death, senility, exhaustion incidental to mitral insufficiency of heart (six months' duration).

WILLIAM BRIMAGE BATE • *Born October 7, 1826*, at Bledoe's Lick, Tennessee. Served in the Mexican War. After a varied career as a clerk, newspaper editor, law student, and member of the Tennessee legislature, he enlisted as a private in the Confederate Army. Later he was elected colonel of the 2nd Tennessee Infantry. On April 6, 1862, while at Shiloh, Bate was on horseback when he was shot through the left leg by a minié ball and suffered two broken bones. Faint from loss of blood, he released the reins and held onto the pommel of the saddle, allowing the horse to return on its own to the rear. He was transported on a cart without springs to Corinth, where he was joined by his wife. The surgeons stated that amputation was mandatory, but supposedly Bate obtained his pistols and prevented the surgery. Later at Columbus, Mississippi, he was seen by another surgeon, who initially also recommended an amputation but then agreed that it was unnecessary. Disabled and unfit for field duty, he was appointed brigadier general and put on garrison duty in Huntsville in October 1862. In March 1863 he was ordered to report for assignment to command a brigade. Bate returned to combat on crutches, which he continued to use until after the war. Unable to mount a horse alone, he had to be lifted into the saddle, and he carried his crutches in one hand while he rode. Although he was quite lame, he did not think that it impaired his usefulness. He was wounded in the battle of Hoover's Gap on June 24, 1863, but did not mention the injury in his report written from a camp near Tyner's Station on July 15, 1863. He was promoted to major general in February 1864. On August 10, 1864, near Atlanta, he was wounded in the knee by a chance minié ball and was taken to the hospital at Barnesville, Georgia. Other sources say that this wound was sustained on August 6 at Utoy Creek. After an absence of two months, Bate rejoined the Army of Tennessee on October 10. He would ride up and down the line using his crutch instead of a sword to urge his men to fight. At the surrender at Durham Station on April 26, 1865, when the call came to stack arms, Bate rode up to what was left of his division, dismounted, and hobbled to the head of his old regiment.[1] Returning to the practice of law, Bate was elected governor of Tennessee and then a U.S. senator. He died March 9, 1905, in Washington, D.C., and was buried in Mount Olivet Cemetery, Nashville, Tennessee.

DEATH CERTIFICATE: Cause of death, primary, la grippe with pneumonia; immediate, heart failure of four days' duration.

1. CSR; *OR*, vol. 10, pt. 1:568, 581, 585; vol. 20, pt. 2:508; vol. 23, pt. 1:611, pt. 2:688; vol. 38, pt. 3:690; vol. 39, pt. 1:826; vol. 52, pt. 2:443; Family Questionnaire (n.d., received Oct. 11, 1922), State of Tennessee, Tennessee Historical Committee, Department of Libraries, Archives and History, Nashville; Park Marshall, *A Life of William B. Bate*, 136, 160, 175; *CV* 2:337; *CMH* 8:292.

CULLEN ANDREWS BATTLE · *Born June 1, 1829,* in Powelton, Georgia. Admitted to the bar in 1852. Battle became lieutenant colonel of the 3rd Alabama soon after the outbreak of hostilities. Due to a wound received at Seven Pines, probably on May 31, 1862, Battle was kept from the field until July 23. He was slightly wounded at Sharpsburg on September 17, 1862. On October 26, he was admitted to a general hospital and furloughed the next day. On April 29, 1863, below Hamilton's Crossing, he was seriously injured when his horse reared and fell into a ditch. On May 1, shortly after his return, he wrenched his back severely in another horse accident while he was leaping a ditch on the Plank Road above Fredericksburg. At Chancellorsville, although still disabled, Battle accompanied his regiment in an ambulance. When he attempted to mount his horse he could not stay in the saddle. Gen. Robert E. Rodes sent him to the rear in his ambulance. Although absent for a while, he participated in the Gettysburg campaign. Appointed a brigadier general in August 1863, he was absent at Tuskegee, Alabama, in November and December, with chronic bronchitis. During the operations south of the James on May 9, 1864, Battle was ready for action if his services were required despite a painful injury to his right foot. He had a thirty-day furlough home to Tuskegee in June because of dysentery and indigestion. At the Battle of Cedar Creek, on October 19, 1864, he was shot in the left knee joint, which injured his kneecap. He was taken to the field hospital, where preparations for amputation of the leg were made. However, the operation was not performed when the surgeons and Battle, fearing capture, learned the day had been lost. After intense suffering, Battle was transferred to the hospital at Richmond, where he remained until furloughed in mid-December 1864. He was never able to return to the field and remained furloughed at home. Battle had to use crutches for two years.[1] After the surrender he again took up the law in Alabama; when elected to Congress in 1868 he was refused his seat. Moving to North Carolina, he became editor of a newspaper and mayor of New Bern. He died April 8, 1905, at Greensboro, North Carolina, and was buried in the Blandford Cemetery at Petersburg, Virginia. Cause of death: Septicemia.[2]

1. CSR; *OR*, vol. 11, pt. 3:650; vol. 25, pt. 1:955–56; vol. 29, pt. 1:877, 885; vol. 36, pt. 1:1084; vol. 43, pt. 1:564, 598; *CMH* 12:388, Ala.; *CV* 13:318.

2. Burial records, Blandford Cemetery, City of Petersburg, Va.

RICHARD LEE TURBERVILLE BEALE • *Born May 22, 1819,* at Hickory Hill in Westmoreland County, Virginia. After entering the law profession, he took up politics and was elected to Congress from Virginia. From 1858 to 1860 he was a member of the upper house of the legislature. He joined the Confederate Army as a first lieutenant of a cavalry company. Beale had severe colic on May 3, 1863, which he thought was from eating bacon gravy, but was able to join his troops in time for the fight at sunrise the next day. Although very ill on the fifth, he did not miss any time from duty and was well by the end of the week. On June 20, 1863, near Middleburg, a piece of shell disabled his right arm. He rode back to the surgeon for treatment and was able to rejoin the regiment the following day. En route to Virginia following the battle at Gettysburg, Beale was sick and had to stay in the rear until the regiment reached Culpeper, whereupon he obtained a ten-day leave of absence. On September 13, 1863, east of Brandy Station, Beale was sitting on his horse watching the battle when a ball struck his right leg. Loss of blood forced him to go to the rear. He was taken to Orange Court-House, where the ball was extracted. He was admitted to the receiving hospital at Gordonsville, Virginia, on September 17 and was transferred the same day to the general hospital in Charlottesville. His wound was complicated by erysipelas and intermittent fever. The final period of his illness was spent under the care of a sister. He arrived home in October and returned to command in November. Still unfit for duty, he was sent back home by R. E. Lee and did not return to the field until late December 1863. After rising through the ranks he was commissioned brigadier general in January 1865. According to a report attributed to W. H. F. Lee, Beale was wounded April 9, 1865, the morning of the surrender at Appomattox, while capturing two federal guns. After the war he returned to the practice of law. On February 18, 1873, Beale was unable to work due to an illness he believed was pneumonia. In May 1888, he experienced back pain, which he concluded was due to his kidneys and liver, and could do only light work. Rheumatic pains in his wrists bothered him during June 1889. Beale died April 21, 1893, in Hague, Virginia, and was buried at Hickory Hill Cemetery.[1]

DEATH CERTIFICATE: RNA

1. CSR; Account book, Richard L. T. Beale to Sue, May 8, 1863, R. L. T. Beale to son, May 11, 1888, and R. L. T. Beale to William, June 13, 1889, and Gen. R. L. T. Beale, "History of the 9th Virginia Cavalry," 69, 94–95, in Beale Family Papers (no. 7754), University of Virginia Library, Manuscript Division, Special Collections Department (hereafter cited as UV); R. L. T. Beale, *History of the Ninth Virginia Cavalry in the War Between the States,* 98–100; Register Book, Medical Department, Receiving Hospital, Gordonsville, Va., June 1, 1863–May 5, 1864, Eleanor S. Brockenbrough Library, MC; *SHSP* 34:243.

WILLIAM NELSON RECTOR BEALL • *Born March 20, 1825,* at Bardstown, Kentucky. Graduated from USMA in 1848. Following service with the U.S. Army on the frontier, he resigned and was appointed a cavalry captain in the Regular Confederate Army in March 1861. He was commissioned a brigadier general in April 1862. Beall was captured at Port Hudson in July 1863. While a prisoner, he was admitted to the Officers' U.S.A. general hospital in Memphis, Tennessee, on July 23, 1863, with anemia and remittent fever. In 1864, Beall was released on parole and, through an agreement between the Confederate and Federal authorities, was allowed to have an office in New York City to sell cotton. The money obtained was used to purchase supplies for Confederates held as prisoners of war.[1] He was finally released by Federals in August 1865 and became a general commission merchant at St. Louis. Beall died July 25, 1883, at McMinnville, Tennessee, and was buried in the Mount Olivet Cemetery in Nashville.

DEATH CERTIFICATE: NAD

1. CSR; *OR*, ser. 2, vol. 7:1117, 1131, 1140.

PIERRE GUSTAVE TOUTANT BEAUREGARD • *Born May 28, 1818,* in Saint Bernard Parish, Louisiana. Graduated from USMA in 1838. Served in the Mexican War. After graduation from West Point, he was assigned to Fort Adams in Rhode Island, where the climate was hard on his health. A chronic throat ailment that had bothered him since boyhood recurred, and he was ill during the winter. In the spring of 1839, Beauregard required treatment in New York for kidney inflammation and was confined to bed for about two months. It was recommended that he go to a warmer climate for his health, and in the fall of 1839, he was transferred to Pensacola, Florida. In March 1847, during the Mexican War, he was kept in bed for several days with a bout of fever and diarrhea. The fever recurred in April, and he was so ill for a few days that he had difficulty getting about. He was reported to have been wounded at Churubusco on August 20, 1847, although some stated he did not participate in the battle. At Chapultepec on September 13, 1847, one musket ball grazed his shoulder and a second wounded him slightly in the thigh. Soon afterward, a third shot hit his side and momentarily stunned him, but his gloves and eyeglass case in his pocket prevented him from being wounded. On the day Mexico City was occupied, Beauregard had the onset of fever and ague, from which he did not recover for weeks. When he returned to New Orleans on June 15, 1848, he was still sick and asked for leave. The fever and ague continued to bother him at monthly intervals, or whenever he was exposed to cold weather. He did not consider himself completely well until after he had taken the water treatment a year later in Biloxi. His health was poor again in October 1858.[1] Resigning his army commission, he was appointed a brigadier general in the Provisional Confederate Army in March 1861. Illness delayed a trip to Montgomery in May, and he was sick when he went to the First Battle of Manassas in July 1861. His appointment as a full general in the Regular Army was dated from July 21, the day of the battle. In January 1862 he was ordered to report to Columbus, Kentucky, but required surgery on his throat before he could leave Richmond. He left on February 2, arrived at Bowling Green on the fourth, and became ill with a cold, fever, and inflammation of the throat on February 7, which confined him to bed and made him unable to continue his trip until the thirteenth. He was ill again in Nashville; when he resumed his travels, he had to stop at Jackson, Tennessee. Arriving there about the middle of February, he was too ill to assume command or to continue on to Columbus. His physicians urged him to rest so as to obtain relief from the chronic throat inflammation and to recover from the results of jaundice. When A. S. Johnston fell at Shiloh on April 6, 1862, Beauregard assumed command, although he was still ill. In June 1862, after repeated recommendations by his physicians to take a rest for his health, he went to Bladon's Springs on the Tombigbee River about seventy-five miles north of Mobile. In August he was assigned to the command of the Department of South Carolina and Georgia. In January 1863, while at Charleston, South Carolina, Beauregard did not think his health could withstand the cold weather if the government sent him to Tennessee. His chronic throat ailment recurred in April 1864; although still ill during May, he believed the water at Weldon, North Carolina, had helped his health. On May 11, he relinquished his sick leave and reported that he was ready and willing to serve the cause to the utter sacrifice of his health. On October 3, 1864, he was assigned to the command of the two military departments known as the Department of Tennessee and Georgia and the Department of Alabama, Mississippi, and East Louisiana. He was confined to quarters with a bad cold in Montgomery on January 28, 1865, and was unable to leave until the thirtieth. By early February he was sick again. Following the war, he had a colorful career in Louisiana as railroad president, supervisor of the state lottery drawing, and state adjutant general. Although Beauregard was very ill prior to his death in New Orleans on February 20, 1893, he appeared to recover and spent his last evening with his family in good spirits. Later, a nurse chanced to go into his room and found him dying. He was buried in the Metairie Cemetery in New Orleans.[2]

DEATH CERTIFICATE: Cause of death, heart disease, aortic insufficiency, and probably myocarditis.

1. T. Harry Williams, *P. G. T. Beauregard: Napoleon in Gray,* 9, 19–22, 26–27, 32–34; Heitman, *Historical Register* 2:14; G. T. Beauregard to Major A. H. Bowman, Oct. 20, 1858, Beauregard Miscellany Letters, Louisiana State University, Louisiana and Lower Mississippi Valley Collections, LSU Libraries (hereafter cited as LSU); *CMH* 1:650.

2. *OR,* vol. 7:880, 889, 893, 895, 906, 912; vol. 10, pt. 1:387; vol. 14:601; vol. 17, pt. 2:599, 601, 623; vol. 36, pt. 2:992; vol. 39, pt. 3:785; vol. 47, pt. 2:1050, 1062, 1113, 1141, 1158; vol. 51, pt. 2:727, 891, 898, 903; vol. 53:271; Williams, *P. G. T. Beauregard,* 63, 115–20, 157, 207; Stanley F. Horn, *Army of Tennessee,* 109, 154; P. G. T. Beauregard to Gen. Sam Cooper, July 17, Aug. 25, 1862, both in P. G. T. Beauregard, Civil War Papers, LSU; Frank E. Vandiver, ed., *Civil War Diary of General Josiah Gorgas,* 98–99, 170; *CV* 1:65.

BARNARD ELLIOTT BEE · *Born February 8, 1824,* in Charleston, South Carolina. Graduated from USMA in 1845. During the Mexican War in 1847 he took part in the siege of Veracruz and was wounded on April 18, 1847, in the assault at Cerro Gordo. He returned in time to be in the field in September. Leaving the Federal army in March 1861, he became a lieutenant colonel of the 1st South Carolina Regulars. In June he was promoted to brigadier general. Bee's brigade was the first to reinforce P. G. T. Beauregard at Manassas Junction, arriving there on July 20, 1861. The next day Bee had dismounted and placed himself to the left of the 4th Alabama. While leading the charge, he was mortally wounded in the abdomen by a bullet. Unconscious, he was carried back to a cabin four miles from the battlefield and died on July 22, 1861. He was buried at Pendleton, South Carolina, in St. Paul's Episcopal Church Cemetery.[1]

1. CSR; *OR*, vol. 2:478, 495; *SHSP* 19:164–67; *CV* 3:7; *Battles and Leaders* 1:213, 237; *CMH* 5:375; John Haskell, *The Haskell Memoirs*, 22.

HAMILTON PRIOLEAU BEE • *Born July 22, 1822*, in Charleston, South Carolina. Served in the Mexican War. He was secretary of the United States and Republic of Texas boundary commission, secretary of the Texas senate, and a member of the legislature. First elected brigadier general of militia in 1861, he was appointed to the same rank in the Confederate Army in March 1862. His early administrative duties poorly prepared him for leading troops. On the morning of January 9, 1864, he was ill and was unable to leave his quarters. At the battle of Pleasant Hill, Louisiana, on April 9, 1864, Bee had two horses killed under him and received a slight wound of the face. He was back on the field the next day. Following the war he moved to Mexico but returned to San Antonio in 1876 when he lost sight in his right eye. Over the years the sight of his remaining eye deteriorated. His health was feeble for some time prior to his death. On October 3, 1897, the day he died, he had retired to his bed as usual. His wife, hearing his heavy breathing, became alarmed, but by the time the doctor arrived, Bee was already dead. He was buried in San Antonio's Confederate Cemetery.[1]

DEATH CERTIFICATE: Cause of death, organic disease of the heart, syncope.[2]

1. *OR*, vol. 34, pt. 1:567, 570–71, pt. 2:849; vol. 48, pt. 2:1286; H. P. Bee to Asbel Smith, June 14, Dec. 7, 1876, H. P. Bee to Guy M. Bryan, Mar. 2, 1894, all in Bernard E. Bee Papers, Barker Texas History Center, UTA; *CMH* 11:225, Tex.; *CV* 5:582–83.

2. San Antonio, Texas Metro Health District, File 255 for 1897, Ledger, 216.

TYREE HARRIS BELL • *Born September 5, 1815*, in Covington, Kentucky. A planter in Tennessee, he raised a company for the 12th Tennessee at the start of the Civil War and was elected its captain. At Shiloh on April 6, 1862, Bell's horse was shot and fell on his leg. This injury disabled him, and he relinquished his command on the seventh. He received severe chest and face wounds at Pulaski, Tennessee, from the explosion of a bombshell; however, he recovered in only a few days. Although the exact date of this injury is uncertain, it probably occurred on September 27, 1864, while Bell was with Nathan Bedford Forrest. Because of his good record, he was commissioned brigadier general in February 1865. In the 1870s he moved to California and did well as a farmer. Returning from a trip in the summer of 1902, Bell became sick while in New Orleans and was taken to the city sanitarium. His physician thought that a blood clot had developed in his brain as a result of the heat, and that it had induced partial paralysis.[1] He died August 30, 1902, and was buried in Bethel Cemetery, near Sanger, California.[2]

DEATH CERTIFICATE: Cause of death, increased intra-cranial pressure.

1. OR, vol. 10, pt. 1:423–24; vol. 39, pt. 1:542–46; CV 6:529; New Orleans Daily Picayune, Aug. 31, 1902.
2. Death certificate.

HENRY LEWIS BENNING • *Born April 2, 1814,* in Columbia County, Georgia. After his admission to the Georgia bar, he was associate justice of the state supreme court and a politician. Without any military background, he was appointed colonel of 17th Georgia Infantry in August 1861 and was promoted to brigadier general to rank from January 1863. In the fight at the Wilderness, on May 6, 1864, Benning was severely wounded in the left shoulder and was carried out on a litter. He was hospitalized in Richmond and Danville, Virginia, during May and was furloughed for sixty days. After receiving extensions of his leave, he returned to duty November 22, 1864, having recovered in a measure from his wound. Following the war he returned to his law practice; he suffered a stroke on the way to court and died on July 10, 1875, in Columbus, Georgia. He was buried there in Linwood Cemetery.[1]

DEATH CERTIFICATE: NAD

1. CSR; SHSP 14:544; CMH 6:395; John Bratton to wife (Betty DuBose Bratton), Nov. 23, 1864, in John Bratton Papers, SHC; William C. Oates, War Between the Union and the Confederacy, 343; Dictionary of American Biography, s.v. "Benning, Henry Lewis."

SAMUEL BENTON • *Born October 18, 1820,* in Williamson County, Tennessee. Attorney and politician, Benton was first captain of the 9th Mississippi; one year later, in 1862, he was colonel of the 37th. On July 22, 1864, during the Battle of Atlanta, he was mortally wounded. A piece of shell struck him over the heart, and he sustained a wound in the foot, which required an amputation. He died in the hospital in Griffin, Georgia, on July 28, before he received his commission as brigadier general to rank from July 26. Initially buried at Griffin, he was later interred in Holly Springs, Mississippi, in Hillcrest Cemetery.[1]

1. CSR of Jacob Hunter Sharp; Samuel Benton subject file, MDAH; Warner, Generals in Gray, 26–27.

ALBERT GALLATIN BLANCHARD • *Born September 10, 1810,* in Charlestown, Massachusetts. He graduated from USMA in 1829. Served in the Mexican War. After duty on the frontier, he left the U.S. Army in 1840 and engaged in a number of private occupations in Louisiana. He entered into Confederate service as a colonel at the start of the war and became a brigadier general in September 1861. In June 1862, because of his advanced age, Blanchard was no longer actively engaged in the field. From June 1862 until February 1863 he commanded the camps of instruction in Louisiana located west of the Mississippi River. After the war he returned to New Orleans and worked as a city surveyor. His death was not unexpected due to his age and failing health. He died in New Orleans on June 21, 1891, and was buried in St. Louis Cemetery No. 2.[1]

DEATH CERTIFICATE: Cause of death, cerebral softening, neurasthenia.

1. OR, vol. 15:760, 979; CMH 10:294, La.; New Orleans Daily Picayune, June 22, 1891.

WILLIAM ROBERTSON BOGGS · Born March 18, 1829, in Augusta, Georgia. Graduated from USMA in 1853. Served in the Mexican War. He resigned from the regular army in early 1861 and was appointed Confederate captain and ordnance officer. Serving as chief of engineers and artillery, he was appointed brigadier general in November 1862. After the war he entered engineering and taught at the Virginia Polytechnic Institute. Boggs died September 15, 1911, at Winston-Salem, North Carolina, and was buried there in the Salem Cemetery. Cause of death: Old age.[1]

1. Internment book, Salem Cemetery Co., Winston-Salem, N.C.

MILLEDGE LUKE BONHAM · Born December 25, 1813, in the Edgefield District, South Carolina. Served in the Florida and Mexican wars. He was sick while at home prior to leaving for New Orleans in June 1847. On August 19, 1847, at Contreras, Mexico, when he was also suffering from diarrhea, the prevailing disease due to the climate, he accidently shot himself in the hand with his own pistol. The bullet entered the palm of the right hand and came out at the wrist, tearing some of the tendons of the two last fingers. The wound initially caused considerable pain, and he could do little more than write his name. Although the hand had healed poorly by October, he did not lose its use, and his health was otherwise good. During the first part of 1858 he had great difficulty with arthritis, which involved multiple joints. A lawyer, Bonham was a member of the United States Congress at the outbreak of the war. He was appointed a major general of the South Carolina state army and then a Confederate brigadier general in April 1861. His military career was interrupted between January 1862 and February 1865, when he was a member of the First Regular Confederate Congress and then the elected governor of South Carolina. After the war he resumed the practice of law and was state railroad commissioner when he died. His death occurred suddenly at White Sulphur Springs, North Carolina, on August 27, 1890, when a blood vessel burst. Bonham was buried in Elmwood Cemetery, at Columbia, South Carolina.[1]

1. M. L. Bonham to Mother, June 29, Aug. 25, Sept. 7, Oct. 17, 1847, Mar. 3, 1858; M. L. Bonham to Miles, Jan. 30, May 15, 1858, all in Milledge Luke Bonham Papers, South Caroliniana Library, Manuscripts Division, University of South Carolina, Columbia (hereafter cited as SCL); Dictionary of American Biography, s.v. "Bonham, Milledge Luke."

JOHN STEVENS BOWEN · Born October 30, 1830, near Savannah, Georgia. Graduated from USMA in 1853. Resigning his army commission after three years, he was an architect in St. Louis at the start of the Civil War. He was captured in May 1861 while a captain in the Missouri militia; when released he was made colonel of the 1st Missouri Infantry, which he had organized. He was promoted brigadier to rank from March 1862. Bowen was wounded at Shiloh on April 6, 1862. He arrived in Corinth the next day completely exhausted, and as soon as he gained sufficient strength, went to Memphis for medical treatment. He rejoined his troops at Corinth in May. By June 1862, he was commanding an outpost near Vicksburg. On July 3, 1863, he became violently ill with dysentery and exhaustion. Following his capture and parole at Vicksburg, he was taken in an ambulance as far as Raymond, Mississippi. After the onset of his illness, Bowen's wife, who had been residing outside of Vicksburg, visited him before his death on July 13, 1863. Years later he was reinterred in the Confederate Cemetery at Vicksburg.[1]

1. CSR; *OR*, vol. 10, pt. 1:390; vol. 15:769; vol. 24, pt. 3:486; *CMH* 9:205, Mo.; Robert S. Bevier, *History of the First and Second Missouri Confederate Brigades*, 223–24.

BRAXTON BRAGG • *Born March 22, 1817,* in Warrenton, North Carolina. Graduated from USMA in 1837. Served in the Florida and Mexican wars. Too sick to remain on duty while in Florida during the spring of 1838, he returned home to recover. His own troops made two attempts to assassinate him in Mexico: one attempt, on August 24, 1847, consisted of a heavily charged twelve-pound shell that exploded two feet from his bed and sent fragments above and below him without causing injury. The second attack was similar and occurred the following October. Again, he was not injured; only his bed was damaged. In 1847, he suffered from two episodes of an unspecified illness. Bragg was very thin, stooped, and had a sickly, cadaverous appearance. He had chronic migraine headaches, stomach trouble, and generally poor health, in part due to chronic dysentery. In 1855, Bragg told a friend that he had taken a mercury preparation each summer because he suffered from his old Florida liver problems. He left the United States Army in 1856 and became a planter in Louisiana. In March 1861 he entered Confederate service as a brigadier general and was promoted to major general in September 1861. His commission as a general in the Regular Confederate Army ranked from April 1862. During the winter and early spring of 1863, Bragg's staff worried that his mental and physical condition would prevent him from eating adequately. As a consequence, they sent his meals to him while he was at his desk working. During May 1863, he was bothered by a boil on his hand. A siege of boils and chronic diarrhea over the next two months culminated in a general breakdown of his physical condition. He reported that he had recovered in July but in fact was in such poor health that he was barely able to continue his duties. Accompanied by Mrs. Bragg, he spent about a week in the middle of August in the hospital at Cherokee Springs, Georgia, in an effort to recuperate. During the last of December 1863, Bragg was at Warm Springs, Georgia; as his health had greatly improved, he was ready for any duty assigned. After the war, he first lived in Alabama and then moved to Galveston, Texas, where he died. On September 27, 1876, he was walking down the street when he suddenly fell to the ground. Carried to a nearby drugstore, he lived for ten to fifteen minutes. An inquest ruled that his death was due to "fatal syncope," possibly induced by organic disease of the heart. There was no evidence of apoplexy. His family physician thought death was due to "paralysis of the brain." He was buried in Magnolia Cemetery in Mobile, Alabama.[1]

DEATH CERTIFICATE: NAD

1. *OR*, vol. 23, pt. 1:623; William P. Snow, *Lee and his Generals*, 341, 357; Grady McWhiney, *Braxton Bragg and the Confederate Defeat* 1:27, 93–94, 97–98, 388–89; Judith Lee Hallock, *Braxton Bragg and the Confederate Defeat* 2:270–71; Kate Cumming, *Kate: The Journal of a Confederate Nurse*, 129, 131; Braxton Bragg to Marcus J. Wright, Dec. 29, 1863, Murray J. Smith Collection, USAMHI; Liddell, *Liddell's Record*, 128; *Galveston News*, Sept. 28, 1876; *CV* 4:102.

LAWRENCE O'BRYAN BRANCH • *Born November 28, 1820,* at Enfield, North Carolina. He served in Florida. He edited a newspaper, was admitted to the bar, and served in the United States Congress from North Carolina. When the Civil War started, he was appointed quartermaster and paymaster general of North Carolina. Resigning these positions, he was made a colonel of the 33rd North Carolina Infantry and was promoted to brigadier general in November 1861. In June 1862 he was having trouble with his bowels. He had brought wood planks, made himself a bed filled with straw, and thought he was doing as well in camp as he would in town. His diet consisted of chicken, fruit, and vegetables. There was little improvement in his condition by late July, and he wrote that if he developed fever, he was going to apply for a leave of absence. At the Battle of Cedar Mountain, Virginia, on August 9, 1862, the weather was intensely hot, and Branch was exposed to the sun all day. He was so feeble due to his diarrhea that he rode in an ambulance, scarcely able to walk fifty yards. However, the excitement braced him, and he felt in better health than at any time since starting the expedition. Two versions exist of Branch's death at Sharpsburg on September 17, 1862. In the first, Gen. A. P. Hill was consulting with James J. Archer, Maxcy Gregg, and Branch when a Federal sharpshooter fired into the group and struck Branch in the head. In the second account, he was killed while leading his brigade. He was buried in the Old City Cemetery in Raleigh, North Carolina.[1]

1. *OR*, vol. 12, pt. 2:223; vol. 19, pt. 1:150, 981, 1001; Lawrence O'Bryan Branch to Nannie, June 23, July 27, Aug. 13, 1862, Lawrence O'Bryan Branch Papers, no. 10057, UV; *CMH* 4:298; Clark, *Histories of Several Regiments* 2:554.

WILLIAM LINDSAY BRANDON • *Born in 1800 or 1802* near Washington, Mississippi. A planter, student of medicine, and major general of militia, Brandon was made a lieutenant colonel of the 21st Mississippi Infantry at the start of the war. About ten days after the battle of First Manassas in July 1861, the wind was blowing through Brandon's tent, and he awoke with a chill. This illness prompted him to take a leave that lasted until the end of August. The rest of the men did not think he would be fit for duty again, and he did not receive the appointment as colonel. At the Battle of Malvern Hill on July 1, 1862, a ball passed through his ankle joint. As he fell, his hand hit a rolling shell, which fortunately did not explode. Not realizing he had been wounded, he jumped up; unable to stay on his feet, he fell again and had to remain on the field until four men were detailed to take him to the rear. Because no bleeding was evident, Brandon did not think the wound was serious. He was put on a horse and taken to a field hospital. His boot was full of fragments of the ankle joint and initially was just bound up. At first he refused whiskey because he would not drink it without water and sugar. However, others convinced him that it was necessary for his condition, and he was given some every half hour. A tourniquet was put in place and an amputation was performed rapidly. The procedure was very painful as there was not enough chloroform to provide complete anesthesia when the arteries were sewn. The doctors thought that, because of Brandon's age, his chances of survival were slight. After being transferred to Richmond, he was taken care of by friends and his servant. President Jefferson Davis even offered the hospitality of his mansion. The operating surgeon had not trimmed off the sharp part of the tibia, and because it was a flap operation, the weight of the muscles of the leg caused great pain. The wound closed by first intention, except at the sides, where the ligatures used to secure the arteries came out. The doctor was surprised that the wound did not suppurate and that there was no discharge. One day Brandon noticed that the pillow he was using to support his stump was covered with a large amount of bright red blood. The doctor took three yards of linen and made three-inch strips of bandage, which were sewn together end to end. The doctor then lifted the leg, which, according to Brandon, hurt like a boil. Lint saturated with tincture of iron was rammed into the wound, while the rest of the tincture was poured into the wound. The bandage was then wrapped as tightly as possible around the stump. Brandon awoke the next morning feeling great pain in the stump. When the doctor removed the bandage he noted that suppuration had been present at the end of the tibia and was pointing. He did not think Brandon could withstand a second operation. Before reexamining the leg, the doctor gave Brandon cognac, then ran his fingers down the shinbone with all of his strength. Brandon heard a popping sound when the collection of pus drained. He improved rapidly after this procedure and was able to go home on furlough. However, finding a comfortable artificial leg proved difficult. One that fit well was still very painful when his weight was put on the point of the stump. Finally he obtained a satisfactory limb from a cabinetmaker in Augusta, Georgia. His knee joint was tender from long disuse, and he went back to the field using crutches, unable to mount or dismount his horse without help. He rejoined the regiment at Lookout Mountain, but because he felt he could not do his field duties, he returned to the hospital in Richmond. Following the September 1863 battle at Chickamauga, Brandon resigned. His decision was based on the poor fit of his artificial leg, his advanced age, and the recurrence of a disease that he had had in 1862 in Virginia caused by irritation from drinking the local lime water. Because of Brandon's crutches, the horse even shied away from him when he tried to mount, and he therefore considered himself more of a hindrance than a help. Appointed brigadier to rank from June 1864, he assumed command of the Reserve Corps for the state of Mississippi on July 23; on October 8, 1864, he took command of the state conscripts. In March 1865 he was confined to the house by an injury to his stump. In spite of his age and his physical disability, Brandon remained active on his plantation for the rest of his life. Until he was eighty-six years of age, he was able to ride sixteen miles to the county seat and back, sometimes making both trips the same day. Brandon died October 8, 1890, at his plantation in Wilkinson County, Mississippi, and was buried in the family burial grounds on the Arcole Plantation, eighteen miles from Woodville, Mississippi.[1]

DEATH CERTIFICATE: NAD

1. CSR; OR, vol. 11, pt. 2:672, 751, 755; vol. 39, pt. 2:724, pt. 3:808; vol. 49, pt. 2:1151; Military Reminiscences of General William L. Brandon, J. F. H. Claiborne Papers, SHC; Robert L. Brandon to Mr. Perry, June 2, 1896, William L. Brandon subject file, MDAH; Steiner, *Physician-Generals in the Civil War*, 21.

WILLIAM FELIX BRANTLEY · *Born March 12, 1830*, in Greene County, Alabama. A lawyer, Brantley entered Confederate service as a captain in the Wigfall Rifles and rose to colonel of the 29th Mississippi. On December 31, 1862, while at Murfreesborough, he was slightly wounded between the shoulders by the concussion of an exploding shell. However, he was back on the field the next day. He was promoted to brigadier general in July 1864. Following the war, he returned to his law practice. While riding down a country road near Winona, Mississippi, on November 2, 1870, Brantley was killed instantly by a hidden assassin using a double-barreled shotgun filled with buckshot. He was buried about three miles north of Tomnolen, Mississippi, in Old Greensboro Cemetery.[1]

DEATH CERTIFICATE: NAD

1. CSR; OR, vol. 20, pt. 1:756, 764–65; S. D. Lee to J. F. H. Claiborne, Aug. 5, 1879, J. F. H. Claiborne Papers, SHC.

JOHN BRATTON · *Born March 7, 1831*, in Winnsboro, South Carolina. Although a practicing physician, he enlisted as a private in the 6th South Carolina Volunteers and was elected a company captain. When state troops were taken into the Confederate Army, he again enlisted as a private but soon had the rank of colonel. On May 31, 1862, Bratton, on foot, led the 6th South Carolina Regiment in the Battle of Seven Pines. Near sundown, he was wounded in the right arm close to the shoulder by a minié ball, which then entered his body. At the same time he was suffering from diarrhea, the prevailing disease due to the climate. Feeling faint, he was unable to get back to the Confederate lines without assistance and was helped off the field into Federal captivity. The progress he and his assistants made under guard was slow until a litter was found and he was taken to the Federal hospital. The surgeon of Gen. David B. Birney, U.S.A., upon being asked by the general to examine Bratton's wound, said it was not fatal. After Gen. Philip Kearny, U.S.A., wrote the prison commandant, Bratton's care and quarters improved. Following his exchange, he joined his brigade on October 28, 1862, at a camp near Culpeper. Later the next year Bratton was ill, but his appetite and a portion of his strength returned by October 1, 1863. He was appointed brigadier to rank from May 1864. Bratton was wounded in the shoulder on October 7, 1864, near New Market Road, Virginia. Although in pain, he rode down his line to determine what was happening. He was back on the field in November.[1] Postbellum, he did not return to the practice of medicine but became a farmer and took an active part in politics, serving as a state senator and U.S. congressman. He died January 12, 1898, at Winnsboro and was buried there in the St. John's Episcopal Church Cemetery.

DEATH CERTIFICATE: NAD

1. CSR; *OR*, vol. 11, pt. 1:858–59, 948; vol. 36, pt. 1:1060; vol. 42, pt. 1:876, 881–82; vol. 46, pt. 1:1277; Dr. James Richmond Boulware Diary, Virginia State Library, Richmond (hereafter cited as VSL); Steiner, *Physician-Generals in the Civil War*, 22; *CV* 8:407; John Bratton to wife, Oct. 28, 1862, Oct. 1, 1863, John Bratton to Betty Dubose Bratton, Nov. 5, 1864, John Bratton Papers, SHC; *The State*, n.p., n.d., 1928, John Bratton Papers, SCL; James Lide Coker, *History of Company G, Ninth S.C. Regiment*, 68–69, 169; *SHSP* 8:556–77, 13:126–28; Elliott, *Richard Heron Anderson*, 118.

JOHN CABELL BRECKINRIDGE • *Born January 15, 1821, near Lexington, Kentucky.* Served in the Mexican War. A lawyer, he held a number of political positions, including vice-president of the United States. In November 1861, after the start of the war, he was commissioned a brigadier. At Shiloh, on April 7, 1862, he was struck twice by spent shells. On April 9, Breckinridge was very sick and not fit for duty. His promotion to major general ranked from April 14. On reaching Tupelo in early May, he obtained a four-week leave and went to Louisiana because he was suffering from a recurring illness. On June 28, 1862, he left in a carriage to rejoin his troops, arriving in time to participate in the engagement at Baton Rouge in August. At Cold Harbor, on June 3, 1864, his horse was killed when a cannonball passed through it, just missing Breckinridge's left leg. Breckinridge was caught beneath the horse when it fell, and several men were required to release him. Although not wounded, he suffered bruises on his thigh and left leg and also injured an old wound, which made him unable to ride. Disabled, he spent a few days in Richmond, and on June 6 he went by railroad to Lynchburg. After returning to the field, he had to go back to Lynchburg on the sixteenth of June, where he remained until able to resume command on the twentieth. He would have gone to see President Johnson on May 3, 1865, but he was too sick and fatigued. After the war he returned to the practice of law. His health continued to be poor, and Breckinridge had one episode of illness after another. During the winter of 1873, he was confined to the house, and while in Lexington in 1874 he had "latent" pneumonia. There was slight improvement during the summer, but he could eat little, and in the autumn of 1874 he coughed up blood. Although better by December, he continued to have difficulty with the lung that had bled earlier. In May 1875, at Lexington, Kentucky, he was attended by Doctors Desha, Gross, Blackburn, and Sayre. Breckinridge was emaciated, anemic, and had slight edema of his feet. On physical examination the left side of the chest and the upper two-thirds of the right chest were normal and there was no abdominal fluid. The lower portion of the right chest was dull to percussion, the intercostal spaces were rounded out, and on measurement the right chest was 1⅞ inches larger than the left. Comparison of percussion of the chest while Breckinridge was both upright and prone revealed that the line of dullness shifted position, suggesting it was due to fluid rather than consolidation. He had been bringing up as much as four quarts of sputum per twenty-four hours. A microscopic examination of the sputum revealed bile pigment and "other evidence of it having come from the liver." The diagnosis of the attending physicians was cirrhosis of the liver (original), subsequent inflammation of the lower lobe of the right lung, adhesions of the liver, diaphragm, and lung, with abscess of liver and lung that had found an outlet through the bronchi. A cannula to drain the area was obtained from one of the local silversmiths. The next morning, May 11, Breckinridge coughed up a little over a pint and a half of material. Chloroform was administered, and an incision was made above the eighth or ninth rib into the pleural cavity. No pus escaped and the lung receded, allowing a finger to be passed into the space so that the diaphragm and adherent lung could be palpated. Because no trochar long enough to reach the area was available, it was decided to wait until the abscess refilled and extended the wall enough to be reached. The procedure was performed on Wednesday morning, but details are not available. By the following Sunday, the sixteenth, his abdomen was distended and Breckinridge was only able to talk in a whisper. The next day, for the first time, he was lying horizontally; tympanites had subsided, and he was breathing normally. The odor in the room was terrible, and the bandages were soaked with discharge. The smell came from the gaping incision that was filled with a white slough that looked like wet cotton. When this material was removed, pus flowed readily. According to Dr. Lewis A. Sayre, a cannula was not required. The wound was covered with oakum (loose hemp jute fiber), which was wetted with carbolic acid and secured with a roller. Breckinridge then washed his hands and face, put on clean linen, combed his own hair, and had breakfast. In a few hours he went into a coma and died suddenly on May 17, 1875. The diagnosis of cirrhosis depends on a gross or microscopic examination of liver tissue and not on an examination of sputum or pleural fluid. The diagnosis therefore is highly suspect from the information available. If he did have cirrhosis, the most likely cause was his prior drinking rather than the trauma resulting from his fall during the war, as has been proposed.[1] His final illness with pulmonary hemorrhage, the large amount of sputum production, and accumulation of fluid in the space around the lung is best explained by a pulmonary abscess and rupture into the pleural space. How much the unsterile examination of the space around the lung might have contributed to the final infection is not clear. He died in Lexington and was buried in the City Cemetery.

DEATH CERTIFICATE: RNA

1. *OR*, vol. 10, pt. 1:389, pt. 2:403, 496; vol. 15:76; vol. 37, pt. 1:766; vol. 49:1277–78; vol. 51, pt. 2:983–84, 1020; vol. 52, pt. 2:745; William C. Davis, *Breckinridge: Statesman, Soldier, Symbol*, 316–17, 437–42, 616–24; *SHSP* 7:317; Douglas S. Freeman, *Lee's Lieutenants* 3:526–27; Lewis A. Sayre, "Operation on General John C. Breckinridge," *American Medical Weekly* 2:605–8.

THEODORE WASHINGTON BREVARD · *Born August 26, 1835, in Tuskegee, Ala-*bama. Admitted to the Florida bar, he was appointed state adjutant and inspector general a year before the war. He organized a battalion of Partisan Rangers and was promoted to colonel of the 11th Florida Infantry. His commission as brigadier to rank from March 1865 was the last such appointment made by President Davis. Following the war he returned to the practice of law. He died June 20, 1882, at Tallahassee, Florida, and was buried in the Episcopal Cemetery.

DEATH CERTIFICATE: RNA

JOHN CALVIN BROWN • *Born January 6, 1827,* in Giles County, Tennessee. He interrupted his practice of law in 1859 because of poor health and made a tour of Great Britain, Europe, Egypt, and the Holy Land. Enlisting in the Confederate Army as a private, he was made colonel of the 3rd Tennessee Infantry in May 1861. Brown's tombstone states that he was wounded at Fort Donelson, but details are lacking and he himself did not mention it in his report. His promotion to brigadier general ranked from August 1862. Brown was shot through the right thigh at Perryville on October 8, 1862. He was in the hospital for three months and reported back for duty at Murfreesborough while still on crutches. He was slightly wounded by spent grapeshot on September 20, 1863, at the Battle of Chickamauga, and was disabled for a day. Near Ezra Church, Georgia, on July 28, 1864, he received another wound, which caused only temporary retirement from the field. In August 1864 he was promoted to major general. On the night of November 30, 1864, at Franklin, Brown was shot from his horse and badly wounded. Disabled for a few months, he rejoined the army in April 1865. There is no evidence that his wounds caused any postwar difficulties. He resumed his law practice but had a varied career, including being governor of Tennessee and a railroad president. He died from hemorrhage from the throat on August 17, 1889, in Red Boiling Springs, Tennessee, and is buried in Maplewood Cemetery in Pulaski, Tennessee.[1]

DEATH CERTIFICATE: NAD

1. CSR; *OR*, vol. 7:346–49; vol. 16, pt. 1:1087, 1122; vol. 30, pt. 2:22, 24, 364, 372, 379; vol. 38, pt. 3:688; vol. 45, pt. 1:654, 686; vol. 47, pt. 3:741; Arthur Middleton Manigault, *Carolinian Goes to War*, ed. R. Lockwood Tower; *CV* 3:36, 242–43; Margaret Butler to author, Dec. 27, 1979.

WILLIAM MONTAGUE BROWNE • *Born July 7, 1823,* in Dublin, Ireland. An immigrant with military service in the English army, Browne helped edit two newspapers before the war. Throughout his life he suffered from poor health. For almost two months before he went to Washington, D.C., in 1859, he was unable to work because he was not well. An attack of bronchitis and a sore throat affected him in the summer of 1860, and rheumatism caused him to be confined for several days during the first part of 1860. He entered Confederate service on the personal staff of President Davis with the rank of colonel. "Camp colic" bothered him in June 1864. He had little field service, and his appointment as brigadier by President Davis ranking from November 1864 was not supported by the Confederate Senate. Following the war, in May 1866, he gave up the editorship of the *Southern Banner* because of lack of time and poor health. The last of the year, because of illness, he had to miss trips during which he had planned to gather news. He blamed his poor health on exposure, fatigue, and anxiety. In the fall of 1867, to regain his strength, he went to Madison Springs to drink iron water at the recommendation of his doctor. Ill health continued to plague him the following year, and in 1869 he was given large amounts of quinine for a severe face pain that his doctor diagnosed as "malaria neuralgia." His left leg was paralyzed in 1873, and he suffered from continuous pain just below his neck in the region of his spine. He received the chair of history and constitutional law at the University of Georgia in 1874. In 1878 he complained of fatigue and languor and reported that his pulse was forty. His continued poor health forced him to miss several faculty meetings. An Atlanta doctor diagnosed his condition as a disordered circulation produced by nervous prostration. For a short period in 1880, an injury to his left foot hampered him so much that he could not take a step. His death on April 28, 1883, in Athens, Georgia, resulted from pneumonia, and he was buried there in the Oconee Hill Cemetery.[1]

DEATH CERTIFICATE: NAD

1. E. Merton Coulter, *William Montague Browne: Versatile Anglo-Irish American*, 1, 30, 66, 106, 129, 136, 145–46, 158–59, 161, 172, 186, 228, 256–57.

GOODE BRYAN · *Born August 31, 1811,* in Hancock County, Georgia. Graduated from USMA in 1834. Resigning from the army soon afterward, he became a planter. During the Mexican War he served as a major of the 1st Alabama Volunteers; he joined the Confederate Army in 1861 as a captain of the 16th Georgia Infantry. On September 28, 1862, Bryan was admitted for observation to the Institute Hospital in Richmond, Virginia, with a diagnosis of chronic hepatitis. In October his wife thought that his health was too feeble for field duty during the winter and wanted him put in command of a new school of instruction. He took part in the First Battle of Fredericksburg in December 1862 and was appointed brigadier general to rank from August 1863. He had general debility and dysentery for three weeks before being hospitalized on June 6, 1864. Furloughed on June 11, he returned and resumed command on August 3. However, he was unable to remain, and on the morning of the twenty-first he left the field again. A surgeon's certificate stated that "because of gouty diathesis, complicated with great disarrangement of the kidneys, acceptance of his resignation is recommended." As a consequence, he resigned in September 1864.[1] He was semiretired for many years after the war. Bryan died at Augusta, Georgia, on August 16, 1885, and was buried in the City Cemetery (Magnolia Cemetery). Cause of death: Paralysis, sick for two months.[2]

1. CSR; *OR*, vol. 21:579, 599; vol. 43, pt. 1:589; CR, 178:150; *CMH* 6:400.
2. Burial records, Magnolia Cemetery, Augusta, Ga.

SIMON BOLIVAR BUCKNER · *Born April 1, 1823,* in Hart County, Kentucky. Graduated from USMA in 1844. He was slightly wounded at Churubusco, Mexico, on August 20, 1847. While in Mexico, along with other officers, he climbed the volcano of Mt. Popocatepetl and had to be brought down with his eyes bandaged because of snow blindness. Buckner was adjutant general of Kentucky when the Civil War started and was appointed a Confederate general in September 1861. Unfortunately for him, he was selected to surrender Fort Donelson to Federal troops. Sickness prevented him from going to eastern Tennessee with James Longstreet in November 1863. He did court-martial duty following his recovery and in February took over command of John B. Hood's old brigade. Following the war, Buckner lived in New Orleans for a few years before moving to Louisville, Kentucky, where he edited a newspaper. In April 1872 he had an acute episode of erysipelas involving his face and was nearly blind for a number of days. In 1887 he was elected governor of Kentucky. At age eighty, he had cataract surgery with good results. A year later, he was very ill and not expected to live. During 1912 and 1913, Buckner's health was poor. He remained active, however, and closed his business affairs on New Year's Day 1914. The following day he had a sudden onset of lethargy and weakness, which improved over the next few days. However, he went into a coma and died on January 8, 1914, on his land near Munfordville, Kentucky.[1] He was buried in the State Cemetery at Frankfort.

DEATH CERTIFICATE: Cause of death, a gradual decline for four months or more. He did have a chronic cystitis, not bad. Duration nine years and five months. Contributory, acute dysentery, nine years ago when cystitis began.

1. Arndt Mathias Stickles, *Simon Bolivar Buckner: Borderland Knight*, 16, 243–44, 312, 418, 423; James L. Morrison, Jr., ed., *Memoirs of Henry Heth*, 64–65; Edwin P. Thompson, *History of the Orphan Brigade*, 356; Horn, *Army of Tennessee*, 292.

ABRAHAM BUFORD · *Born January 18, 1820,* at Woodford, Kentucky. Graduated from USMA in 1841. After serving in Mexico, he resigned from the regular army in 1854 and took up the raising of stock animals. He entered the Confederate Army as a brigadier general to rank from September 2, 1862. During a fight south of Franklin on December 17, 1864, a Federal soldier struck him twice over the shoulder with a saber. Gen. James R. Chalmers killed the soldier with two pistol shots. Apparently little damage was inflicted on Buford, a large man who weighed more than three hundred pounds. He was slightly wounded in the right leg at Richland Creek on December 24, 1864. When he attended S. D. Lee's marriage on February 8, 1865, still weak from this wound, he passed out and fell into the oyster soup, which spilled on his companion. After the Civil War he returned to his home and was the owner of many famous horses. He also served in the Kentucky legislature. Years later, Buford lost everything he had and he committed suicide on June 9, 1884, at Danville, Indiana.[1] He was buried in Lexington, Kentucky, in the City Cemetery.

DEATH CERTIFICATE: Cause of death, suicide by shooting himself through the head.

1. CSR; *OR*, vol. 45, pt. 1:567, 593, 757–58; J. B. Cowan, comp., "Confederate Collection, Casualty List, Forrest Command, 1864," Tennessee State Library and Archives, Nashville (hereafter cited as TSLA); *CMH* 9:228, Ky.; *CV* 9:110, 13:161; James Dinkins, *1862–1865, By An Old Johnnie*, 251; Herman Hattaway, *General Stephen D. Lee*, 151.

ROBERT BULLOCK • *Born December 8, 1828,* in Greenville, North Carolina. Served in the Florida wars. Before the Civil War he was clerk of a county circuit court in Florida. He entered the Confederate Army as a captain of the 7th Florida Infantry. He was in the hospital in October 1863, which caused him to miss the muster roll. Bullock was captured on November 25, 1863, near Chattanooga, Tennessee, and exchanged in March 1864. Wounded near Atlanta on August 3, he took command of the 7th Florida Brigade in September when his commander, Jesse J. Finley, was wounded. After having passed through grades, he was appointed a brigadier general in November. He was severely wounded on the retreat from Nashville near Murfreesborough on December 4, 1864, and hospitalized the following month in Mississippi.[1] Admitted to the Florida bar after the war, he had an active political life until his death on July 27, 1905, at Ocala, Florida. He was buried there in Evergreen Cemetery.

DEATH CERTIFICATE: Cause of death, chronic gastroduodenitis.

1. CSR; *OR*, vol. 39, pt. 2:850; vol. 45, pt. 1:681, 742, 745, 750; *CMH* 11:185–86, 197–98, Fla.

MATTHEW CALBRAITH BUTLER • *Born March 8, 1836,* in Greenville, South Carolina. Lawyer and politician, Butler was commissioned a captain in the Hampton Legion when the Civil War started. He had diarrhea for a few days during the last of July 1861. On June 9, 1863, at the Battle of Brandy Station, a cannonball struck his right foot. The same shell killed one of Gen. J. E. B. Stuart's staff. Butler had to staunch the blood from his wound with his own handkerchief. The injured leg was amputated below the knee. While at home recuperating, he received a telegram from the War Department asking if he could ride a horse. He replied that he could and went back into the field as a brigadier general in September 1863. He succeeded Wade Hampton in brigade command and took part in the fall campaign of 1863. His wound continued to bother him, and in January 1864 he convalesced in South Carolina. On March 30, accompanied by Wade Hampton, he left Columbia for Richmond to discuss his command with Samuel Cooper. He was sick at Bottom Ridge on June 2, 1864. Then, on August 23, while wearing a wooden leg, he fought on horseback. He was promoted major general in September 1864. Butler was ill during the Battle of Bentonville in March 1865, and command of his brigade went to Evander McIvor Law. Butler had hard financial times after the war but was elected United States senator in 1876. In the war against Spain, he was a major general in the U.S. Army. He served as president of a Mexican mining company and as president of the Southern Historical Association. Butler was sick in April 1902. He died on April 14, 1909, in Washington, D.C., and was buried in Edgefield, South Carolina, in the Willow Brook Cemetery behind the Baptist church.[1]

DEATH CERTIFICATE: RNA

1. *OR*, vol. 27, pt. 2:684, 723, 730–31; vol. 33:1125, 1244, 1259; vol. 51, pt. 2:980; M. C. Butler to wife, July 31, 1861, Matthew Calbraith Butler Papers, 1851–1920, Duke University, William R. Perkins Library, Manuscript Department, Durham, N.C. (hereafter cited as DU); M.C. Butler to Lil, Apr. 23, 1902, M.C. Butler Papers, SCL; CSR of P. M. B. Young; *CMH* 5:380; *CV* 3:42, 102; Dabney Herndon Maury,

Recollections of a Virginian in the Mexican, Indian, and Civil Wars, 255; Heros Von Borcke, *Memoirs of the Confederate War for Independence* 2:279–80; Frank M. Myers, *The Comanches: History of White's Battlion, Virginia Cavalry,* 323.

C

WILLIAM LEWIS CABELL • *Born January 1, 1827,* in Danville, Virginia. Graduated from USMA in 1850. In 1851, after being hit in the shoulder by an arrow, he killed the Indian who had inflicted the wound. Resigning from the U.S. Army, Cabell served as quartermaster to Confederate general P. G. T. Beauregard and later was on the staff of J. E. Johnston. At Corinth on October 3, 1862, Cabell was struck in the foot by a spent minié ball; although painful, it did not disable him enough to make him leave the field. Two days later at Hatchie River, his horse became unmanageable and fell on him. Cabell's thigh and hip were seriously injured and his left leg was completely paralyzed. Because he could not walk, he relinquished his command. On November 13, 1862, he arrived at the headquarters of the Trans-Mississippi Department at Little Rock as inspecting officer of the Quartermaster's Department. He was appointed brigadier general to rank from January 1863. In February, when his strength was sufficiently restored, he was put in command of the forces in northwest Arkansas. In March he was sent up-country by T. H. Holmes to put things in order; later, on April 18, he took part in the action at Fayetteville, Arkansas. A report Cabell had written on the series of engagements that occurred from the previous July to September was not sent until December 1863 due to illness. Following the war he was mayor of Dallas, Texas, worked for the railroads, and was one of the supervisors of the Louisiana state lottery. After suffering with bronchitis for ten weeks, which weakened his heart, Cabell died quietly at home in Dallas on February 22, 1911, and was buried in Greenwood Cemetery.[1]

DEATH CERTIFICATE: RNA

1. *OR,* vol. 13:915; vol. 17, pt. 1:401, 403; vol. 22, pt. 1:310, 609, pt. 2:794; Paul J. Harvey, *Old Tige: General William L. Cabell, C.S.A.,* 5; *CV* 16:562–63, 19:179; *Dallas Morning News,* Feb. 23, 1911.

ALEXANDER WILLIAM CAMPBELL • *Born June 4, 1828,* at Nashville, Tennessee. A lawyer, he enlisted in the Confederate Army as a private. He performed staff duties as a major and later was appointed colonel of the 33rd Tennessee. While leading his men at Shiloh on April 6, 1862, he was wounded but did not leave the field. In March 1865 he was commissioned a brigadier. Following the war he returned to the practice of law. Campbell suffered with cancer, which started in his tongue about two years before his death. Although it initially appeared to heal, it spread to the lymph nodes of his neck. He died June 13, 1893, in Jackson, Tennessee, and was buried there in the Riverview Cemetery.[1]

1. *OR*, vol. 10, pt. 1:408–9, 500; vol. 16, pt. 2:770; *CMH* 8:299; Diary 11 (Jan.–Dec. 1893) of Robert H. Cartmell (1828–1915) of Madison Co., Tenn., TSLA.

JAMES CANTEY · *Born December 30, 1818*, in Camden, South Carolina. Following his admission to the South Carolina bar, Cantey served in the state legislature. An officer in the Palmetto Regiment, he was wounded during the Mexican War. At the beginning of the Civil War he was elected colonel of the 15th Alabama Infantry. Cantey was with his command as often as his physical condition would permit but was on sick leave in November and December 1862. His appointment as brigadier general ranked from January 1863. He was at Pollard, Alabama, in March and was assigned with the command of the Army of Tennessee in April 1863. From July to December 1864 he was frequently absent due to illness and was not expected to return. It was generally stated that, because of his poor health, he should not have tried to serve in the army.[1] He returned to his plantation near Fort Mitchell, Alabama, after the war and died there June 30, 1874. Cantey was buried in the family cemetery in the Fort Mitchell County Park.

DEATH CERTIFICATE: NAD

1. CSR; *OR*, vol. 15:1068; vol. 23, pt. 2:702; vol. 39, pt. 2:833; vol. 45, pt. 1:666, 681; *CMH* 12:397, Ala.; Oates, *War between the Union and the Confederacy*, 121–22.

ELLISON CAPERS · *Born October 14, 1837*, in Charleston, South Carolina. He taught at the South Carolina Military Academy after his graduation from that institution in 1857. Elected major of a South Carolina regiment of volunteers, Capers participated in the bombardment of Fort Sumter in April 1861. He was appointed lieutenant colonel of the 24th South Carolina Infantry, which he helped recruit in April 1862. On May 14, 1863, on the Clinton Road outside of Jackson, Mississippi, Capers was wounded. The ball first struck his horse in the shoulder, passed under the skin for six inches, and then entered Capers's leg near the femur, about six inches from his knee. The ball grazed the bone and stopped just at the skin on the underside of the leg. Capers lost so much blood he could not conduct the retreat. After being given a drink of whiskey, he rode his horse a quarter of a mile to the ambulance, which transported him to Canton by midnight. The ball was cut out and the wound dressed by 2:00 P.M. the next day. The muscles in the leg were damaged, and any movement produced pain. Capers was seriously wounded Sunday, September 20, 1863, at the Battle of Chickamauga. He was listed as in command January 1864. At Franklin on November 30, 1864, he was wounded in the foot before reaching the last Federal works and was in the hospital the next day. His report on the battle, dated January 4, 1865, was from Charleston, South Carolina. His appointment as brigadier general ranked from March 1865. After the war he became an Episcopal minister and in 1894 became the bishop of South Carolina. He had a stroke a few months before his death on April 22, 1908, at Columbia, South Carolina, and was buried in Trinity Churchyard.[1]

DEATH CERTIFICATE: NAD

1. *OR*, vol. 30, pt. 2:246; vol. 32, pt. 2:588; vol. 45, pt. 1:686, 733–38; E. Capers to wife, May 17, 1863, E. Capers to Marcus J. Wright, June 17, 1889, Ellison Capers Papers, SCL; *Charleston Evening Post*, June 12, 1861; *CV* 16:289; *CMH* 5:383.

WILLIAM HENRY CARROLL • *Born in 1810* at Nashville, Tennessee. Prior to the war he was a planter and the postmaster of Memphis. He entered the Confederate Army as colonel of the 37th Tennessee Infantry after he had resigned as brigadier general in the provisional army of the state of Tennessee. Appointed to the rank of Confederate brigadier in October 1861, Carroll resigned in February 1863 following a number of charges and a court of inquiry. After leaving the army he moved to Canada; he died in Montreal on May 3, 1868. His remains were later removed to Elmwood Cemetery, Memphis.

DEATH CERTIFICATE: RNA (Passport Services, U.S. Department of State).

JOHN CARPENTER CARTER • *Born December 19, 1837,* in Waynesboro, Georgia. He was practicing law when the war started, and he entered the Confederate service as a captain of the 38th Tennessee Infantry. In command of this regiment, Carter was wounded at Perryville on October 8, 1862. He appeared on a list of those wounded near Murfreesborough in December 1862. In his report on the battle, dated January 14, 1863, he did not mention having been wounded. His commission as brigadier general ranked from July 7, 1864. He was granted a thirty days' leave of absence on a surgeon's certificate in September. Carter was mortally wounded on November 30, 1864, in the assault on the Federal works at Franklin. He died three miles south of the battlefield on December 10. Some sources state the date of death as December 9.[1] He was buried in Rose Hill Cemetery at Columbia, Tennessee.

1. CSR; *OR*, vol. 20, pt. 1:718–19; vol. 45, pt. 1:654, 686, 737; Confederate States Army Casualties: Lists and Narrative Reports, 1861–65, National Archives, M836, roll 1; Warner, *Generals in Gray*, 45; Howell Purdue and Elizabeth Purdue, *Pat Cleburne*, 335.

JAMES RONALD CHALMERS • *Born January 11, 1831,* in Halifax County, Virginia. A practicing lawyer, he was a member of the Mississippi secession convention. He was appointed colonel of the 9th Mississippi Infantry in 1861 and promoted to brigadier general in February 1862. In July 1862 Chalmers asked to be relieved of command of the cavalry due to poor health. He was subsequently ordered to rejoin his infantry brigade. Chalmers was severely wounded on December 31, 1862, in the battle at Murfreesborough. He was borne senseless from the field after being knocked down by a shell fragment. Although he had not fully recovered from his wound, he was ordered to report to Gen. John C. Pemberton on January 12, 1863. This order was revoked, however, and in March he was to assume command of the military forces in the Fifth Military District of Mississippi. From May through early August, he was too sick to take the field or to accomplish all of his duties. On October 11, 1863, during the attack on Collierville, Tennessee, Chalmers was temporarily disabled by a spent ball. In May 1864 he suffered from a rectal fistula and had to be transported by ambulance, as he could not ride a horse. However, because his troops were needed in the field, he declined being relieved from his command and refused the operation suggested by his surgeon. In July 1864, Chalmers and Nathan Bedford Forrest engaged Federal raiders near Pontotoc and Tupelo. He was ordered to proceed to Grenada on September 13, 1864, to assume command of the department.[1] After the war he took a part in the politics of Mississippi and then moved to Tennessee to practice law. He died in Memphis on April 9, 1898, and was buried in Elmwood Cemetery.

DEATH CERTIFICATE: Cause of death, malaria.

1. CSR; *OR*, vol. 17, pt. 2:650; vol. 20, pt. 1:670, 689, 711, 756; vol. 24, pt. 3:623, 625, 659, 875, 1032, 1035; vol. 30, pt. 2:783; vol. 31, pt. 3:829; vol. 38, pt. 4:740, 754; vol. 39, pt. 1:324, pt. 2:835; Robert Selph Henry, *"First with the Most" Forrest*, 511.

JOHN RANDOLPH CHAMBLISS, JR. • *Born January 23, 1833,* in Hicksford, Virginia. He graduated from USMA in 1853. Chambliss resigned from the army within a year of graduation and took up farming. Already a member of a militia group at the outbreak of the war, he became a colonel when they were taken into the Confederate service. Although quite ill at the time, Chambliss was at the head of his brigade as it moved down the turnpike toward Shepherdstown on July 16, 1863. He was commissioned brigadier general to rank from December 1863. At Wickford, Virginia, on February 27, 1864, a doctor found Chambliss had an ulcer on his left heel and gave him a leave of absence. In April Chambliss was commander of the outposts on the lower Rappahannock. He was shot through the body and killed while leading his men during a cavalry battle on Charles City Road north of the James River on August 16, 1864. His body, along with that of V. J. B. Girardey, was left with the Federal troops and recognized by Federal general D. McM. Gregg, a West Point schoolmate. That evening he was buried near the "Potteries" but was disinterred the next day and sent through Confederate lines under a flag of truce. An excellent map of Richmond and its defenses was found by Federal troops on his person, and seventeen copies were made and distributed. He was buried in the family cemetery at Emporia, Virginia.[1]

1. CSR; *OR*, vol. 27, pt. 2:706; vol. 33:1257; vol. 42, pt. 1:242–43, 661, pt. 2:210–11, 215–16, 1189; *CMH* 3:582; Beale, *History Ninth Virginia Cavalry*, 140; *SHSP* 7:427.

BENJAMIN FRANKLIN CHEATHAM • *Born October 20, 1820,* in Nashville, Tennessee. Cheatham had been a colonel in the Tennessee Volunteers during the Mexican War and was a major general of the state militia. His commission as brigadier in the Confederate Army ranked from July 1861. He was slightly wounded at the Battle of Shiloh, probably on April 7, 1862, but did not mention it in his report. His promotion to major general came in March 1862. On August 13, 1864, he was granted a sick leave, which continued until after the Battle of Jonesborough.[1] Following the war he was superintendent of state prisons and postmaster of Nashville, where he died September 4, 1886. He was buried in Mount Olivet Cemetery in that city. Cause of death: Heart disease.[2]

1. CSR; *OR*, vol. 10, pt. 1:389, 437; *Southern History of the War*, 215; *CMH* 8:138.
2. Internment Record Book, Mount Olivet Cemetery, Nashville, Tenn.

JAMES CHESNUT, JR. • *Born January 18, 1815,* in Camden, South Carolina. A lawyer-politician, Chesnut was a United States senator at the start of the war. After serving in staff positions, he was commissioned brigadier general in April 1864. On August 18, 1861, Chesnut had a fever and was given quinine pills. He had improved enough to visit President Davis on the twenty-sixth. In December he was in Richmond with pneumonia. He was found unattended in his room, with a three-day-old uneaten dinner by his bed. A friend and her daughter nursed him back to health. He was sick again in April 1862 and went out against the doctor's advice. The doctor said Chesnut should be salivating in the damp weather after all of the calomel he had taken.[1] After the war he returned to state politics. Chesnut died in the town of his birth on February 1, 1885. He was buried in Knights Hill, the family burial ground, outside of Camden.

DEATH CERTIFICATE: NAD

1. Mary Boykin Chesnut, *Diary from Dixie*, 113, 115, 119, 170, 210.

ROBERT HALL CHILTON • *Born February 25, 1815,* in Loudoun County, Virginia. He graduated from USMA in 1837. Served in the Mexican War. When the Civil War started, he resigned from the United States Army and became a lieutenant colonel in the Adjutant and Inspector General's Department of the Regular Confederate Army. He appeared on the register of the general hospital no. 4, Wilmington, North Carolina, on September 27, 1863, but there are no details. He was back on duty by the middle of October.[1] He had little field duty and was appointed brigadier general in February 1864. After the war he was president of a manufacturing company. Chilton died at Columbus, Georgia, on February 18, 1879, and was buried in Hollywood Cemetery in Richmond, Virginia. Cause of death: Apoplexy.[2]

1. CSR; *OR*, vol. 29, pt. 1:450.
2. Burial Register, Hollywood Cemetery, Richmond, Va.

THOMAS JAMES CHURCHILL • *Born March 10, 1824,* in Jefferson County, Kentucky. Served in the Mexican War. Holding the position of postmaster of Little Rock, Arkansas, when the Civil War started, he recruited the 1st Arkansas Mounted Rifles. Churchill was appointed brigadier general in March 1862. On May 20, 1862, he was sick at Camp Churchill. He had been having an attack of remittent fever for several days but was not willing to take medicine or remain in bed while there was a prospect of an engagement. In addition to the fever, he had a severe cough and acute left pleuretic pain. Because he did not get better, it was felt advisable to move him to a shelter more suitable than his tent, so Churchill requested a leave. He was able to participate in the Battle of Richmond, Kentucky, in August. He was quite seriously ill late in July 1864 and was unable to go back to duty until the first week of August. Churchill was promoted to major general in March 1865. His positions after the war included state treasurer and governor of Arkansas. Churchill died May 14, 1905, at his daughter's home in Little Rock after an illness of several months' duration. He was buried there in Mount Holly Cemetery.[1]

DEATH CERTIFICATE: RNA

1. CSR; *OR*, vol. 16, pt. 1:940; "William M. McPheeters Civil War Diary—June 1, 1863 to June 20, 1865," William M. McPheeters Papers, Missouri Historical Society, St. Louis (hereafter cited as MHS); Timothy P. Donovan and Willard B. Gatewood, Jr., *Governors of Arkansas: Essays in Political Biography*, 68–72; *CV* 15:122–23.

JAMES HOLT CLANTON • *Born January 8, 1827,* in Columbia County, Georgia. Reached Mexico City just after its occupation by American forces. A prewar lawyer-politician, he became colonel of the 1st Alabama Cavalry in 1861. In camp near Corinth, Mississippi, on April 14, 1862, a surgeon stated that for the safe transportation of Clanton to Montgomery, it was necessary for him to have a nurse. No diagnosis was given, but Clanton obtained a fourteen-day leave. On May 28, 1862, he took part in the action near Corinth under Joseph Wheeler. Clanton's appointment as brigadier general ranked from November 1863. He requested a leave on a surgeon's certificate on December 7, 1864, because of an inflammation of the bowels that he thought would become chronic if left untreated. On March 25, 1865, at Bluff Springs, Florida, he was severely wounded in the small of the back and captured by Federal troops. The next day he was paroled. On April 6 he was at Abercrombie's place with six other wounded Confederate soldiers. He had recovered sufficiently to travel by April 22, 1865. Following the war he returned to the law and politics. He was killed in a street duel in Knoxville, Tennessee, on September 27, 1871. Clanton was hit in the right shoulder by the charge from a double-barreled shotgun. The shot broke his arm, and he had to support his right hand with his left in order to fire his own pistol. His attacker then fired the second barrel. Clanton was carried into the Lamar House, dead from fifteen or more slugs in his chest. He was buried in Oakwood Cemetery at Montgomery, Alabama.[1]

DEATH CERTIFICATE: NAD

1. CSR; *OR*, vol. 10, pt. 1:853; vol. 49, pt. 1:136–37, 280–81, 285, pt. 2:118, 258, 450–51, 498; *Memphis Daily Appeal*, Sept. 29, 1871; *Knoxville Free Press and Herald*, Sept. 29, 1871; Allen J. Going, "Shooting Affray in Knoxville with Interstate Repercussions: The Killing of James H. Clanton by David M. Nelson, 1871," *East Tennessee Historical Society's Publications* 27:39–48.

CHARLES CLARK • *Born May 24, 1811,* at Lebanon, Ohio. He took sick leave in April 1845 while a captain of militia at Camp Wilkins, Louisiana. He fought in Mexico in spite of a statement from Dr. Stone of New Orleans, who claimed that Clark was unfit because one of his lungs was almost gone from tuberculosis. His prewar career included teaching, farming, politics, and being brigadier and major general of Mississippi troops. With the transfer of state troops to the Confederacy, Clark was commissioned brigadier general in May 1861. At Shiloh on April 6, 1862, he was severely wounded in the right shoulder. Aides helped him seek treatment.

After his wound improved, he went home on leave. In a month he was back in Corinth, and he reported to duty at Vicksburg in the middle of July 1862. On August 5, during the battle at Baton Rouge, a ball passed through his right thigh and fractured the bone. Because the wound was thought to be mortal, and any motion caused severe pain, he was left on the field at his own request. The next morning he surrendered and was taken care of by Federal surgeons. They sent him on a gunboat to New Orleans, where he stayed in private quarters. Dr. Stone attended him again. Clark's family and sick wife joined him to help with his care. He had a single iron bed specially outfitted to lift him so that air would circulate around and under his body. Blood poisoning and sloughing of bone complicated his injury. The surgeon cut into the wound to remove the bone fragments without benefit of an anesthetic. Then, by the order of Federal general Benjamin F. Butler's staff surgeon, Clark and his family were forced to move to a boardinghouse. His release from Federal captivity was delayed because of the supposed execution of Federal soldiers by the Confederates. In April 1863 he was exchanged and had to be carried aboard ship. When he first arrived in Mississippi, he was confined to a wheelchair. A surgeon's certificate in October reported that the gunshot wound in the upper third of the right femur made the leg shorter than the left. Clark asked to resign from the military service that month because of his physical disability. After leaving the army, he was elected governor of Mississippi in 1863 and served until 1865. He was riding horseback by 1868, needing help only to mount. For years he walked with a limp due to a stiff leg. Later he slipped on icy pavement and tore the adherent ligaments. Once the initial pain went away, he had improved motion of the extremity. He then relied mainly on his cane, not requiring crutches as often. A chronic cough Clark had for years continued to be a problem, and he would take whiskey or brandy toddies when it was severe. He was active as a circuit judge, but in November 1877 his physical condition worsened. On one occasion he held court in his bedroom because he could not get out. He developed fever, congestion of the lungs, and mild delirium while residing at his plantation "Doro" in Bolivar County, Mississippi. Toward the end he became wildly delirious and was given sedation until he became unconscious. He died quietly on December 18, 1877, and was buried in "Doro" Plantation cemetery.[1] Cause of death: Pneumonia.[2]

1. CSR; OR, vol. 10, pt. 1:389, 408, 415; vol. 15:14, 54–55, 76, 78, 80, 83; ser. 2, vol. 4:594, 708; Annie E. Jacobs, "Master of Doro Plantation," 9, 57–58, 63–66, 75–77, 85, 92½, 160, 186, 237–39, 249, typescript, MDAH; Charles Martin Cummings, "Seven Ohio Confederate Generals: Case Histories of Defection" (diss.), 113, 558, 565.
2. Mrs. Vera Speakes, great granddaughter, Benoit, Miss.

JOHN BULLOCK CLARK, JR. • *Born January 14, 1831, at Fayette, Missouri.* Practicing law in Missouri when the war started, Clark entered the Confederate Army as a lieutenant. He was wounded during the Battle of Wilson's Creek on August 10, 1861. At Elkhorn Tavern in March 1862, he held the rank of colonel and was in command of troops. Appointed brigadier general in March 1864, Clark was slightly wounded in the arm in the battle of Jenkins' Ferry, Arkansas, on April 30. In his report of the engagement, he did not mention the injury, and there was no evidence that he left the field.[1] Following the war he returned to the practice of law and politics, serving in Congress for ten years. He died in Washington, D.C., on September 7, 1903, and was buried there in Rock Creek Cemetery.

DEATH CERTIFICATE: Cause of death, primary, paralysis of one year's duration; immediate, asthena and syncope of thirty-six hours' duration.

1. *OR*, vol. 8:305; vol. 34, pt. 1:537, 810–11; vol. 53:424; Confederate States Army Casualties, roll 3.

HENRY DELAMAR CLAYTON • *Born March 7, 1827,* in Pulaski County, Georgia. A prewar lawyer-politician, he entered Confederate service as a colonel of the 1st Alabama Infantry. On August 8, 1861, at Pensacola, Clayton was sick and unable to command. He served with his regiment at the batteries during the bombardment at Pensacola in November. His right shoulder was injured by a projectile on December 31, 1862, at the Battle of Murfreesborough, and he was furloughed home until he recovered, some three months later. His promotion to brigadier general ranked from April 1863. At Chickamauga on September 20, 1863, Clayton was struck by spent grapeshot and was forced to dismount for a short time. Apparently he did not have to leave his command. In July 1864 he was appointed major general. Following the war he again practiced law and was a planter. His Murfreesborough wound impaired his health for the rest of his life and supposedly contributed to his death. He died October 13, 1889, at Tuscaloosa, Alabama, and was buried in the Fairview Cemetery at Eufaula, Alabama.[1]

DEATH CERTIFICATE: NAD

1. CSR; *OR*, vol. 1:469; vol. 6:492; vol. 30, pt. 2:364, 400, 402; Preston C. Clayton to author, Jan. 10, 1980.

PATRICK RONAYNE CLEBURNE • *Born March 17, 1828,* near Cork, Ireland. He served in the British Army before emigrating to the United States. He studied law while working as a pharmacist and established a profitable law practice. On May 24, 1856, Cleburne was shot in the back during a street fight. Before collapsing, he shot one of his attackers. He was carried across the street to a building. Blood streamed from his mouth, his eyes were glassy, and his breathing faint. The bullet had hit Cleburne three inches above the crest of the ileum and to the right of the spine. It traveled upward at a forty-five-degree angle and finally lodged underneath the skin and rested on the ensiform (xiphoid) cartilage. As no blood appeared to come from the wound entrance, it was probed and the clot broken up until blood flowed freely to the floor. Judging from the vomited blood, which contained a little food, and the location of the ball, the doctor concluded that the stomach had been perforated. Because the bullet would not cause trouble where it had lodged, the doctor left it alone, hoping the fistulous tract would close spontaneously. It was uncertain for about a week whether Cleburne would live. Later the bullet was removed without benefit of an anesthetic, and the site healed rapidly. He never completely recovered from the effects of this wound. In January 1861, Cleburne felt better than he had in the summer, although his lungs had not been well since the injury in 1856. He caught cold at the slightest provocation, and an hour's debate would sometimes cause his mouth to fill with blood. His weight was never more than 135 pounds. (Dr. Charles Nash reported that Cleburne had weighed about 180 pounds in 1852.) He was elected colonel of the 15th Arkansas when the war started and was promoted to brigadier general in March 1862. At Richmond, Kentucky, on August 30, 1862, Cleburne had stopped to talk to Col. L. E. Polk, who had been wounded and was being carried to the rear, when a ball passed through his left cheek, carried away some teeth, and emerged from his open mouth. Unable to talk as a consequence of this wound, Cleburne would have been useless on the field, so he was taken to the nearby home of a citizen. The wound left only a thin scar, which was covered by his whiskers. A few weeks later he was back on the field. At Perryville on October 8, 1862, he was wounded near the ankle by a cannon shot that killed his horse. However, he was able to remain in command. Ten days later he was recovering rapidly. On September 10, 1863, Gen. D. H. Hill was unable to make the movement required of his troops because Cleburne had been sick in bed all day. Early in June 1864 Cleburne was ill for several days, but by the twelfth he was well and had resumed his full duties. He was killed at the Battle of Franklin on November 30, 1864, when a minié ball struck him in the left side of the abdomen. Cleburne was on foot at the time of his death, two of his horses having been killed earlier. He was initially buried at Franklin, but his remains were later removed to Helena, Arkansas, and buried in Maple Hill Cemetery.[1]

1. CSR; *OR*, vol. 16, pt. 1:934, 946, 1087, 1121; vol. 30, pt. 2:28, 138, 300; vol. 45, pt. 1:654, 685; Charles Edward Nash, *Biographical Sketches of General Pat Cleburne and General T. C. Hindman*, 10, 64–70, 202; Irving A. Buck, *Cleburne and his Command*, 107, 110, 290–93; Thomas A. Head, *Campaigns and Battles of the Sixteenth Regiment, Tennessee Volunteers*, 377–79; Purdue, *Pat Cleburne*, 40, 89, 195, 252.

THOMAS LANIER CLINGMAN • *Born July 27, 1812*, at Huntsville, North Carolina. Clingman was a lawyer and involved in politics. Resigning from the United States Senate, he was appointed colonel of the 25th North Carolina Infantry in August 1861 and brigadier in May 1862. On August 7, 1862, Clingman could not ride a horse or walk because of an inflamed foot. However, he thought he would be able to ride within three days. On the eighteenth he was ordered to assume command of the troops at Wilmington, North Carolina. In September 1862 he was on sick leave. The next month Robert E. Lee stated that Clingman should remain in North Carolina, where he would probably be of more service than in northern Virginia. During an expedition to New Bern, North Carolina, on February 1, 1864, Clingman's troops were halted in a line of battle when the Federal artillery fired upon them. A shell exploded nearby, and Clingman was hit by several shell fragments. Only bruised, he remained on the field. In May 1864 Clingman was in command of his own brigade. At Second Cold Harbor on May 31, a portion of a shell took away the front of his hat and slightly wounded him on the forehead. Stunned for a minute, but not disabled, he remained on the field. He was severely wounded in the leg on August 19, 1864, at the battle on the Weldon Railroad. He was absent in North Carolina in October, still suffering severely. In January his leave was extended, and it was reported he would not be able to return. While the army was at Smithfield in early 1865, Clingman visited his brigade. Although on crutches, he asked to command the rear guard. This was denied him as he was physically unable to perform the duties. However, he rejoined the command and was with them in the retreat and at the surrender of the army at Greensboro on April 26, 1865. After the surrender he returned to his law practice. His mind had been gradually weakening for years prior to his death. He died November 3, 1897, at Morgantown, North Carolina, and was buried in the Riverside Cemetery in Asheville, North Carolina.[1]

DEATH CERTIFICATE: NAD

1. CSR; *OR*, vol. 9:477, 480; vol. 19, pt. 2:689; vol. 36, pt. 3:842; vol. 42, pt. 1:858, 940; T. L. Clingman to James A. Seldon, Oct. 15, 1864, W. H. S. Burgwyn Papers, NCSA; CSR of Collette Leventhorpe; Clark, *Histories of Several Regiments* 4:487, 495, 499, 5:198; *CMH* 4:300; *SHSP* 24:306.

HOWELL COBB · *Born September 7, 1815,* in Jefferson County, Georgia. He entered politics following his admission to the bar and was a congressman, Speaker of the House, governor of Georgia, and finally secretary of the treasury in President Buchanan's administration. Cobb was commissioned a brigadier general in February 1862, after serving for a period in the Provisional Confederate Congress. On June 14, 1862, Robert E. Lee appointed Cobb to act as the negotiator with Federal officers for prisoner exchange. In July, a few days after the Battle of Malvern Hill, he was ill in Richmond with a throat infection. Although Cobb was too sick for active field duty, Robert E. Lee wanted him to continue the prisoner-exchange talks. Granted a thirty-day leave on July 12 to recover his health, he arrived in Athens, Georgia, four days later. He returned to duty in good health and remained so throughout September. By October 6, 1862, Cobb's foot had become so infected that he could not put on a boot, and he left his post in mid-October. However, he returned to duty and was assigned to the command of the District of Middle Florida in November. In September 1863 he was appointed a major general and assigned the job of organizing the Georgia militia at Atlanta. On October 9, 1868, he died in the lobby of New York City's Fifth Avenue Hotel. He had been walking toward the stairs when he grasped his chest and collapsed on the floor, dead. He was buried in Oconee Hill Cemetery, at Athens.[1]

DEATH CERTIFICATE (INQUEST): Compression of the brain.

1. *OR*, vol. 14:677; vol. 28, pt. 2:348–49; ser. 2, vol. 4:773, 807; Horace Montgomery, *Howell Cobb's Confederate Career*, 63, 65–66, 75–76, 132; Richard Taylor, *Destruction and Reconstruction*, 213.

THOMAS READE ROOTES COBB · *Born April 10, 1823,* in Jefferson County, Georgia. Following his graduation from the University of Georgia, he practiced the law. Utilizing his astute legal mind, he prepared a number of volumes on various aspects of Georgia law. Before the war his weight tended to fluctuate between 155 to more than 190 pounds, depending on the amount of energy expended. He organized Cobb's Legion and was elected colonel at the start of the war. Disturbed by what he interpreted as mistreatment from the Confederate command in July 1862, he smoked excessively and lost weight. He received his brigadier general stars in November. On December 13, 1862, at the First Battle of Fredericksburg, Cobb was mortally wounded. There are at least two versions of his fatal wounding and the type of projectile. In the first account, a musket ball fired from some 150 yards away hit him in the thigh. In the second, and probably more accurate, version, he was wounded on a sunken road near a house at Marye's Hill by fragments of a random cannon shot. The shell went through the house and exploded on the side of the building where Cobb was standing. A fragment grazed his right thigh and embedded itself in his left thigh, breaking the bone and lacerating the femoral artery. Knocked to the ground, he raised himself on one elbow and asked for a tourniquet. None was available, so a handkerchief was used instead. He was carried on a litter to an ambulance, which took him to a hospital behind the hill. En route he asked that the handkerchief be tightened. The first surgeon who reached him did what he could to stop the flow of blood. Cobb suffered a great deal of pain and did not recover from the blood loss and shock, although stimulants were given. He became unconscious and died. He was buried in the Oconee Hill Cemetery in Athens.[1]

1. CSR; *OR*, vol. 21:547, 555, 570, 582, 590; William B. McCash, *Thomas R. R. Cobb: The Making of a Southern Nationalist*, 14, 308; E. J. Eldridge to Dr. E. D. Newton, April 2, no year, Carlton-Newton-Mell Collection, and J. H. Lumkin to daughter (Calie), Dec. 30, 1862, Joseph Henry Lumkin Papers, both in University of Georgia, Hargrett Rare Book and Manuscript Library, Athens (hereafter cited as UG); *SHSP* 10:450–51; *CV* 7:309; *CMH* 6:403.

PHILIP ST. GEORGE COCKE · *Born April 17, 1809*, in Fluvanna County, Virginia. Graduated from USMA in 1832. He remained in the army for only two years following graduation before returning to Virginia, where he developed a national reputation as an agricultural expert. When the war started, he was appointed a brigadier general in the Virginia service. Transferred to the Confederate Army as a colonel, Cocke was promoted to brigadier in October 1861. After eight months of service, he left on sick leave. On arrival home in Powhatan County, Virginia, he alternated between excitement and depression and took no interest in his surroundings. Upset because of his inability to be at his post, he would despondently say he was unfit for duty and was only a burden to his country and family. Finally he wrote his resignation. On the evening of December 26, 1861, he sent his family to a social affair and stayed home alone. Returning after one hour to see if he was all right, they found his body on the ground outside of the house. He had shot himself in the temple with a pistol. His body was first buried on his estate and later moved to Hollywood Cemetery, Richmond.[1]

1. *CMH* 3:585; J. D. Powell to Wm. N. Pendleton, Jan. 3, 1862, W. N. Pendleton Papers, SHC.

FRANCIS MARION COCKRELL · *Born October 1, 1834,* near Warrensburg, Missouri. A lawyer, Cockrell entered the war in command of a company of Missouri militia. At Corinth, in October 1862, he received a wound from a shell fragment but was able to remain on the field. In a fight at Vicksburg on May 18, 1863, he was struck by a shell fragment; as it did not cause serious injury, he stayed on the field. On July 1, 1863, at Vicksburg, a mine exploded not far from the parapet where he was standing and blew Cockrell and others into the air. He fell some distance down the hill without any serious injury. After having been promoted through grades, he was appointed a brigadier general in July 1863. On June 19, 1864, at Kennesaw Mountain, he was wounded in both hands by a piece of shell. Several fingers were broken, two or three nails were knocked off his left hand, and the third finger of his right hand was fractured at the second joint. While his hands were being dressed at the field hospital, he inquired of the surgeon if his right finger would be stiff. When he replied that it undoubtedly would be, Cockrell told him that as he would do a lot of writing if he lived through the war, he wanted the finger set in the curved shape it would be in when he held a pen. When Cockrell insisted, the surgeon set the finger in a curved shape. He resumed command of the Missouri brigade on August 8. At Franklin on November 30, 1864, he was shot four times: twice in the right arm, once through the left leg, which just missed the bone, and once in the right ankle, which broke a small bone. Cockrell had been wounded while in the front line, and when he found he could walk on his right leg, he hobbled off the field. It was not until the surgeon was working on his right ankle that he discovered that he had been wounded in the left leg as well. On the first of February 1865, the Missouri brigade was ordered to Mobile. Before reaching the city, General Cockrell rejoined the brigade, still suffering from his wounds. Following the surrender of the Confederate forces, Cockrell still had not fully recovered.[1] He returned to his law practice and was elected to the United States Senate from Missouri. His death occurred on December 13, 1915, at Washington, D.C., and he was buried probably in Sunset Hill Cemetery, in Warrensburg. DEATH CERTIFICATE: Cause of death, primary, myocarditis and diffuse nephritis of four years' duration; immediate, acute dilatation (heart).

1. CSR; *OR,* vol. 38, pt. 3:904, 916; Ephraim McD. Anderson, *First Missouri Confederate Brigade,* 327, 352, 412; Samuel G. French, *Two Wars: An Autobiography of General Samuel G. French,* 203, 205, 208; *CMH* 9:125, 155, 197, 208, Mo.; Bevier, *History Ninth Virginia Cavalry,* 201, 215; Oscar Kraines, "Incorruptible Cockrell: Presidential Troubleshooter and Senate Watchdog" (typed copy, Missouri Historical Society), 14–16.

ALFRED HOLT COLQUITT · *Born April 20, 1824,* in Monroe, Georgia. Served in the Mexican War. Admitted to the bar, he entered politics. He was elected colonel of the 6th Georgia Infantry at the start of hostilities and was promoted to brigadier general in September 1862. After the Civil War he returned to Georgia, where he was elected governor twice and United States senator in 1882. Colquitt developed paralysis on July 27, 1892. Two weeks later he was able to go home, but his recovery was slow. He returned to Washington, D.C., in March 1893 and was able to attend to his duties. During the night of March 19, 1894, he became ill and could not talk. His physician did not think it was a new episode but rather a continuation of an old throat problem. Unable to take nutrition and unresponsive to strong stimuli, he died March 26, 1894. His throat problem and inability to take nutrition were probably secondary to his cerebral vascular accident.[1] He was buried in Rose Hill Cemetery at Macon.

DEATH CERTIFICATE: Cause of death, hemiplegia of eighteen months' duration; immediate cause, cardiac failure.

1. Newspaper, Atlanta, Ga., n.i., Mar. 27, 1894, and newspaper, Washington, D.C., n.i., Mar. 20, 1894, Alfred H. Colquitt Collection, UG.

RALEIGH EDWARD COLSTON • *Born October 31, 1825,* in Paris, France. Colston was sent to the United States in his early teens and entered the Virginia Military Institute. Following his graduation, Colston remained as a professor of French until the start of the war, when he was made colonel of the 16th Virginia. He was promoted brigadier general in December 1861. In June 1862 he had an attack of "Peninsular" fever and malaria, so his physician sent him on leave. His recovery was slow, and he did not return until December, when he was assigned to the command of a brigade.[1] Following the war he went to Egypt in 1873 and served in the Egyptian army, spending a number of months in the desert. He fell from a camel on one trip, which produced partial paralysis of his left leg and thereby caused him to leave the expedition. Halfway back on the more than five-hundred-mile trip through the desert, he had to be carried in a litter suspended between two camels. He was taken to the Red Sea and transported first by steamer, then by rail to Cairo. Colston went to Europe for medical treatment, which consisted of hydrotherapy and electrotherapy. After six months he had improved enough to walk two to three miles. His health was poor in 1875, and his gums were sore from taking calomel. During April 1876, despite sulphur baths, Colston required assistance to walk. He was in Geneva, Switzerland, for a medical consultation in September 1876 and had improved enough that he could walk for two or three hours. However, the cold weather produced bronchial symptoms. Exertion caused difficulty in 1878, and he was unable to get on or off a donkey without help. Dysfunction of his intestinal tract and urinary bladder caused him additional trouble. He returned to the United States in 1879.[2] Although Colston did not have his usual yearly attack of chills in 1885, he intermittently had great difficulty walking, straightening up, or even turning over in bed. On one occasion he was cupped all over his back and twelve ounces of blood were removed. Ice bags seemed to help his "sciatica lumbago" more than any other treatment. He was able to go to his office part time but was too ill to work on his lectures. In March 1891, when the news of Joseph E. Johnston's illness appeared in the paper, Colston was too crippled to travel across Washington, D.C., to visit him. As time went on, his disabilities increased. In April 1894 he was dismissed from his position as a clerk in the office of the surgeon general because of poor health. (He had been performing his duties from his bed at home.) He had been paralyzed from the waist down for more than a year and suffered with his bowels, poor appetite, and multiple joint pain. By late summer of that year, Colston's pain and weakness increased to the point that he required two strong men to lift him. In the fall, he was in the Lee Camp Soldiers' Home in Richmond. Although he could not eat, he was taken out of doors occasionally. He died at the Confederate Soldiers' Home on July 29, 1896, and was buried in Hollywood Cemetery.[3]

DEATH CERTIFICATE: RNA

1. *OR*, vol. 18:807; Raleigh E. Colston biographical notes; Special Orders no. 153, July 3, 1862; R. E. Colston to Louise (wife), Nov. 20, 1862, R. E. Colston Papers, all in SHC; *SHSP* 25:346.

2. Raleigh E. Colston biographical notes, R. E. Colston to wife, May 9, 1874, Daughter to Ma (Mrs. R. E. Colston), Apr. 11, Sept. 17, 1876; R. E. Colston to Stone Pacha, Mar. 27, 1878, R. E. Colston Papers, SHC.

3. R. E. Colston to daughter, Jan. 8, 27, Mar. 3, Apr. 26, Sept. 19, Oct. 20, Dec. 22, 1885, Jan. 4, Feb. 22, Aug. 8, Oct. 25, 1894; Daniel Lamont to Joshua Nicholls, Apr. 25, 1894, and John W. Walsh to Sir (Confederate Veterans Association), June 9, 1894, R. E. Colston Papers, SHC; R. E. Colston to Jos. E. Johnston, Mar. 19, 1891, Joseph E. Johnston Papers, College of William and Mary, Earl Gregg Swem Library, Williamsburg, Va. (hereafter cited as CWM); *SHSP* 25:351.

JAMES CONNER • *Born September 1, 1829*, in Charleston, South Carolina. A lawyer, Conner was a United States district attorney in 1856; when the war started, he joined the Hampton Legion as a captain. At Mechanicsville on June 26, 1862, his leg was broken by a rifle ball. This wound kept him from any duty for two months, and he spent part of the time with relatives near Petersburg. Unfit for field duty, he was assigned as one of the judges of the military court of the Second Corps. On April 1, 1863, he returned to the army at Camp Gregg, Virginia. Conner was colonel of the 22nd North Carolina at Gettysburg in July. He was appointed brigadier general in June 1864. Conner was again wounded in the left leg on October 13, 1864, during a skirmish near Cedar Creek. The troops had charged too far forward and he rode out to reorganize them. A shell exploded ten feet in front of him, a fragment passing through his knee and shattering the bone. Unconscious, he was carried on a litter to an ambulance, which took him to a field hospital. That night the leg was amputated close to the hip. He was never able to return to active duty, but his amputation did not prevent him from reestablishing his law practice after the war.[1] He died June 25, 1883, in Richmond, Virginia, and was buried in Magnolia Cemetery, Charleston, South Carolina.[2]

DEATH CERTIFICATE: Cause of death, bronchitis.

1. CSR; *OR*, vol. 11, pt. 2:836, 839, 899; vol. 27, pt. 2:290; vol. 43, pt. 1:579; James F. J. Caldwell, *History of a Brigade of South Carolinians*, 159; William W. Hassler, ed., *General to His Lady: The Civil War Letters of William Dorsey Pender to Fanny Pender*, 224; *CMH* 5:386; Clark, *Histories of Several Regiments* 2:168–70; newspaper clipping, n.p., July 18, 1901, James Conner Papers, SCL.

2. Death certificate.

PHILIP COOK • *Born July 31, 1817*, in Twiggs County, Georgia. Served in the Florida wars. A graduate of the University of Virginia Law School, he joined the 4th

Georgia Infantry as a private in 1861. Cook was wounded by a shell fragment on July 1, 1862, in the Battle of Malvern Hill. Later promoted to the rank of colonel, he was listed as in command in December. At Chancellorsville on May 2, 1863, he received a minié ball in his left leg just below the knee. The tibia was damaged, and on May 3, four inches of the bone had to be excised. He recovered first in a hospital in Richmond and then at home. On October 13, 1863, he asked for leave on surgeon's certificate from the general hospital in Macon, Georgia. He rejoined his command at Orange Court-House and in 1864 went to Petersburg. His promotion to brigadier general ranked from August 1864. Wounded in the right elbow during the assault on Hare's Hill on March 25, 1865, he rode to the rear with his arm dangling by his side. He was admitted three days later to a general hospital in Petersburg. The arm was badly broken, and it was feared for a while that it would have to be amputated. Cook was captured on April 3, 1865, and lay in the hospital until July 30.[1] After the war he restarted his law practice, served in the United States Congress, and was Georgia's secretary of state at the time of his death on May 21, 1894. He died at Atlanta and was buried in Rose Hill Cemetery, Macon.

DEATH CERTIFICATE: Cause of death, pneumonia.

1. CSR; *OR*, vol. 21:1072; vol. 25, pt. 1:947, 970; vol. 46, pt. 1:382; CR, 764:53; Gary W. Gallagher, ed., *Extracts of Letters of Major-General Bryan Grimes, to his Wife*, comp. Pulaski Cowper, 99; *CMH* 6:406.

JOHN ROGERS COOKE • *Born June 9, 1833*, at Jefferson Barracks, Missouri. Following his graduation from Harvard in 1855, he was commissioned directly into the old army as a second lieutenant. He resigned his commission at the start of the war and rose to become colonel of the 27th North Carolina in April 1862. He was reported to have been wounded at Sharpsburg on September 17, 1862, but details are lacking. It is known that he did not leave the field. He was commissioned brigadier general in November. In the First Battle of Fredericksburg, on December 13, 1862, Cooke was severely wounded by a bullet that entered over his left eye. Although a glancing blow, it purportedly broke the skull. He was carried down the lines on a litter and then taken by ambulance to the home of a friend some three miles to the rear. In late February of 1863 there was still concern about his wound, but he was back on the field by April. At the battle of Bristoe Station on October 14, 1863, his shinbone was shattered. In March 1864 he was detailed to a court of inquiry. Having recovered from the wound to his shinbone, he returned to duty about the middle of April. At Spotsylvania Court-House in May 1864, he was wounded in the leg but led an attack from horseback. Later, on the lines in front of Richmond, he lay in his tent suffering from his wounds and neuralgia.[1] Following the war he became a merchant at Richmond, Virginia, where he died April 10, 1891, and was buried in Hollywood Cemetery.

DEATH CERTIFICATE: Cause of death, pyemia.

1. CSR; *OR*, vol. 18:1022, 1045; vol. 21:555, 570–71, 626; vol. 29, pt. 1:427, 431–32, 435; vol. 33:100; J. E. B. Stuart to Mrs. J. E. B. Stuart (telegram), Dec. 14, 1862, J. E. B. Stuart collection (no. 7442), UV; J. E. B. Stuart to J. R. Cooke, Feb. 28, 1863, Cooke Family Papers, VSL; William W. Hassler,

A. P. Hill: *Lee's Forgotten General*, 178; *SHSP* 18:324–25; *CMH* 4:302; Clark, *Histories of Several Regiments* 2:434–38; *CV* 14:181.

DOUGLAS HANCOCK COOPER • *Born November 1, 1815,* in Amite County, Mississippi. At the start of the Mexican War he was a farmer and served during that conflict as a captain of the 1st Mississippi Rifles. His appointment as United States agent of the Choctaw Nation in Indian Territory in 1853 helped determine much of his activities during and after the Civil War. Appointed colonel of the First Choctaw and Chickasaw Mounted Rifles, he was commissioned brigadier general in Confederate service in May 1863. In the middle of October 1862, he was so ill that he could hardly dictate his reports and was confined to bed with a painful and dangerous disease. No specific diagnosis was provided. Cooper did his best to ready the troops for the march on Fort Scott; however, they were attacked by Federal troops on the morning of October 22. Cooper's report on these events was delayed until the middle of December, in part due to his continued ill health.[1] After the war he conducted Choctaw and Chickasaw claims against the Federal government in regard to their removal from their original homelands. He died at Old Fort Washita, Chickasaw Nation, Indian Territory, on April 29, 1879, and was buried at Fort Gibson, Oklahoma, in an unmarked grave.

DEATH CERTIFICATE: NAD

1. *OR,* vol. 13:48, 332, 334–36.

SAMUEL COOPER • *Born June 12, 1798,* in Dutchess County, New York. Graduated from USMA in 1815. Served in the Florida and Mexican wars. He remained in the United States Army following his graduation from West Point until the start of the Civil War. Receiving his appointments to brigadier general and general in the Confederate Army at the outbreak of hostilities, Cooper served as adjutant and inspector general during the war. Although he was left in Charlotte, North Carolina, because he was physically unable to go on any longer, he wanted to be included in the surrender arrangements in April 1865. After the war he became a planter near Alexandria, Virginia. Ill health plagued him for two to three years before his death. At about 6:00 A.M. on December 3, 1876, he had chest pain and died before a doctor could arrive. He was buried in Christ Church cemetery at Alexandria.[1]

DEATH CERTIFICATE: RNA

1. *OR,* vol. 47, pt. 3:842; *Alexandria Gazette,* Dec. 4, 1876.

MONTGOMERY DENT CORSE • *Born March 14, 1816,* at Alexandria, Virginia. Served in the Mexican War. Working in the banking business and as a militia officer in 1861, he was later made colonel of the 17th Virginia Infantry. On August 30, 1862, at the Second Battle of Manassas, Corse was slightly wounded in the thigh just as he was handed a captured Federal flag. However, he continued on duty. He fought at Boonsboro and was wounded in the mouth on September 14, 1862. The scar left by this wound was never noticeable because it was covered by his mustache. Three days later, at the Battle of Sharpsburg, Corse was severely wounded in the foot and for a time lay within the enemy lines. He was rescued by an advance of Gen. Robert A. Toombs's brigade and rode back to be examined by the surgeon. Later appointed brigadier general, he was given brigade command in the Army of Northern Virginia in November. At Drewry's Bluff on May 16, 1864, a spent ball struck him across the loins without inflicting a wound. Fever incapacitated him in August, and he had to go to Richmond to recuperate. Although he returned to the Howlett Line in September, he was back in Richmond during October and November on sick leave. He returned in December and was captured April 6, 1865, at Sayler's Creek. After the war he again entered the banking business. Corse and a friend were standing in the Virginia state capitol when the floor collapsed in April 1870. His friend was killed and Corse was struck on the head. In 1872, during U. S. Grant's second inauguration, Corse noticed blurring of his vision, which his physician diagnosed as cataracts. Surgery was performed on one eye without benefit of an anesthetic. Although the operation itself was successful, Corse contracted a cold, which caused his vision to be markedly diminished. The other eye was operated on in September 1887, using cocaine for an anesthetic. The surgery was a partial success: Corse was able to see enough to get about, but not well enough to read or to write. He died in the town of his birth on February 11, 1895, and was buried there in St. Paul's Cemetery.[1]

DEATH CERTIFICATE: Cause of death, debility incident to old age.

1. CSR; *OR*, vol. 19, pt. 1:905; vol. 21:1034–36; vol. 46, pt. 1:1268; Montgomery D. Corse, "Biography of General Montgomery Corse," 29, 32–33, 67–71, Lloyd House, Alexandria, Va. (hereafter cited as LH); Corse to wife, Nov. 5, 1864, Montgomery Corse letters, LH; Robert K. Krick, *30th Virginia Infantry*, 58–59, 65; *CMH* 3:588; *SHSP* 8:538–41.

GEORGE BLAKE COSBY • *Born January 19, 1830,* in Louisville, Kentucky. He graduated from USMA in 1852. In a skirmish with Indians near Lake Trinidad, Texas, on May 9, 1854, he was severely wounded. Leaving the U.S. Army in 1861, he became a staff major in the Confederate service. Cosby was captured at Fort Donelson in February 1862. Federal general R. W. Johnson wrote Federal general H. W. Halleck that Cosby's wife was his niece, and as Cosby's health was too feeble to stand prison confinement, he requested a parole for him. Paroled in May, he was on Simon B. Buckner's staff in August 1862. He was promoted to brigadier general in January 1863. Following the war he moved to California, where he engaged in farming and held different state and federal jobs. About ten years before his death he had an attack of paralysis, and he spent his later years as an invalid. Drugs ceased to alleviate his pain; in fact, the opiates may have contributed to depression. Cosby committed suicide June 29, 1909, at Oakland, California, by opening a gas valve. He was buried in City Cemetery, Sacramento.[1]

DEATH CERTIFICATE: Cause of death, asphyxiation by gas (suicide).

1. CSR; *OR*, vol. 7:160, 336; vol. 15:905; H. B. Lyon to wife, Mar. 30, Apr. 13, 1862, in H. B. Lyon letters, Microfilm, 2 rolls, Murray State University, Forrest C. Pogue Special Collections Library, Murray, Ky. (hereafter cited as MSU); *CMH* 9:230, Ky.; *Oakland Times*, June 30, 1909.

WILLIAM RUFFIN COX • *Born March 11, 1832,* at Scotland Neck, North Carolina. Admitted to the bar in Tennessee, he was in practice when he was commissioned a major of the 2nd North Carolina at the start of the war. On May 3, 1863, during the Battle of Chancellorsville, Cox was wounded five or six times but remained with his regiment as long as he could. He was listed as in command in June 1863. On November 7, 1863, during operations on the Rappahannock near Kelly's Ford and Wheatley's Ford, Cox was wounded in the right shoulder and face. He was admitted to the receiving hospital at Gordonsville, Virginia, on November 8, 1863, and transferred the same day to Richmond. Three days later he was granted a leave of absence. Cox was given the temporary rank of brigadier general in May 1864, and on June 4 he was assigned to command.[1] After the war he held a number of political positions, including a period in Congress. He died December 26, 1919, at Richmond and was buried in Oakwood Cemetery, in Raleigh, North Carolina. DEATH CERTIFICATE: Cause of death, chronic cardiorenal disease contributed to by senility.

1. *OR,* vol. 25, pt. 1:948; vol. 27, pt. 3:922; vol. 29, pt. 1:616, 633; vol. 36, pt. 3:873–74; Receiving Hospital, Register Book, Gordonsville, Va., June 1, 1863–May 5, 1864, p. 318, Eleanor S. Brockenbrough Library, MC; CR, 178:82; *CMH* 4:303; Gary W. Gallagher, *Stephen Dodson Ramseur,* 64.

GEORGE BIBB CRITTENDEN • *Born March 20, 1812,* at Russellville, Kentucky. Graduated from USMA in 1832 and resigned from the U.S. Army one year later. In 1835 he went to Texas, and while serving in the Texas Army was taken prisoner by the Mexicans and held for nearly a year. After service in the Mexican War, he remained in the United States Army until 1861. Appointed brigadier general in the Confederacy in August 1861 and major general in November, he resigned his commission the following October. He played little part in the rest of the war. He returned to civilian life and later became librarian of the state of Kentucky. He died November 27, 1880, at Danville, Kentucky, and was buried in the State Cemetery at Frankfort.
DEATH CERTIFICATE: NAD

ALFRED CUMMING • *Born January 30, 1829,* at Augusta, Georgia. He graduated from USMA in 1849, after which most of his duty in the U. S. Army was spent on the frontier. Upon entering Confederate service in June 1861, he was commissioned lieutenant colonel of the 10th Georgia Infantry. While leading his regiment at the Battle of Crew's Farm on July 1, 1862, Cumming was hit by a shell fragment. Stunned, he was borne from the field. On September 17 he was wounded at Sharpsburg; hospitalization was required through October, the same month he was promoted to brigadier general. Still disabled, he convalesced at his home in Georgia. Cumming was listed as in command of a brigade in the Western Division in the Department of the Gulf in April 1863. While leading his troops at the Battle of Jonesborough on August 31, 1864, he was severely wounded in the hip joint and in both hands. By February 1865 he had not recovered enough to raise himself from his bed and believed that it would be many months before he could perform

military duties of any description. He was not in command of his brigade in March 1865 in the action at Bentonville.[1] After the war he farmed at Rome, Georgia, where he died December 5, 1910. He was buried in Summerville Cemetery at Augusta.
DEATH CERTIFICATE: NAD

1. CSR; *OR*, vol. 11, pt. 2:672, 723; vol. 15:1069; vol. 38, pt. 3:694–96, 765; vol. 39, pt. 2:833; vol. 47, pt. 1:1057; *CMH* 6:409.

JUNIUS DANIEL • *Born June 27, 1828,* at Halifax, North Carolina. He graduated from USMA in 1851. Although admitted to the military academy in 1846, he was delayed graduation for a year because of severe injuries sustained during artillery practice. He resigned from the army in 1858 and managed his father's plantation. In 1861 he weighed about two hundred pounds. At the start of the war he was made colonel of the 14th North Carolina Infantry. Daniel was absent due to illness in September 1861 but returned by November. On June 30, 1862, near Malvern Hill, a Federal shell exploded near where he was riding, and he fell from his horse. He was soon able to get up and walked to a nearby gatepost, where he remained until he had recovered from the shock. After going to the rear to secure another horse, he returned to the battle. He received his brigadier stars in September 1862. Because of sickness, Daniel had to give up his command on July 21, 1863, at Darkesville. In August he was in a general hospital in Charlottesville, Virginia, with "hepatitic derangement" but was able to return to duty the next month. He was shot through the abdomen in the battle of Spotsylvania Court-House on May 12, 1864, and died the next day.[1] He was buried at Halifax, North Carolina, in the Old Colonial Churchyard Cemetery.

1. CSR; *OR*, vol. 27, pt. 2:564, 571; vol. 36, pt. 1:1030, 1073; Bryan Grimes to wife, May 14, 1864, Bryan Grimes Papers, SHC; Clark, *Histories of Several Regiments* 3:165; *SHSP* 8:92, 18:340–49; *CMH* 4:306.

HENRY BREVARD DAVIDSON • *Born January 28, 1831,* at Shelbyville, Tennessee. He graduated from USMA in 1853. Because of his bravery as a private during the Mexican War he received an appointment to West Point. He served on the frontier until he entered the Confederate Army in 1861 as a major in the Adjutant and Inspector General's Department. Following his commission as brigadier general in August 1863, he had field command until the end of the war. He moved to California and became engaged as a civil engineer and railroad agent. His death occurred on March 4, 1899, near Livermore, California, and he was buried at Oakland.
DEATH CERTIFICATE: RNA

JOSEPH ROBERT DAVIS • *Born January 12, 1825,* at Woodville, Mississippi. A lawyer-politician, Davis entered the Confederate Army in 1861 as a captain and was later appointed lieutenant colonel of the 10th Mississippi Infantry. His brigadier general commission ranked from September 1862. He was wounded during the charge on July 3, 1863, at Gettysburg. Later that month Davis was in Richmond with typhoid fever, and there was some question as to how long he would be away from his command. He was furloughed on July 30 with an engorged liver and general debility. On August 22 he was well enough to take a note from President Davis to Robert E. Lee at a camp near Orange Court-House. By October Davis was back on the field with his brigade. The first week in August 1864 he left on sick leave. On September 30 he was listed as in command of his brigade.[1] He resumed the practice of law after the war. Davis died at Biloxi, Mississippi, on September 15, 1896, and was buried in the Biloxi (City) Cemetery. Cause of death: Albuminuria.[2]

1. CSR; *OR*, vol. 27, pt. 3:1030, 1049; vol. 29, pt. 1:431, pt. 2:660–61; vol. 42, pt. 2:1273, 1309.
2. Internment records, Biloxi Cemetery, Miss.

WILLIAM GEORGE MACKEY DAVIS • *Born May 9, 1812, at Portsmouth, Virginia.* A practicing lawyer in Florida when the war started, he recruited the 1st Florida Cavalry and was elected colonel. He was commissioned brigadier general in November 1862. In March 1863 he was on leave in Richmond because of a chronic vesicular eruption of his skin. His health, which had never been good, had been particularly poor since October 1862; however, he had continued on duty except for this one absence. He requested to resign in April 1863 because he thought his health would not improve due to his age. His doctor reported that he had a chronic lichen planus condition of his skin, which was an inflammatory disease associated with pain and itching. In his case it was manifest by frequent episodes of papules followed by severe and obstinate excoriation.[1] Davis resigned in May from the military service and ran blockade runners for the rest of the war. After the war he returned to his law practice. He died March 11, 1898, at Alexandria and was buried in Remington, Virginia, on the Ott farm.

DEATH CERTIFICATE: RNA

1. CSR; *OR*, vol. 23, pt. 2:662; *CMH* 11:199, Tex.

JAMES DEARING • *Born April 25, 1840,* in Campbell County, Virginia. He resigned from West Point in April 1861 without graduating and entered the Confederate Army as a lieutenant. During June and July 1862, he was sick with chills and fever. He convalesced in Richmond and was not back until late August. Passing through grades and being transferred to the cavalry, he was promoted brigadier in April 1864. His health was poor in July. He had two attacks of chills, fever, and headache in September 1864, and on the thirtieth he was too ill to take the field during the Richmond campaign. However, Dearing was with his troops in late October. Pursuing Federal troops near Jetersville on April 5, 1865, he was slightly wounded in the arm but did not leave the field. Dearing was mortally wounded during a pistol duel with Federal general Theodore Read, whom he killed on April 6, 1865, at High Bridge, Virginia. It is not clear whether he was wounded by Read or shot accidentally through the lungs by one of his own men. He was taken first to a nearby house and then to the Ladies' Aid Hospital (old City Hotel) at Lynchburg, Virginia. He survived until the twenty-second and was buried the next day in Spring Hill Cemetery, at Lynchburg.[1]

1. *OR*, vol. 42, pt. 1:947, pt. 3:1159, 1162; vol. 51, pt. 2:1083; William L. Parker, *General James Dearing CSA*, 28, 30, 75, 83, 90; *CMH* 3:590; Special Staff of Writers, *History of Virginia: Virginia Biography* 5:352, 6:70; Asbury Christian, *Lynchburg and Its People*, 235; Lyon Gardiner Tyler, ed., *Encyclopedia of Virginia Biography* 5:963; *News* (Lynchburg, Va.), extra Sat. evening, Apr. 22, 1865, Jones Memorial Library, Lynchburg, Va.; Diuguid's Burial Records, roll No. 3, 929.3D, Book 7, 222, Jones Memorial Library, Lynchburg, Va.; Myers, *Comanches*, 377, 380.

ZACHARIAH CANTEY DEAS • *Born October 25, 1819*, in Camden, South Carolina. Served in the Mexican War. A well-to-do cotton broker, he recruited the 22nd Alabama Infantry in 1861 and was elected colonel of the regiment. Deas was hit by several balls at Shiloh on April 7, 1862, and, because of the blood loss, was compelled to retire from the field. By late May he was back to duty. His commission as brigadier general ranked from December 1862. In July 1864, Deas was absent due to sickness but returned on August 6. He was slightly wounded at Franklin on November 30, 1864, but was listed as in command of his brigade on December 10. Deas was with his troops during the Carolina campaign in early February 1865, but on the second day of the skirmish at Columbia, South Carolina, he became ill and had to leave the field. He had not returned by the end of March.[1] After the war he moved to New York City, became a broker again, and finally became a member of the stock exchange. He died March 6, 1882, in New York City and was buried in Woodlawn Cemetery in New York.

DEATH CERTIFICATE: Cause of death, primary, chronic Bright's disease; immediate, cerebral apoplexy.

1. *OR*, vol. 10, pt. 1:468, 539, 540, 543, 855; vol. 38, pt. 5:951, 953; vol. 45, pt. 1:664; vol. 47, pt. 2:1107, 1147; *CMH* 11:401, Ala.; *CV* 18:420.

JULIUS ADOLPH DE LAGNEL • *Born July 24, 1827*, in Newark, New Jersey. Served in the Mexican War. He was commissioned as a second lieutenant of artillery directly into the United States Army in 1847. Resigning from the army in 1861, he joined the Confederate artillery as a captain. At Rich Mountain, during the attack of a large Federal force on July 11, 1861, his horse was shot from under him. He volunteered his help with the remaining piece of artillery and was shot in the side by a minié ball. Hiding until the Federal troops left, de Lagnel found shelter with a local resident while he recovered. Disguised as a herder, he was captured when he tried to return to the Confederate lines. He was released to be exchanged on December 13, 1861. During March 1862 he was in command of a battery. Although commissioned brigadier general in April, he declined the position. In late July and August 1862, de Lagnel was sick and had to take a leave. For the remainder of the war he served in the Ordnance Bureau. Following the war he was involved in the

Pacific steamship service. He was a bridegroom at eighty-two years of age. For the last two months of his life he was ill; two weeks before his death he suffered from a severe attack of heart disease. His death on June 3, 1912, in Washington, D.C., was attributed to heart disease. He was buried in St. Paul's Cemetery in Alexandria, Virginia.[1]

DEATH CERTIFICATE: RNA

1. CSR; *OR*, vol. 2:244, 260, 270, 271; vol. 9:69; vol. 11, pt. 3:384; vol. 13:874; vol. 32, pt. 3:592; *CMH* 3:691; Warner, *Generals in Gray*, 71; *Washington Post*, June 4, 1912.

JAMES DESHLER • *Born February 18, 1833,* at Tuscumbia, Alabama. Graduated from USMA in 1854. He served on the frontier and apparently left the army in 1861 without formal notice. He entered Confederate service as a captain of artillery in 1861. At the battle of Allegheny Mountains, West Virginia, on December 13, 1861, Deshler was wounded in both thighs. He remained in the trenches until the end of the day. After a leave of absence, he was assigned to the position of chief of Ordnance and Artillery in April 1862. He was commissioned brigadier general in July 1863. At the Battle of Chickamauga on September 20, 1863, he was killed instantly when a three-inch shell passed through his chest while he was examining the cartridge boxes. He was buried in Oakwood Cemetery, Tuscumbia.[1]

1. CSR; *OR*, vol. 5:460, 464; vol. 30, pt. 2:143, 156, 188–89; *CMH* 12:403, Ala.

GEORGE GIBBS DIBRELL • *Born April 12, 1822,* at Sparta, Tennessee. A merchant and farmer when the war started, he enlisted in Confederate service as a private. In 1862 he recruited and commanded as colonel the 8th Tennessee Cavalry. About May 18, 1863, he was unable to accompany his troops because of an accident. Dibrell had been run over by a horse and was so badly injured that he had to remain behind for several days. Although in great pain, he tried to follow his troops and just avoided being captured. During the Knoxville winter campaign, probably on December 21, 1863, Dibrell was wounded at Clinch River. His appointment as brigadier general ranked from July 1864. In a report by Joseph Wheeler after the surrender in April 1865, in which he congratulated his officers, he stated that Dibrell had been wounded twice during the long series of campaigns.[1] After the war he held a number of positions, including merchant, congressman, railroad president, and coal-mine developer. He died May 9, 1888, at the city of his birth and was buried there in the Old City Cemetery.

DEATH CERTIFICATE: NAD

1. *OR*, vol. 47, pt. 1:1132; Thomas Jordan and John P. Pryor, *Campaigns of Lieutenant-General N. B. Forrest, and of Forrest's Cavalry*, 283; *CV* 9:320.

THOMAS PLEASANT DOCKERY • *Born December 18, 1833,* probably in Montgomery County, North Carolina. Dockery joined the Confederate service as a colonel of the 5th Arkansas State Troops and later became colonel of the 19th Arkansas Infantry. He was captured at Vicksburg. Following his parole, he was appointed brigadier general in August 1863. For the rest of the war he was engaged in an unsuccessful attempt to organize troops in Arkansas. He had lost everything in the war, so afterward he took up civil engineering. Dockery died February 26, 1898, at New York City and was buried in the City Cemetery at Natchez, Mississippi.[1] DEATH CERTIFICATE: Cause of death, rheumatoid endocarditis and pulmonary edema.

1. Death certificate.

GEORGE PIERCE DOLES • *Born May 14, 1830,* in Milledgeville, Georgia. He was a businessman in Georgia before the war and joined a militia company in 1861. He was elected colonel in May 1862, after the company entered Confederate service as part of the 4th Georgia Infantry. Doles was wounded by a shell at the Battle of Malvern Hill on July 1, 1862, but signed the regimental muster rolls in July and August. The following November he was commissioned brigadier general. Near Bethesda Church, on June 2, 1864, while supervising the entrenchment of his line, Doles was killed when a Federal sharpshooter's bullet went through his left chest. He was buried at Milledgeville in Memory Hill Cemetery.[1]

1. CSR; *CMH* 6:412.

DANIEL SMITH DONELSON • *Born June 23, 1801,* in Sumner County, Tennessee. He graduated from USMA in 1825 and resigned from the United States Army soon afterward. He became a planter, Tennessee politician, and member of the militia. At the start of the war, he was made a brigadier general of state troops and received the same rank in the Confederate service in July 1861. Late in 1862 he was sick but had recovered enough to return to duty in January 1863. Donelson was in command of the Department of East Tennessee until April 1863, when he was granted a leave of absence. His health had been quite bad for several months prior to his arrival in East Tennessee, and he had been confined to his room almost all of the time. According to the doctor's certificate, Donelson was incapable of performing his duties because of chronic diarrhea and extreme prostration. His appetite was poor, and he took no nourishment. The reduction in his weight was proportional to his loss of strength. He died April 17, 1863, at Montvale Springs, Tennessee, from chronic diarrhea. Donelson was buried in the Presbyterian Cemetery, Hendersonville, Tennessee.[1]

1. CSR; *OR,* vol. 23, pt. 2:744–45, 787; CSR of Otho French Strahl.

THOMAS FENWICK DRAYTON • *Born August 24, 1808,* probably at Charleston, South Carolina. He graduated from USMA in 1828. Drayton remained in the old army for eight years following graduation, then took up farming, politics, and railroad construction. Appointed a Confederate brigadier general in September 1861, he had a lackluster military career. Following the war he again took up farming and later became an insurance agent. He died February 18, 1891, at

Florence, South Carolina, and was buried in Elmwood Cemetery at Charlotte, North Carolina.

DEATH CERTIFICATE: NAD

Dudley McIver DuBose • *Born October 28, 1834,* in Shelby County, Tennessee. Following his graduation from law school, he was admitted to the bar in 1857. He entered the Confederate Army as a lieutenant and was commissioned a colonel of the 15th Georgia Infantry in January 1863. DuBose was wounded at the Battle of Chickamauga on September 19, 1863. However, he retained his command and participated in the subsequent operations.[1] He reached the rank of brigadier general in November 1864. After the war he returned to the practice of law and politics. He died March 2, 1883, at Washington, Georgia, and was buried there in Rest Haven Cemetery.

DEATH CERTIFICATE: NAD

1. CSR; *OR,* vol. 30, pt. 2:519.

Basil Wilson Duke • *Born May 28, 1837,* in Scott County, Kentucky.[1] A practicing lawyer at the start of the war, he entered the Confederate service as a private in the company of his brother-in-law, John H. Morgan. He was later appointed second lieutenant and then colonel. As Duke rode through the Federal line at Shiloh on the afternoon of April 6, 1862, he was shot and fell from his horse. He was in the act of striking an enemy on his right with his saber when another soldier on his left placed a gun to Duke's shoulder and pulled the trigger. The weapon was an old-fashioned Brown Bess musket, loaded with a ball and three buckshot. One of the buckshot entered Duke's left shoulder; the ball struck the spinal process and tore its way through his right shoulder blade. Duke attributed his erect position in the saddle in keeping the ball from severing his spinal column. He was back in July 1862 and participated in John H. Morgan's subsequent raids. As Morgan's rear regiment was crossing Rolling Fork on December 29, 1862, it was attacked by Federal troops. Duke fell from his horse severely wounded in the head by a shell, which killed his aide-de-camp. Capt. Thomas Quirk is credited with saving General Duke from capture. The stream was very swollen, and it was thought impossible to take the wounded officer across the river. Quirk took the apparently lifeless body in his arms and carried Duke across the water on his horse. He then took a carriage, filled it with bedding, and brought Duke back to the South. Duke was absent from his command through March 1863. Captured later with John H. Morgan and others, he was imprisoned in the Ohio Penitentiary, where severe conditions impaired his health. He was promoted to brigadier general in September 1864. Two months after he was paroled at the end of the war, he set about raising a bargeload of cotton sunk in the Savannah River below Augusta. Duke superintended the work for ten to fourteen days and slept each night on low ground near the water. He contracted the fever so common in that part of the country, which was probably malaria. After two weeks in bed in Augusta, Duke finished his business and returned to Kentucky in very bad health.[2] Resuming the practice of law, he had an active and varied life as politician and author. He died September 16, 1916, at New York City and was buried in the City Cemetery in Lexington, Kentucky.

DEATH CERTIFICATE: Cause of death, primary, arteriosclerosis, chronic nephritis and endarteritis obliterans; contributory, operation, amputation thigh.

1. Death certificate.

2. OR, vol. 20, pt. 1:157; General Basil W. Duke, *Personal Recollections of Shiloh*, 14–15; idem, *Reminiscences of General Basil W. Duke, C.S.A.*, 125, 339, 397–98; idem, *A History of Morgan's Cavalry*, 339, 353, 474; *CV* 5:16–17.

JOHNSON KELLY DUNCAN • *Born March 19, 1827*, at York, Pennsylvania. He graduated from USMA in 1849. Served in the Florida wars. He had home leave in September 1852; then, after his arrival in Fort Preble, Maine, in mid-December, he was ill for a few weeks. Duncan resigned from the army in 1855 and held engineering positions in Louisiana. Although a Northerner by birth, he was appointed colonel of artillery in the Confederate Army at the outbreak of war. Commissioned brigadier general in January 1862, he was in charge of the coastal defenses in and near New Orleans when it fell to Federal forces in April. On November 15, 1862, he became ill with typhoid fever. He was carried along in an ambulance, but when his condition worsened, he was left in Knoxville. Despite the illness, Braxton Bragg appointed him his chief of staff on November 20. Duncan died at Knoxville on December 18, 1862. His wife, who was pregnant at the time of his death, wore mourning for the next fifty-six years and never visited his grave in the McGavock Cemetery at Franklin, Tennessee.[1]

1. CSR; *OR*, vol. 20, pt. 2:403, 411, 457, 508; Cummings, "Seven Ohio Confederate Generals," 319–20, 345, 575–77.

JOHN DUNOVANT • *Born March 5, 1825*, at Chester, South Carolina. He received a severe wound at Chapultepec on September 13, 1847, and was discharged by reason of a certificate of disability on December 7. Dunovant obtained a direct commission to captain in the regular U.S. Army in 1855. In November 1860 he was at the Planter's House in St. Louis with a broken leg. He resigned soon after the start of the Civil War and went from major of militia to colonel of the 1st South Carolina Regulars. On the regimental returns for the months of June and July 1861, Dunovant was absent sick, but he returned in August. In June 1862 he was dismissed from the service for drunkenness but was reappointed as a colonel of the 5th South Carolina Cavalry. Soon after arriving in Virginia in 1864, he was detached with his regiment on temporary duty under the command of General Fitzhugh Lee. During an engagement near the James River on May 28, 1864, he was wounded in the left hand by a pistol ball and was admitted to the Jackson Hospital in Richmond the same day. He reported for duty July 8, before the wound had healed and with his arm in a sling, which he wore until his death. On August 22, 1864, Dunovant was appointed brigadier general and ordered to report to Wade

Hampton for assignment to the command of Matthew C. Butler's brigade. He was killed at the head of his troops on October 1, 1864, on the Vaughan Road. When he was shot, he tumbled forward from his horse and died almost instantly. After the body was picked up, an indentation was discovered in his forehead, which was concluded to be the site of his mortal wound. However, on further examination he was found to have been shot in the chest. The wound on the forehead appeared to have been made by a root or a log located on the causeway where he fell. Supposedly he was killed by Sgt. James T. Cancy, a U.S.A. Medal of Honor winner, but this has been questioned. He was buried in the family plot three miles from Chester.[1]

1. CSR Mexican War; CSR; *OR*, vol. 42, pt. 1:636, 948, pt. 2:1195; *CV* 8:33, 16:183–84; Morrison, *Memoirs of Henry Heth*, 149; Richard J. Sommers, *Richmond Redeemed: Seige at Petersburg*, 563.

E

JUBAL ANDERSON EARLY • *Born November 3, 1816*, in Franklin County, Virginia. He graduated from USMA in 1837. Served in the Florida and Mexican wars. Lewis Addison Armistead was dismissed from West Point for supposedly hitting Early over the head with a mess plate. Early resigned from the army after serving in Florida and took up law and politics. He served as a major of the Virginia Volunteers in the war with Mexico, where he developed rheumatism following a severe cold. As a result, he walked bent over. He took a leave to recuperate and spent most of the time with his father in the Kanawha River valley. He was aboard a steamboat sailing along the Ohio River en route to Mexico when a boiler exploded, causing him injury; he suffered cuts on his feet and burns. Early entered the Confederate service as a colonel and was commissioned brigadier general in July 1861. He was wounded twice on May 5, 1862, at the Battle of Williamsburg, Virginia. Weak from loss of blood and suffering from excruciating pain, he finally had to leave the field and retired to a redoubt. When he was taken to a hospital at Williamsburg, it was found that one wound was just a scratch, whereas the minié ball that struck him near the shoulder joint had flattened when it passed around his back to the opposite shoulder blade. After recuperating in Richmond, Lynchburg, and, finally, in Franklin County, he returned to duty June 29. When Early took command on July 1, he was still so feeble from the effect of his wound that he was unable to mount his horse without assistance. One month later, at the Battle of Cedar Mountain (August 9), he still had to be helped onto his horse. Early fought at the Second Battle of Manassas on August 29, 1862. On September 19, 1864, at Winchester, he was not feeling well. The following month, ill with rheumatism and in general poor health, he was not able to make the steep ascent up Three Top Mountain to the signal station. When Robert E. Lee surrendered,

Early was on his way from southwestern Virginia in an ambulance. He was very sick, having had a hemorrhage from his lungs, which he thought was the result of a bad cold. As soon as he could travel, he left for the Trans-Mississippi. Between August and October of 1865, while in Texas, Early had three episodes of chills and fever.[1] Following the war, after a period in Cuba and Canada, he returned to his law practice. He also participated in the Louisiana lottery and wrote extensively. On February 15, 1894, he missed a step and fell down the stairs at the Lynchburg post office. After resting a while he was taken home in his buggy; however, he insisted that he be taken back to town, where he remained until evening. His doctor found no broken bones, but Early's speech was incoherent and he had severe back pain. He remained confused but was able to go out a few times during the next couple days. He was confined to the house after this incident and died quietly on March 2, 1894. He was buried in Spring Hill Cemetery at Lynchburg.[2] DEATH CERTIFICATE: Cause of death not given by attending physician.

1. CSR; OR, vol. 11, pt. 1:567, 603, 608, pt. 2:607, 611; vol. 12, pt. 2:227, 556, 703; Millard K. Bushong, *Old Jube: A Biography of Jubal A. Early,* 4, 55, 57, 59, 70, 252, 280; G. Moxley Sorrel, *Recollection of a Confederate Staff Officer,* 56; Freeman, *Lee's Lieutenants* 1:185; "Military Reminiscences of Major Campbell Brown, 1861–1863," 67–68, Campbell Brown-Ewell Papers, TSLA; J. A. Early to Dr. H. McGuire, Oct. 30, 1865, Hunter Holmes McGuire Papers (no. 9320), UV; *SHSP* 18:249, 37:145.

2. *CV* 2:113; *News* (Lynchburg), Mar. 3, 1894, Jones Memorial Library, Lynchburg, Va.

JOHN ECHOLS · *Born March 20, 1823,* in Lynchburg, Virginia. A lawyer and politician before the war, he entered Confederate service as a lieutenant colonel and was soon made a colonel. At the First Battle of Kernstown, Virginia, on March 23, 1862, Echols was wounded and taken from the field in an ambulance. A musket ball had entered near his shoulder, passed through the arm, and shattered the bone. He was at Staunton in mid-April recovering from his wound. His promotion as brigadier general ranked from April. In mid-1862 he was assigned to command a brigade of the Army of West Virginia. However, he was unable to command in September and October 1862 because of illness and was given a leave for his health in November. He reported for duty in the Department of Western Virginia in February 1863. On June 30, Echols requested leave because of the uncertain state of his health, which he said had been precarious for the past year. However, by September 23, 1863, he was ready to garrison the Narrows in the event of a Federal advance, and fought in the Battle of Droop Mountain, West Virginia, in November. On June 3, 1864, Robert E. Lee requested that Echols be relieved of command of his brigade because of poor health. For some years he had had an organic affliction of his heart, and on July 19, 1864, he was given a leave of absence on surgeon's certificate. In August he assumed command of the District of Southwest Virginia. After the war he became a businessman in Virginia and Kentucky. Prior to his death on May 24, 1896, at Staunton, Virginia, he had been in declining health for some months. He was buried at Staunton in the Thornrose Cemetery.[1] DEATH CERTIFICATE: Cause of death, kidney disease.

1. CSR; *OR*, vol. 12, pt. 1:381, 393; vol. 19, pt. 1:667, 1074, 1090, pt. 2:713; vol. 25, pt. 2:640; vol. 29, pt. 1:528, pt. 2:744; vol. 51, pt. 2:981–82; *CMH* 3:591–93; *CV* 4:316–17.

MATTHEW DUNCAN ECTOR • *Born February 28, 1822,* in Putnam County, Georgia. Admitted to the Georgia bar in 1844, he later moved to Texas, where he was elected to the state legislature. He enlisted as a private when the war started. Within a short time he was appointed adjutant of Gen. J. L. Hogg's brigade and was then elected colonel of the 14th Texas Cavalry. His commission as brigadier general ranked from August 1862. Ector was struck four times at Chickamauga in September 1863, but did not leave the field. Following the battle he was ordered to Mississippi with his brigade. Near New Hope Church, Georgia, on June 2, 1864, Ector was slightly wounded. He was well enough by the tenth to ride the picket line with Gen. Samuel G. French. Ector was directing part of the artillery fire beside the Turner's Ferry Road in front of Atlanta on July 27, 1864, when a shell fragment hit his lower left thigh. The wound necessitated a midthigh amputation and put an end to his active field service. During the last days of the war, he took part in the defense of Mobile.[1] Returning to Texas after the war, he again took up the practice of law and became a judge. He died October 29, 1879, at Tyler, Texas, and was buried in the Greenwood Cemetery at Marshall, Texas.

DEATH CERTIFICATE: NAD

1. CSR; *OR*, vol. 30, pt. 2:240, pt. 4:689; vol. 38, pt. 3:904, 910; French, *Two Wars,* 201–2, 219; *CMH* 11:227, Tex.

STEPHEN ELLIOTT, JR. • *Born October 26, 1830,* in Beaufort, South Carolina. Before the war he was a planter and politician. He was captain of the Beaufort Volunteer Artillery when it became a company in the 11th South Carolina Infantry in June 1861. At Fort Beauregard on November 7, 1861, he was wounded in the leg by a fragment of a rifled gun when it exploded on the thirty-second discharge. During the bombardment of Fort Sumter on December 11, 1863, Elliott was slightly wounded in the head and ankle. In a few days his head wound was almost healed, but he had to be careful of his footing on rough ground. After passing through grades, he was promoted to brigadier general, ranking from May 1864. Following the explosion of the mine in the Battle of the Crater on July 30, 1864, Elliott was badly wounded by a rifle ball in the upper left lung. His wife and father came to join him. His arm was paralyzed for some time, and he obtained a furlough from a Petersburg general hospital on August 17. After being incapacitated for field service for several months, he joined Gen. Joseph E. Johnston's army near Bentonville, North Carolina, and on March 19, 1865, he was wounded in the arm. In late March Elliott was compelled to retire from active service and return home because of his recent wound as well as the reopening of the wound received at the Crater.[1] He survived the end of the war by only a few months and died February 21, 1866, at Aiken, South Carolina. Elliott was buried in the St. Helena's Episcopal Church Cemetery at Beaufort.

DEATH CERTIFICATE: NAD

1. CSR; Confederate States Army Casualties, roll 3; *OR*, vol. 28, pt. 1:177, 643–44, pt. 2:546–47, 555; vol. 40, pt. 1:790; CR, 145:133; Stephen Elliott, Jr., to mother, Dec. 14, 1863, Stephen Elliott, Jr., Papers, SCL; *CMH* 5:390; Chesnut, *Diary from Dixie*, 426; Warner, *Generals in Gray*, 81–82; Hagood, *Memoirs of the War of Secession*, 365.

ARNOLD ELZEY (JONES) • *Born December 18, 1816*, in Somerset County, Maryland. He graduated from USMA in 1837, dropping the Jones from his name while there. Served in the Florida and Mexican wars. When the Civil War started, he resigned from the old army and joined the Confederate service as a colonel. Elzey was hospitalized in Richmond in January 1862, but the reason was not listed. At the Battle of Cross Keys, Virginia, on June 8, 1862, his horse was shot from under him and he was slightly wounded in the leg by a rifle ball. Within a week he was back to duty. Late on the evening of June 27, 1862, during the engagement of Cold Harbor, Elzey was wounded again. A minié ball entered the right side of his face just above the mouth and passed transversely through his head and out behind his left ear. Disabled, he was taken to the rear in an ambulance by his aide. Later he was granted a leave to recuperate. He was in Richmond in November, looking miserable and requiring a second operation on his jaw. In December 1862 he was placed in command of the Richmond defenses. In May 1863 he was doing all that his poor physical state would permit. On June 2, 1863, Elzey was too ill to see the secretary of war, and he was unable to leave his bed during July. He was given a thirty-day leave of absence on July 29, 1864. Elzey was assigned as chief of artillery of the Army of Tennessee in September 1864 and relieved from duty in February 1865.[1] After the war he lived on a farm. He died February 21, 1871, at Baltimore, Maryland, and was buried there in Green Mount Cemetery. Cause of death: Inflammation of bowels.[2]

1. CSR; *OR*, vol. 11, pt. 2:607, 610; vol. 12, pt. 1:714, 728, 782, 784; vol. 18:794, 953, 1091; vol. 27, pt. 3:996; vol. 38, pt. 5:1031; vol. 39, pt. 2:872; vol. 40, pt. 3:814; vol. 47, pt. 2:1208; Lou to brother, Nov. 14, 1862, Louis T. Wigfall Family Papers, University of Texas at Austin, E. C. Barker Texas History Center (hereafter cited as UTA); Taylor, *Destruction and Reconstruction*, 84; Freeman, *Lee's Lieutenants* 3:41; *CMH* 2:157, Md.

2. Burial record no. 18355, Green Mount Cemetery, Baltimore, Md.

CLEMENT ANSELM EVANS • *Born February 25, 1833*, in Stewart County, Georgia. A lawyer at a young age, he was a judge and a state senator before the war. Following his enlistment in the Confederate service in 1861, he was appointed colonel of the 31st Georgia Infantry, ranking from May 1862. His stomach and bowels were out of order on November 23, 1861, and he planned to take a big blue pill that night and Epsom salts the next day. During the battle at Cold Harbor on June 27, 1862, he received a slight flesh wound in the leg. After reaching Gordonsville in late July, he had a chill and became ill with typhoid. The last of September he returned to the field. He was wounded at Chancellorsville on May 3, 1863, but there are few details except that it did not keep him from his duties. He had dysentery in late May and early June, and although not too sick, he felt puny and lost weight. Evans was slightly wounded in the side at Gettysburg on July 1, 1863, but it was not serious enough to force him from the field. A shell fragment had struck him near where the ribs joined his backbone. After dark he went to the hospital and had the wound dressed. Although he could hardly mount his horse, he remained on the field. The wound healed rapidly. On July 13, during the retreat, he suffered abdominal pain. Later in the summer he had almost daily headaches, a complaint he apparently had every summer. In late November, while coming back from Orange Court-House, he had severe pain associated with fever in his back, chest, and throughout his body. He thought he was going to develop pneumonia, but his symptoms improved during the next few days. In May 1864 in the Wilderness he was wounded slightly, but it was enough to draw blood. He had a bad headache, and although his face wound was healed, his knee still bothered him on May 15. His commission as brigadier general ranked from May 1864. At the Battle of Monocacy, Maryland, on July 9, 1864, Evans was severely wounded. His men carried him on a blanket back across the river to a house. He had been hit by two balls: one passed through his left arm and the other lodged in his left side. After dark the surgeon probed the wound and took out the bullet. Not wanting to be captured, Evans went with the army in its demonstration against Washington and on its return south. He was admitted to the receiving hospital in Gordonsville, Virginia, on the eighteenth and was transferred to a general hospital in Richmond the same day. On July 23 he started a circuitous route through the Carolinas to return to his home in Georgia. The minié ball that had hit him in the left side carried with it a number of pins which were so deeply imbedded that they were not all extracted for a number of years. Although not fully recovered, he returned to duty in the middle of September 1864. A minister of the Methodist church after the war, Evans retired after twenty-five years because of problems resulting from his old wounds. He died July 2, 1911, at Atlanta and was buried there in the Oakland Cemetery.[1]

DEATH CERTIFICATE: Cause of death, primary, interstitial nephritis, chronic of probably a year or more; contributing, arteriosclerosis.

1. CSR; *OR*, vol. 11, pt. 2:596; vol. 19, pt. 2:639; vol. 29, pt. 1:398, pt. 2:684; vol. 37, pt. 1:348, 351; *Battles and Leaders* 2:313–17; CR, 178:170; *CV* 12:54; G. W. Nichols, *A Soldier's Story of his Regiment (61st Georgia)*, 117–19, 181; Gordon, *Reminiscences*, 312; Robert Grier Stephens, Jr., *Intrepid Warrior: Clement Anselem Evans*, 86, 109, 111, 114, 150–52, 163, 169, 174, 179, 221–23, 226, 237, 295, 397–98, 426–31, 450.

NATHAN GEORGE "SHANKS" EVANS • *Born February 3, 1824*, in Marion, South Carolina. Graduated from USMA in 1848, after which he served on the frontier. He resigned from the U.S. Army in 1861 and entered Confederate service as adjutant general of South Carolina troops. On April 11, 1861, the morning of the attack on Fort Sumter, he joined John Dunovant soon after the battle commenced in spite of the fact that he had been sick in bed for several days prior. He was commissioned colonel of the 4th South Carolina during the summer. Accused of drunkenness at the Battle of Leesburg on October 21, 1861, he replied that he was not drunk but sick and that he had rested on account of his poor physical condition only when he thought the battle was over. His promotion to brigadier general ranked from that date. On April 16, 1864, Evans had a serious fall from his horse and three days later had to give up his command because of the injury. He was back in the field with his troops by May 2.[1] Following the war he became a high school principal at Midway, Alabama, where he died on November 23, 1868. He was buried in the Tabernacle Cemetery at Cokesbury, South Carolina.

DEATH CERTIFICATE: NAD

1. *OR*, vol. 1:36; vol. 35, pt. 2:436, 441, 443; vol. 36, pt. 2:942; James L. Conrad, "From Glory to Contention: The Sad History of 'Shanks' Evans," *Civil War Times Illustrated* (hereafter cited as *CWTI*), 22:32–38; Haskell, *Memoirs*, 12.

RICHARD STODDERT EWELL • *Born February 8, 1817,* at Georgetown, Washington, D.C. He graduated from USMA in 1840. Served in the Mexican War. While at West Point, he was hospitalized in March 1840 with a sore throat that he thought was the result of the changing weather. He was uncomfortable from both the pain and the remedy, which consisted of applying cayenne pepper and spirits of turpentine. Although his appetite was excellent, he was able to take only small amounts of spooned victuals. In November 1841, while at Fort Wayne, Cherokee Nations, he shaved his head because his hair was falling out. Malaria was first mentioned as a diagnosis in October 1843. His illness recurred over the years; unwell in September 1845, Ewell ate only a concoction of raw tomatoes, onions, salt, sweet potatoes, and dried beef. During the winter of 1847, while near the Rio Grande, he was again quite sick. In July 1850 he helped take a group of recruits to New Mexico, but because of diarrhea he had to remain in an ambulance most of the trip. He had a badly inflamed finger in 1856. Three years later he was wounded during a skirmish with the Apaches. In late 1860 Ewell had vertigo, nausea, and dyspepsia and ate only a restricted diet. He was exceedingly debilitated, experienced occasional attacks of the ague, and had violent pain in his head accompanied by a sick stomach. Ewell believed that he could not withstand another season in Arizona because the last one had almost done him in. While on court-martial duty he received recommendations by two surgeons to leave as soon as possible. Obtaining a sick leave in late January 1861, he left by ambulance for San Antonio and then returned to the East. Ewell apparently recovered rather quickly, for on April 25, 1861, after resigning from the United States Army, he was appointed lieutenant colonel in the state of Virginia. During the war his unusual eating habits continued, and he frequently ate nothing but frumenty, a preparation of wheat. His nervousness did not allow him to sleep in a normal position, and he spent nights curled around a camp stool. On the night of May 31–June 1, 1861, he received a flesh wound in the shoulder during a Federal cavalry raid on his Fairfax Court-House headquarters. Although the wound was not severe, it kept him from taking to the saddle for several days. He was commissioned brigadier general in the Confederate Army in June 1861 and major general in January 1862. In May 1862 he had a bad headache and declared that he had never suffered so much from dyspepsia in his life. His horse was killed at Cold Harbor on June 27, 1862, and Ewell limped from a spent ball that had entered his boot. The ball had flattened itself on a tree before hitting him. On July 20, along with a great part of the army, he suffered from exposure and malaria of the Chickahominy swamps. A minié ball hit near the center of his patella (kneecap) while he was kneeling on the ground observing the fighting at Groveton on August 28, 1862. Found after dark by Campbell Brown, Ewell was conscious but in a great deal of pain. Brown rode off to find a surgeon and returned after Ewell had already been carried off the field on a litter. Although Ewell had requested amputation before being removed from the field, the physicians refused, thinking the leg might be saved. He was moved from the first field hospital to a second where he stayed until it came under fire. About 8:00 A.M. he was carried another four miles to "Buckner's House." Dr. Hunter McGuire, using chloroform, amputated just above the knee at about two o'clock in the afternoon. Since one surgeon had objected to the surgery, the leg was first opened along the track of the ball to determine if amputation was justified. On examination, the patella was found to have been split in two and the head of the tibia knocked into several pieces. The ball had followed the bone marrow for six inches, fragmenting the bone into several splinters before finally splitting into two pieces. Following surgery, Ewell's pulse was weak, and Dr. McGuire didn't expect him to live because of exhaustion and his generally poor condition. When McGuire left, he gave Campbell Brown a bottle of brandy and told him to give Ewell a small amount every fifteen minutes, being careful not to nauseate him and not to awaken him if he was asleep. Ewell displayed improvement by two or three A.M. After a week the Federal cavalry came into the area, which made it necessary for Ewell to be moved. In order for him to be transported by rail, he had to be carried on a litter for fifty miles. Twelve men alternated carrying the litter while one shielded Ewell with an umbrella. Ewell thought that grapes and other fruit coupled with Madeira wine contributed to his recovery. By November he was well enough to go to a private home in Richmond. On Christmas Day his crutches slipped on icy pavement and he fell, reopening the wound and knocking off another inch of bone. He was still flat on his back on January 7, and his health had not improved enough for him to get about by the end of the month. In March 1863 his leg had still not healed. He could not ride on horseback, but he did go out in a carriage at times. As it was very unpleasant when he sat up to write, he had to lie down occasionally to rest. In April 1863 President Davis did not consider Ewell well enough to resume the duties of field command. He was promoted to lieutenant general, however, and when he returned to the army in May he was able to perform some active service. Because of the shape of his stump and his poorly made wooden leg, he was frequently bothered by abrasions of the skin and by small abscesses. Once, while talking with another officer, Ewell forgot about his amputated leg and started to walk. He fell and struck the poorly healed stump, which caused extensive bleeding. On June 14, 1863, at his quarters on the Millwood Road, he was hit squarely in the chest by a spent ball, which inflicted no more than a bruise. By that time he was managing his leg better and was able to mount his horse. He was struck again at Gettysburg on July 1, 1863, but this time he was hit on his wooden leg. He was still a cripple, looked sickly, and fell off his horse occasionally. As soon as he dismounted, he had to be put on crutches. On November 26, 1863, Ewell was absent because of chills, fever, and pain in his stump, probably due to osteomyelitis. His leg was in such a condition that he was unable to command, and he was hospitalized in Charlottesville. By December he had resumed command, but Robert E. Lee thought Ewell was still too feeble to be on the field. In the middle of January 1864, he was bruised when his horse slipped on the snow and rolled over. On May 27, 1864, he had something of "the nature of scurvy" with severe diarrhea and had to travel in an ambulance. He remained in his tent for a few days but recovered rapidly, returning to duty on the thirtieth. In June both Ewell and Dr. Hunter McGuire thought that he was in as good a physical condition as at any recent time. However, Robert E. Lee felt field duty would be too much for him, so he suggested that it would be better for Ewell to be in command of the defenses of Richmond. During the siege of Petersburg, Ewell fell from his horse and was badly bruised and bleeding. He was sent to Richmond, but within two to three hours he was back on the line. He returned swathed in bandages from the crown of his bald head to his shoulders, with only two little apertures for his eyes and two small breathing spaces. Ewell was captured April 6, 1865. In May, while a prisoner, he suffered severely with neuralgia; one eye was partly closed as a result. In addition, his dyspepsia continued to bother him, and although he could not drink coffee, he did quite well with tea. After the war he lived on a farm in Tennessee. In 1866 Ewell was using a suitable artificial limb and, with the assistance of a cane, was getting along well. Although he no longer had infections of his stump, he was never free from boils, which started in 1864, and he continued to have severe attacks of neuralgia. His eyes had been affected by the neuralgia, and when he awoke in the mornings, he could only open one eye. In January 1872, an acute respiratory infection afflicted the Ewell household near Spring Hill, Tennessee. Ewell was sick for a couple weeks. He attributed his bad health to having put on blue infantry pants during the cold weather after having worn a much thicker pair. His wife took care of him until she became ill and died. Ewell died soon afterward on January 25, 1872, supposedly with typhoid pneumonia. He was buried in the Old City Cemetery, Nashville.[1]

DEATH CERTIFICATE: NAD

1. *OR*, vol. 2:62–63; vol. 12, pt. 2:645, 679, 704, 710–11; vol. 23, pt. 2:753; vol. 25, pt. 2:824–25; vol. 29, pt. 1:827, pt. 2:861, 899; vol. 36, pt. 1:1074, 1276, pt. 3:846, 863, 897–98; Hunter McGuire, "Clinical Reports on Gun-Shot Wounds of Joints," *Richmond Medical Journal* 1:260–65; "Military Reminiscences of Major Campbell Brown, 1861–1863," 67–68, 101–3, Campbell Brown-Ewell Papers, TSLA; *MSHW*, vol. 2, pt. 3:242; Percy Gatling Hamlin, *"Old Bald Head" (General R. S. Ewell): The Portrait of a Soldier*, 32, 54–56; idem, *The Making of a Soldier: Letters of General R. S. Ewell*, 34, 40, 61, 96–99, 108, 112, 115–18, 123, 127–30, 134, 137–38, 150–51; Paul E. Steiner, *Medical-Military Portraits of Union and Confederate Generals*, 278, 287, 290; R. S. Ewell to Thomas Jordan, June 1, 1861, M. L. Bonham Papers, SCL; William G. Bean, *Stonewall's Man Sandie Pendleton*, 128–29, 176; Archie E. McDonald, ed., *Make Me a Map of the Valley: The Civil War Journal of*

Stonewall Jackson's Cartographer, 183, 187; Sir Arthur J. L. Fremantle and Frank A. Haskell, *Two Views of Gettysburg*, 66–67; Freeman, *R. E. Lee* 3:207; idem, *Lee's Lieutenants* 3:23; Sorrel, *Confederate Staff Officer*, 268; Morrison, *Memoirs of Henry Heth*, 81–82; Taylor, *Destruction and Reconstruction*, 37, 78; Gordon, *Reminiscences*, 157; *SHSP* 10:259; *Memphis Daily Appeal*, Jan. 27, 1872.

F

JAMES FLEMING FAGAN • *Born March 1, 1828*, in Clark County, Kentucky. During the Mexican War he was a lieutenant and afterward served one term in the Arkansas legislature. He recruited men for the war in 1861 and was elected colonel of the 1st Arkansas Infantry. Fagan rose to the rank of brigadier general in September 1862 and then to major general in April 1864. After the war he was a farmer and politician. He died September 1, 1893, at Little Rock, Arkansas, and was buried there in Mount Holly Cemetery.
DEATH CERTIFICATE: NAD

WINFIELD SCOTT FEATHERSTON • *Born August 8, 1820*, near Murfreesborough, Tennessee. A lawyer and politician, he served in Congress for four years. When the war started he was elected colonel of the 17th Mississippi Infantry. Twice in 1861 he was sick while in camp near Leesburg, the first time on September 2 and the second on October 15. He gave up his command for a short time on each occasion. Featherston's promotion to brigadier general ranked from March 1862. In early April, Featherston was assigned to brigade command but due to illness was unable to command on May 31 during the Battle of Seven Pines. He was wounded in the shoulder at Frayser's Farm on June 30, 1862. He was absent sick October 27. On January 19, 1863, he was relieved from duty with the Army of Northern Virginia and ordered to report for duty at Jackson, Mississippi. He was given a forty-day sick leave on January 3, 1865, but was back in command by the middle of February. Postbellum he returned to politics and the practice of law and finally became a judge. He died May 28, 1891, of paralysis at his residence at Holly Springs, Mississippi, and was buried there in the Hillcrest Cemetery.[1]
DEATH CERTIFICATE: NAD

1. CSR; *OR*, vol. 11, pt. 1:950–51, 957, pt. 2:759, 786, 870, pt. 3:425; vol. 12, pt. 2:601; vol. 17, pt. 2:846; vol. 19, pt. 2:683–84; vol. 47, pt. 2:1177, 1273; Pvt. Robert A. Moore, *A Life for the Confederacy*, 56, 61, 67, 70; *Holly Springs South* (Holly Springs, Miss.), June 3, 1891.

SAMUEL WAGG FERGUSON • *Born November 3, 1834*, in Charleston, South Carolina. He graduated from USMA in 1857. Ferguson resigned from the U.S. Army in 1861 and served on the staff of Gen. P. G. T. Beauregard. While at Vicksburg he had a severe, protracted attack of bilious dysentery. In August 1862 he obtained a sick leave and borrowed a buggy to drive to Ditchley. He returned on the twenty-second to participate in a battle but then went back to Ditchley to be married on the twenty-fifth. Poor health continued, and since he had developed jaundice, his leave was extended. He did not start back to Vicksburg until November 1862. Reaching the dividing line between Ditchley and the adjoining plantation, he came to a fence across the road. While attempting to remove it, he climbed up and injured his arm when the fence fell with him. Because the arm was so swollen, the doctor did not realize it had been dislocated. After another week, Ferguson started again for Vicksburg. He arrived at Jackson, applied to a medical board, and was given leave for a severe contusion involving the elbow joint; the dislocation was again missed. It was not until Dr. Chopin at P. G. T. Beauregard's headquarters in Charleston examined Ferguson that the correct diagnosis was made. The doctor told him he had an anterior dislocation of the radius, which was very unusual without the bone being broken. Four weeks after the injury, the dislocation was finally reduced without difficulty using chloroform. Ferguson reported back to duty in Mississippi in February 1863, but the elbow was so stiff he couldn't use a saber at all and had difficulty using a pistol. He was appointed brigadier general from July 1863. East of Pearl River on February 24, 1864, he ambushed part of Sherman's troops. He received a slight wound in the shoulder which did not even cause him to dismount. He was sick for a short time in late March and early April 1865. Following the war he studied law and served on the Mississippi levee and then the River Commissions. Ferguson died at the State Hospital in Jackson, Mississippi, on February 3, 1917, and was buried in Greenwood Cemetery at Jackson.[1]

DEATH CERTIFICATE: RNA

    1. CSR; OR, vol. 32, pt. 1:367, 380; "Memories of General Samuel W. Ferguson," 99, 101, 102, 105–11, 139, Samuel W. Ferguson Papers, DU; Journal of S. W. Ferguson, Brigadier General of Cavalry, C.S.A., 17, 19, Samuel W. Ferguson Papers, MDAH; Craig Mathews to Mrs. Charlotte Capers, Aug. 25, 1951, Samuel J. Gholson subject file, MDAH.

CHARLES WILLIAM FIELD • *Born April 6, 1828*, in Woodford County, Kentucky. He graduated from USMA in 1849. Field resigned from the U.S. Army when the war started and was commissioned colonel of the 6th Virginia Cavalry in May 1861. He was promoted brigadier general to rank from March 1862. At the battle of Second Manassas on the night of August 29, 1862, Field was severely wounded. He remained in bed recuperating for nearly a year. In May 1863, Field was assigned superintendent of the Bureau of Conscription in Richmond and was still on crutches when he reported for duty. He was admitted to the hospital in Richmond in October 1863 because of the old wound. On February 12, 1864, he was sent to Tennessee for assignment to duty with the division that had been John B. Hood's. However, because of Field's badly crippled condition, James Longstreet assigned him to the smaller division previously commanded by Simon B. Buckner. He joined the division at Bull's Gap, East Tennessee, about March 13, 1864. During the charge in the Wilderness on May 6, he was slightly wounded twice but continued in command.[1] After the war he was engaged in a number of occupations, including service in Egypt, businessman, and doorkeeper of the U.S. House of Representatives. He died at Washington, D.C., on April 9, 1892, and was buried in Loudon Park Cemetery, Baltimore.

DEATH CERTIFICATE: Cause of death, primary, lithemia; immediate, angina pectoris. Duration of his last illness was eight days.

1. CSR; CR, 178:68, 181:13; *OR*, vol. 12, pt. 2:646, 671; vol. 25, pt. 2:824; vol. 31, pt. 2:726; vol. 32, pt. 2:802; *CMH* 9:236; *SHSP* 14:542–63.

JOSEPH FINEGAN • *Born November 17, 1814,* in Clones, Ireland. He came to America as a young man and became a planter and lumber mill operator in Florida. In 1861 he was placed in charge of Florida's effort to raise and train troops. Finegan was commissioned as a Confederate brigadier general in April 1862. In January 1865 he requested transfer to a climate more agreeable to his health and age, even though he had not been absent from duty even one week. In March he was assigned to duty in Florida.[1] Following the war he served in the Florida state senate for a short time and was a cotton broker in Georgia. He returned to Florida a few years before his death. Finegan died at Rutledge, Florida, October 29, 1885, and was buried in the Old City Cemetery, Jacksonville.

DEATH CERTIFICATE: RNA

1. *OR*, vol. 46, pt. 2:1128, pt. 3:1327.

JESSE JOHNSON FINLEY • *Born November 18, 1812,* in Wilson County, Tennessee. He served in the Florida wars. After becoming a lawyer, he held political positions in Arkansas, Florida, and Tennessee and became a Florida judge in 1852. He resigned his position as a Confederate district judge for the state of Florida in April 1862 and enlisted in the army as a private. Rising rapidly in rank, he was appointed a brigadier general in November 1863. On May 14, 1864, during the Battle of Resaca, Finley was wounded. His disability lasted until after Joseph E. Johnston's army had reached Atlanta. At Jonesborough, on August 31, 1864, he was severely wounded by a shell fragment which killed his horse. He declined to be sent to the rear by train until all of his wounded men were embarked, and consequently narrowly escaped capture. In October 1864, he was at home in Jackson County, Florida, recuperating from his wound. Although the wound was only partially healed, Finley attempted to rejoin his brigade soon after the army was ordered to North Carolina. His journey was interrupted by Federal troop movements.[1] After the war he returned to politics and the practice of the law. He died November 12, 1904, in Lake City, Florida, and was buried in what is now referred to as "the Old Cemetery" at Gainesville.[2]

DEATH CERTIFICATE: RNA

1. CSR; *CV* 13:37; *CMH* 11:185, 202, Fla.
2. Burial monument.

JOHN BUCHANAN FLOYD • *Born June 1, 1806,* in Montgomery County, Virginia. A planter and lawyer, he was governor of Virginia from 1848 to 1852 and U.S. Secretary of War from 1857 until he resigned in December 1860. Poor health plagued him before the war. Floyd entered Confederate service as a brigadier general in May 1861. He was slightly wounded in the right forearm on September 10, at Carnifix Ferry, West Virginia. A letter from his headquarters on September 12, 1861, had to be signed by his adjutant because the injury prevented him from holding a pen. Although Floyd considered the wound insignificant, the poor weather and more than usual soreness of his arm prevented him from visiting Robert E. Lee's camp on September 27. His health was again poor during November 1861, but he was on the field.[1] His poor performance at Fort Donelson prompted the loss of his commission in March 1862 without a court of inquiry. The cause of his death on August 26, 1863, near Abingdon, Virginia, was not clear. He was buried near Abingdon in the Sinkingspring Cemetery.

DEATH CERTIFICATE: RNA

1. CSR; *OR*, vol. 5:148–49, 980; vol. 51, pt. 2:297, 300, 318, 383; Coulter, *William Montague Browne*, 66; Vandiver, *War Diary of Josiah Gorgas*, 60.

JOHN HORACE FORNEY • *Born August 12, 1829*, at Lincolnton, North Carolina. He graduated from USMA in 1852. Forney served in the United States Army until the start of the war, when he entered Confederate service as colonel of the 10th Alabama Infantry. He was severely wounded in the arm on December 20, 1861, at Dranesville, Virginia, and had to leave the field. His promotion to brigadier general ranked from March 1862. When he arrived to assume command of the Department of Alabama and West Florida in April 1862, his wound and general health was such that he could not return to duty. Taking another leave of absence on a surgeon's certificate, he did not return to take command until May. Although Forney was in command and became a major general in October, his health was far from good. Still having trouble with the wound while in Mobile, he was again given a leave in mid-November 1862. Forney finally relinquished command of the District of the Gulf on December 14, 1862. The arm continued to discharge and cause pain until he had surgery. Following the operation, the pain and discharge ceased; however, the arm remained irritated and swollen. In January 1863, Forney thought there might still be bone fragments or imbedded foreign material in his arm that should be removed. A surgeon was requested and presumably performed additional surgery. Forney was back in February 1863, and in April was ordered to take command of Dabney H. Maury's division. In April 1864, many men of his division were afflicted with the "camp state"; his chief surgeon suggested they stop at the Sulphur Springs. Forney did not improve as rapidly as he had hoped but thought he would be better in a few days. He was ordered to proceed to Shreveport in May for assignment to duty.[1] Following the war, he took up residence in Alabama, where he was a farmer and engineer. He died September 13, 1902, in Jacksonville, Alabama, and was buried there in the City Cemetery.

DEATH CERTIFICATE: NAD

1. CSR; *OR*, vol. 5:491; vol. 6:663, 880; vol. 15:899; vol. 20, pt. 2:403, 423; vol. 23, pt. 2:636; vol. 24, pt. 3:720, 758; vol. 34, pt. 3:808; vol. 52, pt. 2:361, 379, 579; *CMH* 12:405, Ala.

WILLIAM HENRY FORNEY • *Born November 9, 1823,* in Lincolnton, North Carolina. Served in the Mexican War. A lawyer and member of the Alabama state legislature before the Civil War, he entered the Confederate service as a captain of the 10th Alabama Infantry. Forney was wounded in the shinbone at Dranesville, Virginia, on December 20, 1861, but within two months was back on the field. At the Battle of Williamsburg on May 5, 1862, his right arm was fractured near the shoulder by a ball. Taken to William and Mary College, which had been converted into a hospital, Forney was captured by Federal troops when they occupied Williamsburg. He was admitted July 30 to the Federal hospital at Fort Monroe, Virginia, and was exchanged after four months of captivity. He was slightly wounded in the leg on May 3, 1863, at the Battle of Salem Church. Forney led his regiment again at Gettysburg on July 2, 1863; when charging the enemy lines he received flesh wounds of the arm and chest. He continued on until another ball fractured his right arm, at the same site as the still unhealed wound received at Williamsburg. Another ball, which struck his left heel after he had fallen, produced his most severe wound. On the retreat from Gettysburg, it was necessary to leave him behind, and he was captured by the Federal troops on July 5. He was admitted to the Letterman general hospital in Gettysburg. After transfer to a hospital in Baltimore, Forney underwent excision of the posterior portion of the os calcis. Simple dressings were applied. He was one of the officers selected on June 24, 1864, to be sent to Hilton Head and was carried as far as Port Royal for this purpose. A prisoner for thirteen months, he was still on crutches at the time of his exchange. He was on home leave because of his wounds from September through October 1864. Upon return to duty, Forney was placed in charge of Cadmus M. Wilcox's Alabama brigade. His commission as brigadier general ranked from February 1865, and he was paroled at Appomattox Court-House.[1] Following the war he resumed the practice of law and politics. He died January 16, 1894, at Jacksonville, Alabama, and was buried there in the City Cemetery.

DEATH CERTIFICATE: NAD

1. CSR; *OR,* vol. 11, pt. 1:592–93; vol. 27, pt. 2:619; vol. 35, pt. 2:147–48; vol. 46, pt. 1:1278; vol. 51, pt. 1:94; *CMH* 12:407, Ala.; *CV* 7:364; *SHSP* 7:284.

NATHAN BEDFORD FORREST • *Born July 13, 1821,* in Bedford County, Tennessee. He was seriously ill with typhoid fever in 1840 but made a complete recovery. Two of his brothers and three sisters died with typhoid at the same time. After returning home from the Republic of Texas in 1841, he had fever and dysentery. Recovery took a number of months. During a March 1845 street fight at Hernando, Mississippi, Forrest was wounded by a pistol shot. He wounded three of his attackers; although arrested, he was released. In 1852 he received a severe contusion of his shoulder in a steamboat explosion near Galveston. Although quite rich at the start of the war as a planter and slave trader, Forrest enlisted as a private in the 7th Tennessee Cavalry. Using his own money, he raised a battalion of mounted troops and was elected lieutenant colonel in October 1861. On the twenty-first of that month, he had chills and was too sick to do much until November 4. On December 28, 1861, at Sacramento, Kentucky, he was bruised but not disabled when his horse collided with that of a Federal officer. At Fort Donelson on February 15, 1862, Forrest was slightly injured when a solid cannonball passed just behind his legs and through his horse. His feet were covered in blood and temporarily numb. On April 8, 1862, after the Battle of Shiloh, he received a wound which was thought to be mortal. The ball from an Austrian rifle had entered just above his left hip, transversed the large muscles of the back, and lodged against the spinal column. His right leg, numbed by the injury, hung useless in the stirrup. By riding on horseback and in a spring wagon, he arrived at Corinth where he was furloughed to Memphis on a surgeon's certificate. He returned to duty in three weeks; however, his wound had become swollen and painful. The ball was finally removed without an anesthetic. He was confined to bed for two weeks and returned to the field early in June. The next month he was promoted to brigadier general. His wound continued to give him pain for at least six months. Forrest had his right shoulder dislocated when he was unhorsed at Munfordville, Kentucky, on September 17, 1862. Disabled, he went with the wagon train to Bardstown, Kentucky, on September 22. However, he remained in command and on September 25 was charged with military operations in middle Tennessee. On February 3, 1863, during an assault on Fort Donelson, he received another injury when his horse fell. This disability was brief. An attempt to assassinate him was made on June 13, 1863, at Columbia, Tennessee, by his former artillery officer, Lt. Andrew Wills Gould. Gould shot Forrest at close range with a large caliber pistol, but Forrest was able to stab his assailant with a knife. The bullet entered just above his left hip joint and struck the outer edge of the pelvic bone below the anterior superior spinous process. It was deflected upward and passed back through his body without having touched either his intestines or any large blood vessels. Although the doctors wanted to remove the ball, Forrest refused. He lost a lot of blood but soon recovered; on the morning of June 25 he left his sick bed and took to the saddle. Forrest's next combat wound occurred on September 11, 1863, at Tunnel Hill, Georgia, prior to the Battle of Chickamauga. Faint from pain and loss of blood, he took a drink of whiskey at the surgeon's urging and did not leave the field. In December 1863 he was made a major general although he was ill and fatigued. During the April 12, 1864, attack on Fort Pillow, he was bruised again when his horse fell. The contusions and exhaustion restricted his activity for a few days, but he did not relinquish his command. Following the Battle of Brice's Cross Roads on June 11, he had a fainting spell, fell from his horse, and was unconscious for a period of thirty to sixty minutes. Later in the month he suffered from boils. Forrest's third combat wound was received in the Battle of Tupelo on July 15. He was shot in the right foot near the base of the great toe. This proved to be the most painful wound of all. The ball ranged backward through his sole producing a flesh wound. When the severe hemorrhage was finally stopped, he mounted his horse and rode in front of his men. Healing of this wound was delayed, as Forrest

was in poor health at the time and was plagued with boils. He requested leave to go to Columbus because of the wound, but S. D. Lee wanted him to remain in command. Forrest rode around the camp in a farm buggy, looking sick and as thin as a rail, with his injured foot projecting over the front. He was incapacitated for some time, and when he took the field on August 9, he was still riding in a buggy. In October 1864 he requested a leave of absence because of failing strength, but it was not granted. He received saber bruises about the head, shoulders, and arms on April 1, 1865, at Ebenezer Church, Alabama. These wounds were painful but not incapacitating; the next day, at Selma, he was on the field again. On April 8, his arm was still in a sling. Following the war he returned to his plantation and continued to have bad health. In later years his wife thought he had an unusual appetite and a great craving for various foods. In view of his symptoms, it has been speculated that he might have had diabetes mellitus. During 1873 he had chronic diarrhea, and in the summer of 1877, because of continued poor health, he took the waters at Hurricane Springs in middle Tennessee. In September he spent most of the time on his back and was unable to get up without help. When he returned to Memphis, he had to be carried from his carriage to his residence. He weighed little more than a hundred pounds before he died.[1] Forrest's symptoms were compatible with diabetes mellitus as has been suggested or a gluten-sensitive enteropathy. He died in Memphis on October 29, 1877, and was initially buried there in Elmwood Cemetery. Later he was reinterred in Forrest Park, Tennessee.
DEATH CERTIFICATE: Cause of death, chronic diarrhea.

1. CSR; *OR*, vol. 10, pt. 1:924; vol. 16, pt. 2:864, 876, 980–81; vol. 30, pt. 1:446; vol. 31, pt. 3:876–77; vol. 32, pt. 1:610; vol. 39, pt. 2:671, 715–17, 749, pt. 3:807; vol. 41, pt. 2:1016; vol. 52, pt. 1:29; John Allen Wyeth, *Life of General N. B. Forrest*, 18, 32, 53–54, 79–82, 240, 454–55; Jordan, *N. B. Forrest*, 19–20, 22–24, 27–28, 51, 84, 147–49, 159, 185, 227; Eric William Sheppard, *Bedford Forrest: The Confederacy's Greatest Cavalryman*, 92, 119–20, 296, 298; Brian Steel Wills, *A Battle from the Start*, 84, 274–78; Frank A. Smith, "Forrest-Gould Affair," *CWTI* 9:32–37; Henry, *"First with the Most" Forrest*, 162–64, 316, 329–30, 459–60; Jill L. Garrett, *Obituaries from Tennessee Newspapers*, 120; Steiner, *Medical-Military Portraits*, 297–336; *SHSP* 7:455, 458, 477; *CV* 4:387, 5:83.

JOHN WESLEY FRAZER • *Born January 6, 1827*, in Hardin County, Tennessee. He graduated from USMA in 1849. His prewar duty in the U.S. Army was routine and similar to most other West Point graduates. He did not resign until March 1861, and then he took positions, first as captain, then as lieutenant colonel of the 8th Alabama Infantry. He was absent because of sickness from October 18, 1861, through February 1862. A physician who examined him at Columbus, Kentucky, on February 3, 1862, reported that Frazer was unfit for active duty because he had little use of his right leg and could not ride. The cause and the nature of the disability were not described. In March he was ready to rejoin his regiment.[1] He was commissioned brigadier general in May 1863. Frazer surrendered at Cumberland Gap on September 9, 1863, and was still a prisoner at the end of the war. Afterward he became a farmer in Arkansas and later a businessman in New York City, where he died on March 31, 1906. He was buried at Clifton Springs, New York.

DEATH CERTIFICATE: RNA

1. CSR.

SAMUEL GIBBS FRENCH • *Born November 22, 1818,* in Gloucester County, New Jersey. He graduated from USMA in 1843. During the Mexican War, French was wounded at Buena Vista on February 23, 1847. While mounting his horse with his left foot in the stirrup, he was struck by a musket ball in the upper right thigh. Initially he felt as though he had been hit by a club and did not feel pain. He was assisted onto the horse so he could help direct the artillery fire. While riding back he was stopped twice by surgeons who probed the wound, but they were unable to find the ball. The first night he spent in a hacienda, but the second day he was taken by wagon to a camp at Saltillo and was left alone on the ground in a tent. The surgeons could not find the ball, and French, confined to a cot for over forty days, became emaciated. At last French himself pointed to where the ball was located. One of the surgeons cut down on the area without anesthesia, making a hole large enough for his finger and a large steel hook. Within three days after the ball had been removed, French could sit up. He arrived in New Orleans in May 1847 and in a few days was getting around on crutches. After being given an indefinite leave, French went to Washington, D.C., where he went to another doctor in July. The leg was bandaged; as the wound was healing poorly and a sinus tract had developed, it was recommended that he remain on his back for three weeks. Finally French poured something with a turpentine odor into the wound; within a day it was inflamed and the bandage soaked in blood. However, the wound healed following this, and in three weeks he was on crutches again and able to put his foot on the ground for the first time in six months. In January 1848 he was assigned as an assistant quartermaster. Having married well, he resigned from the U.S. Army in 1856 and became a planter. He was commissioned a Confederate brigadier general in October 1861 and major general in August 1862. On April 19, 1863, French was sick when the guns of Stribling's battery at Hill's Point were lost to Federal troops. He believed that medicine he had taken contributed to his illness. He had remittent fever complicated by dysentery in July 1863. The fever and tenesmus subsided to some extent with the usual remedies, but he was very debilitated. Taking sick leave, he left camp on August 4, spent the next two months with friends in Columbus, Georgia, and later was in Warm Springs. He returned in October 1863. French's report on the Battle of Franklin, fought November 30, 1864, was delayed because of problems with his eyes, which also resulted in his absence from December 16, 1864, until February 1865. Even with the care of specialists, his eyes did not improve until years later.[1] After the war he returned to the life of a planter. He died April 20, 1910, at Florala, Florida, and was buried in St. John's Cemetery at Pensacola.

DEATH CERTIFICATE: Cause of death, senility.

1. CSR; *OR,* vol. 18:325–26, 328, 1000; vol. 30, pt. 4:722, 733; vol. 45, pt. 1:709; French, *Two Wars,* 80–82, 85–87, 90–94, 183, 297, 302; Claudius W. Sears Diaries, MDAH.

DANIEL MARSH FROST • *Born August 9, 1823,* in Schenectady County, New York. He graduated from USMA in 1844. Served in the Mexican War. In 1852, while pursuing marauding Indians in Texas, he was seriously wounded and almost lost the sight in one eye.[1] The next year he resigned from the army and became a businessman in St. Louis. A brigadier general in the Missouri militia, Frost surrendered Camp Jackson at St. Louis to Federal troops in 1861. Following his parole, he was made a brigadier general in Confederate service in March 1862. He took only a small part in the Civil War and, unannounced, left for Canada. As a consequence, he was removed from army rolls in December 1863. After the war he returned to St. Louis and took up farming. Frost died October 29, 1900, in St. Louis County and was buried in Calvary Cemetery in St. Louis. Cause of death: Heart disease.[2]

1. J. Thomas Scharf, *History of St. Louis City and County,* 502.
2. Calvary Cemetery, Catholic Cemeteries of the Archdiocese of St. Louis, St. Louis, Mo.

BIRKETT DAVENPORT FRY • *Born June 24, 1822,* in Kanawha County, (West) Virginia. A one-year student both at the Virginia Military Institute and at West Point, Fry participated in the Mexican War and later went to Nicaragua. He was involved in the cotton industry when the Civil War started and was made colonel of the 13th Alabama Infantry. On May 31, 1862, at the Battle of Seven Pines, he was wounded in the right hand. After an absence of six weeks he returned to the field. His right arm was shattered near the shoulder at Sharpsburg on September 17, 1862, and the surgeons advised amputation. (Some sources reported that it was the left arm.) When it was explained to him that his chances of living without the operation were one in three hundred, he told the surgeons that he would take the chance. A medical board examined him on February 27, 1863, stated that he had an affliction of the humerus, and recommended a leave of absence. He rejoined his command in time for the battle at Chancellorsville, where he was wounded on May 2, 1863. Despite his injury, Fry commanded either his regiment or the brigade until Gettysburg. On July 3 at Gettysburg, he was again hit on the right shoulder by a shell fragment. He continued on the field until a shot in the thigh fractured his bone. Captured by Federal troops, he lay in a field hospital for six days. He was taken to the hospital at Fort McHenry; then, in October 1863, he was sent to the Federal prison on Johnson's Island. By special exchange, he returned to the army in Virginia in March 1864. In May he was made a brigadier general although he was absent from May through August, again because of sickness. Upon his return, he was assigned to duty at Augusta, Georgia, on September 14.[1] After the war and a period in Cuba, Fry was a businessman in Alabama, Florida, and Virginia. He died January 21, 1891, in Richmond, Virginia, and was buried in Oakwood Cemetery at Montgomery, Alabama.

DEATH CERTIFICATE: Cause of death, diarrhea and hemorrhage of bowels.

1. CSR; *OR,* vol. 11, pt. 1:970; vol. 19, pt. 1:1027, 1054; vol. 27, pt. 2:608, 651; vol. 39, pt. 2:835; *CV* 8:536; *CMH* 12:409, Ala.; *SHSP* 7:92–93.

G

RICHARD MONTGOMERY GANO • *Born June 17, 1830,* in Bourbon County, Kentucky. Educated at a number of institutions, Gano practiced medicine and was a politician in Texas before the Civil War. He joined the Confederate service as part of John Hunt Morgan's command and became a colonel of the 7th Kentucky Cavalry. In April 1863 he was diagnosed as having valvular heart disease with hypertrophy and was pronounced unfit for active service. He attempted to either resign or be transferred to a less active post because of poor health, and was ordered to the Trans-Mississippi Department. In January 1864 Gano took a sick leave but returned in March. In the battle on the Moscow and Camden Road in Arkansas on April 14, he received a flesh wound of the left arm that left some permanent disability. On July 27, 1864, while in command of a detachment from his brigade, he attacked the 6th Kansas Cavalry near Fort Smith. Supposedly on September 19, 1864, during the battle of Cabin Creek, Indian Territory, his left arm was broken by a minié ball, which left him with a stiff elbow for the rest of his life. However, he does not mention it in his report of the battle.[1] He did not receive his brigadier general commission until March 1865. After the end of the war he returned to Texas, where he became a minister in the Christian church. He died March 27, 1913, in Dallas, Texas, and was buried there in Oakland Cemetery.

DEATH CERTIFICATE: Cause of death, uremic poisoning.

1. *OR,* vol. 34, pt. 1:783, pt. 2:876, pt. 3:766; vol. 41, pt. 1:29, 31, 788–91; Duke, *History of Morgan's Cavalry,* 386; *Dallas Morning News,* Mar. 28, 1913; S. B. Maxey to S. S. Anderson, Feb. 13, Mar. 6, 1864, and Tom P. Ochiltree to Gano, Mar. 16, 1864, Letter Book "A," 65, 109, 114, Samuel Bell Maxey Papers, Texas State Library, Archives Division, Austin (hereafter cited as TXSL); Steiner, *Physician-Generals in the Civil War,* 50.

FRANKLIN GARDNER • *Born January 29, 1823,* in New York City. Graduated from USMA in 1843. He served in the Mexican War. He was made a lieutenant colonel of infantry in the Regular Confederate Army in March 1861 and brigadier general in April 1862. His appointment to major general was not confirmed until June 1864. Following the war he was a planter in Louisiana. He died April 29, 1873, near Vermillionville (now Lafayette), Louisiana, and was buried there in St. John's Cathedral Cemetery.

DEATH CERTIFICATE: NAD

WILLIAM MONTGOMERY GARDNER • *Born June 8, 1824,* in Augusta, Georgia. Graduated from USMA in 1846. He was wounded at Contreras, Mexico, on August 19, 1847, and in the Battle of Churubusco on August 20, 1847. He left the United States Army in January 1861 and became a lieutenant colonel of the 8th Georgia. On July 21, 1861, during the battle of First Manassas, Gardner was severely wounded in the leg and lingered between life and death. In spite of his severe wound, his commission as brigadier general ranked from November 1861. He was still confined to the house, unable to walk, in February 1862; since the wound remained open with bone fragments protruding, his physician had little hope that Gardner could bear weight on the limb for several more months. In April, Gardner was able to stand and walk a little with the assistance of crutches even though the wound had not yet completely healed. Still unable to ride a horse, he traveled around in a buggy. He obtained consultation on his leg in Charleston in November 1862, and an operation was performed to partially restore use of the limb. During 1863, Gardner received further extensions of his furlough. On September 19, he was assigned to a Georgia brigade, and in October he was ordered to assume command of the Department of West Florida. In February 1864 he returned from sick leave. P. G. T. Beauregard expressed doubts about Gardner's ability to physically withstand duty in the field, as he had recently undergone surgery in Augusta. In March, because of his physical condition, he requested to be relieved of command of the forces in the field and returned to the command of his subdistrict. He was finally physically fit for duty in April. In the middle of 1864, he was assigned to the command of military prisons.[1] Following the war he returned to Georgia. He died at the home of his son in Memphis, Tennessee, on June 16, 1901, and was buried in Elmwood Cemetery at that city.

DEATH CERTIFICATE: Cause of death, malaria and age.

1. CSR; OR, vol. 2:477, 490; vol. 5:954; vol. 28, pt. 2:397, 470; vol. 29, pt. 2:775; vol. 30, pt. 4:668; vol. 35, pt. 1:323, 326, pt. 2:332; vol. 40, pt. 3:805; Heitman, *Historical Register and Dictionary* 2:22; *CMH* 6:417.

SAMUEL GARLAND, JR. • *Born December 16, 1830, in Lynchburg, Virginia.* A graduate of the Virginia Military Institute, lawyer and captain of a Virginia militia company, he was commissioned colonel of the 11th Virginia Infantry at the beginning of the war. Garland was wounded by a ball through the elbow at Williamsburg, Virginia, on May 5, 1862, but refused to leave the field. He was able to participate in the Battle of Seven Pines at the end of the month. The same month he received his promotion as a brigadier general. At Fox's Gap at South Mountain on September 14, 1862, while holding off a Federal attack, he was struck by a rifle shot and died on the field. He had been urged to go to a safer place just before he was mortally wounded.[1] Garland was buried in the Presbyterian Cemetery in Lynchburg.

1. CSR; OR, vol. 11, pt. 1:567, 578; vol. 19, pt. 1:140, 146, 1020, 1026, 1045; John Lipscomb Johnson, *University Memorial,* 270; *CMH* 3:595.

RICHARD BROOKE GARNETT • *Born November 21, 1817, in Essex County, Virginia.* He graduated from USMA in 1841. Served in the Florida wars. Leaving the United States Army in May 1861, he became a major in the Regular Confederate Army and was made a brigadier general in the Confederate Army the following November. Late in June 1863, while ill with a fever, he was accidently kicked on the ankle by a horse and had to travel in an ambulance. On July 3, while at Gettysburg, Garnett was too sick to walk, yet despite orders to the contrary, he insisted on leading the charge of his brigade from horseback. It has been stated that he wore his old blue overcoat in spite of the fact that it was a very hot day. Instead, he probably wore a new gray uniform that he had purchased in Richmond two weeks earlier. Garnett was hit in the head by a rifle ball and fell dead from his horse during the assault on Cemetery Hill. Other reports say he was killed by grapeshot and almost cut in half. He had been riding to the rear of his advancing line, trying to keep it closed, when he was shot within twenty-five paces of the stone wall. Garnett's body was picked up by Federal troops when they retook the area.[1] Initially buried at Gettysburg, it is believed that his body was later moved with other Confederate unknowns to Hollywood Cemetery in Richmond, Virginia, where he has a marker.

1. OR, vol. 27, pt. 1:440, pt. 2:310, 320, 363, 387; James I. Robertson, Jr., *18th Virginia Infantry*, 21–23; *SHSP* 4:108, 31:230, 33:26–29; *CV* 12:7, 23:391; *CMH* 3:597.

ROBERT SELDEN GARNETT • *Born December 16, 1819*, in Essex County, Virginia. He graduated from USMA in 1841. Served in the Mexican War. Following his resignation from the U.S. Army, he was appointed brigadier general in the Confederate Army in June 1861. Garnett was the first general officer on either side to die in battle during the Civil War. On June 10, 1861, because of superior Federal forces, he had to evacuate his positions on Rich Mountain and on Laurel Hill. He was pursued by the Federal troops, and a fight occurred on the Cheat River on July 13. Riding with an aide, he was in direct view of the Federal troops at a ford about half a mile north of Corrick's Ford. As he turned to see if his men were following, a bullet hit him in the back. Dying, he fell from his horse into the water, and as the Federal troops arrived, he drew his last breath.[1] He was ultimately buried in Green Wood Cemetery, Brooklyn, New York.

1. CSR; OR, vol. 2:223, 247, 287; *CMH* 3:598; Warner, *Generals in Gray*, 374; Freeman, *Lee's Lieutenants* 1:35–37.

ISHAM WARREN GARROTT • *Born in 1816* in either Wake or Anson County, North Carolina. Before the war he was a lawyer in Alabama and took an active part in state politics. He helped recruit the 20th Alabama Infantry and was elected its colonel. Garrott's commission as brigadier general ranked from May 1863. On June 17, 1863, at Vicksburg, while he was aiming a rifle, a bullet pierced his heart. He expired immediately.[1] He was buried in the Confederate Cemetery at Vicksburg.

1. OR, vol. 24, pt. 2:329, 351; *CMH* 12:411, Ala.

LUCIUS JEREMIAH GARTRELL • *Born January 7, 1821*, in Wilkes County, Georgia. A lawyer, he resigned from the United States Congress at the beginning of the war and helped organize the 7th Georgia Infantry. When he was elected to the Confederate Congress, he resigned his commission as colonel and served in the House of Representatives until 1864. Later he reentered the Confederate Army and was commissioned brigadier general in August. At Coosawhatchie, South Carolina, on

December 9, 1864, Gartrell was slightly wounded by a shell fragment before he reached the battlefield. He was temporarily relieved from duty and sent back to Augusta.[1] Following the war, he returned to Atlanta, Georgia, and practiced law and participated in politics. He died in that city on April 7, 1891, and is buried there in Oakland Cemetery.

DEATH CERTIFICATE: Cause of death, inanition.

1. *OR*, vol. 44:446, 945, 978; *CMH* 6:418.

MARTIN WITHERSPOON GARY • *Born March 25, 1831*, in Cokesbury, South Carolina. When the war started, he entered the Confederate Army as a captain, having previously been a lawyer and politician in South Carolina. Gary served as a colonel during most of the war, and he was promoted to brigadier general in May 1864. After the war he returned to politics. During the summer of 1879, Gary's health was poor and his long-standing neuralgia bothered him. He took six baths at Warm Springs and twenty-one at Hot Springs but noted improvement only in his complexion. In 1880 he spent another two and a half months at the springs. On April 6, 1881, he was ill but attended a meeting the next day. On the day before his death, he was very ill with severe nausea and vomiting. After being given morphine, he became unconscious and did not respond to stimuli. The cause of death was supposedly uremia.[1] He died April 9, 1881, in Edgefield County, South Carolina, and was buried in the Tabernacle Cemetery in Cokesbury.

DEATH CERTIFICATE: NAD

1. M. W. Gary to Robert Burns, May 20, 1879, and M. W. Gary to Hugh, July 15, 18, 22, Aug. 8, 1879; newspaper clipping (n.i., n.d.), 1880; *Augusta Daily Chronicle and Constitutionalist*, Apr. 10, 1881; *Edgefield (S.C.) Advertiser*, Apr. 14, 1881, in Martin W. Gary Papers, SCL.

RICHARD CASWELL GATLIN • *Born January 18, 1809*, in Lenoir County, North Carolina. He graduated from USMA in 1832. Served in the Florida and Mexican wars. On September 21, 1846, he was wounded during the storming of the works at Monterey, Mexico. From 1846 to 1848 he was on recruiting duty. He terminated his service with the U.S. Army in May 1861 and took a commission as colonel in the Regular Confederate Army. Two months later he was made a brigadier general. In late September 1861, Gatlin's health was so bad that he remained in bed and could not keep up with his correspondence. There was some improvement in his condition during January 1862; however, by the middle of March he was so ill that he was confined to bed and prevented from taking the field. On March 19, due to poor health, Gatlin was relieved from duty at his own request. Although still sick in May, his strength was sufficient for him to attend to his duties, and he asked to be assigned to the Inspector General's Office. He resigned in September 1862, but subsequently served as adjutant and inspector general of North Carolina.[1] After the war he took up farming. He died September 8, 1896, at Mount Nebo, Arkansas, and was buried in the National Cemetery at Fort Smith, Arkansas.

DEATH CERTIFICATE: NAD

1. CSR; *OR*, vol. 4:578–79, 659; vol. 9:445; vol. 51, pt. 2:316, 327, 452, 486, 503, 506, 525; Heitman, *Historical Register and Dictionary* 2:22; Clark, *Histories of Several Regiments* 4:414; *CMH* 4:308.

SAMUEL JAMESON GHOLSON • *Born May 19, 1808,* in Madison County, Kentucky. Following his admission to the bar, he was active in state and national politics and was a United States district judge when the Civil War started. Gholson enlisted as a private but was soon elected captain of a company. On February 13, 1862, before the surrender of Fort Donelson, he was wounded in the body and sent home. By that summer he was on the field again. He was wounded in the left thigh at the Battle of Corinth in October 1862. By January 1863, the wound had become infected. There were several abscesses with associated inflammation of the tendons and lymphatics of the hip. By the middle of the summer, Gholson was able to return to the field. His appointment as brigadier general ranked from May 1864. On July 7, 1864, in the battle around Jackson, Mississippi, he was wounded again but was absent only a short time. In October 1864, his health too poor for field duty because of the July wound, he asked for duty in Mobile or somewhere in a warm climate. During the battle of Egypt, Mississippi, on December 28, 1864, Gholson was wounded and his left arm amputated. Captured, he was left under the care of the assistant surgeon of the 2nd New Jersey Cavalry. Returning to Mississippi after the war, he again took an active part in politics. He was ill for some time before his death on October 16, 1883, at Aberdeen, Mississippi.[1] He was buried there in the Odd Fellows Cemetery.

DEATH CERTIFICATE: NAD

1. CSR; *OR*, vol. 39, pt. 1:246, pt. 2:690; vol. 45, pt. 1:851, 857, 862–63, pt. 2:747; vol. 52, pt. 2:462; James A. Bailey to J. F. H. Claiborne, Apr. 27, 1877, in J. F. H. Claiborne Papers, SHC; Dunbar Rowland, *Mississippi* 1:787–89, newspaper clipping, n.i., Samuel J. Gholson subject file, MDAH; *CMH* 12:255, Miss.

RANDALL LEE GIBSON • *Born September 10, 1832,* near Versailles, Kentucky. Following graduation from law school, he traveled abroad before the war. He was appointed colonel of the 13th Louisiana Infantry in August 1861 and brigadier general in 1864. When the war was over he returned to the practice of law in New Orleans and took an active part in politics and civil affairs. Before his death, Gibson was told by his physician that his gout was attacking his kidneys and that he required a change in climate. He had gone to the Park Hotel in Hot Springs, Arkansas, for his health; there he became weaker, appeared to go to sleep, and died December 15, 1892. It was reported he died from heart disease. He was buried in the City Cemetery at Lexington, Kentucky.[1]

DEATH CERTIFICATE: NAD

1. *New Orleans Daily Picayune,* Dec. 16, 1892.

JEREMY FRANCIS GILMER • *Born February 23, 1818,* in Guilford County, North Carolina. He graduated from USMA in 1839. As part of the U.S. Army, Gilmer served at many posts, and he resigned in June 1861 to enter Confederate service as a captain of engineers. After a gunshot fractured a bone in his right arm at

Shiloh on April 7, 1862, he was sent to Georgia to regain his health. The wound had almost healed by June, but he had severe rheumatism of his neck, hand, and body. He required dental work in Savannah soon afterward. On August 4, 1862, Gilmer was made chief engineer of the Department of North Virginia. The rheumatism continued to bother him during October, especially in the previously injured right arm and shoulder. He was not able to raise the arm and took iodine of potassium and applied chloroform until it blistered the skin. In August 1863, Gilmer was promoted from colonel to major general and reported for duty with the defenses of Charleston. His health had improved by October when he returned to Charleston following a trip to Savannah. Although his eyes, which had been bothering him, improved by late November, Gilmer was hospitalized in Savannah during December 1863 when their condition made it unsafe for him to be outdoors except in the most favorable weather. His services were required in Savannah in the middle of February, but Gilmer was unable to take the field again because of his eyes. The problem with them did not seem to interfere with his frequent letters to his wife, however. In early March 1864, he took a good dose of paregoric and salts for a head cold. He planned to meet a surgeon in Atlanta that same month for some undisclosed reason. During May 1864, Gilmer was in the hospital at Savannah. Still suffering from eye trouble in July, he planned to travel to Richmond as soon as he thought he could be of any service. During July and August he was concerned with the defense of Mobile and in January 1865 was at the Engineer Bureau of the War Department in Richmond.[1] After the war he was president of the Savannah Gas Light Company. He died in that city on December 1, 1883, and was buried there in Laurel Grove Cemetery.

DEATH CERTIFICATE: Cause of death, valvular disease of the heart.

1. CSR; *OR*, vol. 10, pt. 1:391; vol. 28, pt. 2:297, 566; vol. 35, pt. 1:601; vol. 39, pt. 2:705, 755; vol. 46, pt. 2:1013; vol. 51, pt. 2:1029; *CMH* 4:309; Jeremy F. Gilmer to Mrs. J. F. Gilmer, June 7, Oct. 2, 22, 30, 1862, Oct. 4, Nov. 22, 1863, Feb. 22, Mar. 5, 1864, Jeremy F. Gilmer Papers, SHC.

VICTOR JEAN BAPTISTE GIRARDEY · *Born June 26, 1837,* in Lauw, France. His family moved to the United States from France when he was a young boy. Although apparently living in Georgia at the start of the war, Girardey enlisted in Louisiana. During most of the war he had staff duties, and he received his appointment as brigadier general in August 1864. On August 16, 1864, at Deep Bottoms, Virginia, Girardey was killed by a bullet that hit him in the forehead. His body, along with that of John Randolph Chambliss, Jr., was left in Federal hands.[1] He was buried in the Magnolia Cemetery in Augusta, Georgia.

1. CSR; *OR*, vol. 42, pt. 2:210, 215, 1217; *CV* 13:207.

STATES RIGHTS GIST · *Born September 3, 1831,* in Union District, South Carolina. A practicing lawyer before the war, he was made a brigadier general in the South Carolina militia in 1859. Leading his troops at First Manassas, he was wounded on July 21, 1861. He went to Richmond, where he recovered through the next month. In March 1862 he was commissioned brigadier general in the Confederate service. Gist was wounded in the hand near Atlanta on July 22, 1864, and was sent to the hospital. He had not returned during August, but he did take part with his command in the skirmish on September 6 near Jonesborough. On November 30, 1864, at the Battle of Franklin, Gist waved his hat and rode off into the smoke after ordering the charge. He was mounted on his horse "Joe Johnston," which became skittish under fire. When the horse was hit in the neck, it started plunging, so Gist had to dismount. Charging on foot, he was shot through the chest and died about half past eight that night in a field hospital.[1] Gist was buried at Franklin, but his remains were later moved to Trinity Episcopal Churchyard in Columbia, South Carolina.

1. CSR; *OR*, vol. 38, pt. 3:708, 894, 916, 919, pt. 5:900, 911; vol. 45, pt. 1:654, 686, 737; William Hawkins to sister, July 23, 1864, Elijah T. D. Hawkins Papers, DU; E. Capers to Sir, Jan. 29, 1880, Ellison Capers Papers, SCL; "Uncle Wily" Howard (his body servant), "Narrative of His Slave. Death of General States Rights Gist," n.d., SCL; *CMH* 5:26.

ADLEY HOGAN GLADDEN • *Born October 28, 1810,* in Fairfield District, South Carolina. Served in the Florida and Mexican wars. During the Mexican War at Belen Gate on September 13, 1847, he was severely wounded in the leg and spent November in Mexico City recovering. The following month he was present sick in San Angel but was absent sick in Mexico City during March and April 1848. On his return from Mexico he went to New Orleans, served as a member of the Louisiana secession convention, and was appointed colonel of the 1st Louisiana Regulars. In September 1861 he was commissioned a brigadier general. On the morning of April 6, 1862, at Shiloh, Gladden was struck by a cannon shot. The wound necessitated amputation of his arm on the field. He was taken to P. G. T. Beauregard's headquarters near Corinth and survived only a few days, dying April 12, 1862.[1] He was buried in Magnolia Cemetery at Mobile, Alabama.

1. CSR Mexican Service; CSR; *OR*, vol. 10, pt. 1:536, 538, 568; *CMH* 10:301, La.; Manigault, *Carolinian Goes to War*, 318; Warner, *Generals in Gray*, 107.

ARCHIBALD CAMPBELL GODWIN • *Born in 1831* in Nansemond County, Virginia. Godwin returned to Virginia at the start of the Civil War after a career as a miner and rancher in California. Appointed a major in the Confederate Army, he served at the Libby Prison and at the prison at Salisbury, North Carolina. He later recruited and led the 57th North Carolina Infantry. Godwin was in private quarters in Richmond in October 1862 with jaundice. After a short furlough, he returned to duty on November 1. On May 4, 1863, near Fredericksburg, Godwin was wounded slightly in the knee but was back in service in June. He was captured at Rappahannock Station, Virginia, on November 7, 1863. Because of chronic diarrhea he was admitted to the Hammond General Hospital, U.S.A., Point Lookout, Maryland, on April 27, 1864. Soon afterward he was exchanged. Godwin was admitted to the Charlottesville hospital with bubo simplex on June 17, 1864, but returned to duty on the twenty-ninth. In August he was promoted to brigadier general and assigned to command the brigade formerly commanded by Robert F. Hoke. Godwin was killed on September 19, 1864, in Winchester, Virginia, when, while praising his men, he was struck on the head by a shell fragment.[1] He was buried there in the Stonewall Cemetery.

1. CSR; *OR*, vol. 27, pt. 2:482–85; vol. 43, pt. 1:552, 995; Clark, *Histories of Several Regiments* 3:410, 421.

JAMES MONROE GOGGIN • *Born October 23, 1820*, in Bedford County, Virginia. After an unsuccessful period as a student at West Point, he had a variety of occupations in Texas, California, and Tennessee. When the Civil War started, he entered the Confederate Army as a major of the 32nd Virginia Infantry and was promoted to brigadier general in December 1864. For some reason the appointment was canceled, and he reverted to staff duties. After the war he returned to Texas and died in Austin on October 10, 1889. He was buried in Oakwood Cemetery in that city. Cause of death: Heart disease.[1]

1. Burial records, Oakwood Cemetery, Austin, Tex.

GEORGE WASHINGTON GORDON • *Born October 5, 1836*, in Giles County, Tennessee. A graduate of the Nashville Western Military Institute, he became drillmaster of the 11th Tennessee Infantry in 1861. After passing through grades, he was made colonel of the regiment in December 1862. Gordon was wounded in the right thigh at Murfreesborough on December 31, 1862, and was taken to the hospital there as a prisoner. After being exchanged, he was back on the field by at least July 1863. Gordon's commission as brigadier general ranked from August 1864. He was wounded and captured again on November 30, 1864, while at Franklin, and was not released until July 24, 1865. After he was captured he was supposedly injured when struck on the shoulder by a Federal gun butt.[1] On his return to civilian life, he settled in Memphis; after becoming an attorney, he held a number of city, state, and national offices. He died in Memphis on August 9, 1911, and was buried there in Elmwood Cemetery.

DEATH CERTIFICATE: Cause of death, primary, uremia; contributing factor, nephritis.

1. CSR; *OR*, vol. 20, pt. 1:914, 940; vol. 30, pt. 2:110; vol. 45, pt. 1:654; *CV* 7:72, 12:396; Dinkins, *By An Old Johnnie*, 238.

JAMES BYRON GORDON • *Born November 2, 1822*, in Wilkesboro, North Carolina. A businessman, farmer, and politician, he entered Confederate service as a private in the Wilkes Valley Guards. He was a lieutenant, captain, and major before finally being promoted to colonel of the 1st North Carolina Cavalry in 1863. In September he was appointed brigadier general. Near Warrenton Road, Virginia, on October 14, 1863, he was wounded but continued on the field. A bullet had cut the skin of his nose and severed a small blood vessel, which bled profusely. He was in command two days later. At Meadow Bridge, Virginia, on May 12, 1864, Gordon was wounded in the arm. He was admitted to the hospital at Richmond that same day and died six days later.[1] He was buried in St. Paul's Episcopal Church Cemetery in Wilkesboro.

1. CSR; *OR*, vol. 29, pt. 1:448; vol. 51, pt. 1:250; CR, 178:614; Clark, *Histories of Several Regiments* 1:427, 456; *CMH* 4:312.

JOHN BROWN GORDON • *Born February 6, 1832,* in Upson County, Georgia. Although trained in law, he was in the coal mining business at the start of the war. His Confederate service began as a captain of the "Raccoon Roughs." He was sick in his quarters with diarrhea from February 21 to March 28, 1862. On July 1, at Malvern Hill, he was blinded for a short time when dirt from an exploding shell hit him in the eyes. At Sharpsburg, on September 17, 1862, Gordon was wounded five times. First he was shot through the calf of the right leg, and then he was hit higher up in the same leg, but as he suffered no broken bones, he was able to continue on the field encouraging his men. Later in the day, a ball pierced his left arm and tore the tendons and flesh, but he remained on the field, blood running down his fingers. A fourth ball ripped through his shoulder, leaving a wad of clothing in the wound. Gordon still stayed on the field, although weak from loss of blood and scarcely able to stand. After he had gone only a short distance, he was struck in the face by a ball, which just missed the jugular vein when it passed out. Unconscious, he fell forward with his face in his cap and almost drowned in his own blood. Speaking about this wound after the war, Gordon said that it felt as if the top of his head was gone and that only part of one jaw along with part of his tongue was left. He was borne on a litter to the rear and recalled nothing until given stimulants that night. His wounds were so serious that the surgeon had little hope for his recovery. After he was carried farther to the rear, he was taken across the Potomac River. He soon developed erysipelas, and his wife was sent for to help take care of him. Because Gordon's jaw had to be wired shut, his wife gave him brandy and beef tea. Years later he recalled that the doctors told Mrs. Gordon to paint the arm above the wound three to four times a day with iodine. She obeyed the doctors by painting the arm, he thought, three hundred to four hundred times a day! Gordon's face had not yet healed by the time he returned to duty. In November 1862 he was promoted to brigadier general. On April 11, 1863, he was ordered to take command of Alexander R. Lawton's former brigade. He was wounded over the right eye by a piece of shell or ball from a loaded shell on August 25, 1864, near Shepherdstown. Being in front of the skirmish line, he turned his horse around and slowly rode back with the wound bleeding freely. Gordon went to the rear, and after having the wound dressed, returned in about thirty minutes. On March 25, 1865, he received a flesh wound of the leg at Fort Stedman. He was paroled at Appomattox Court-House. After the war, Gordon was a leader in Georgia state politics and was a United States senator and governor. He had a severe attack of inflammatory rheumatism in 1879 and was very sick during the last of March. In May of the following year, he was uncertain of his health, as he had been ill on two occasions. During his last years he had a series of injured joints, broken bones, and periods of sickness. Prior to his death in Miami, Florida, he had a severe chill, which was thought to be malaria. This was followed by a fever to 105 degrees Fahrenheit associated with nausea and vomiting. In the evening his temperature decreased and he felt better. On the following day, however, the fever recurred and was accompanied by a weak pulse and persistent hiccoughs. Stimulants were given parenterally without effect. His temperature went up again on the eighth, and he became delirious. On the day of his death, January 9, 1904, he became semicomatose.[1] He was buried in Oakland Cemetery, at Atlanta.

DEATH CERTIFICATE: RNA

1. CSR; OR, vol. 25, pt. 1:813; vol. 43, pt. 1:570–71; vol. 46, pt. 1:1277; John B. Gordon to W. G. Lewis, Aug. 21, 1886, W. G. Lewis Papers, SHC; Allen P. Tankersley, *John B. Gordon: A Study in Gallantry*, 185, 371–75; Ralph Lowell Eckert, *John Brown Gordon: Soldier, Southerner, American*, 35–37, 199, 220, 331; Gordon, *Reminiscences*, 74–75, 88–92, 411; Nichols, *Soldier's Story*, 180; CV 2:272, 12:57.

JOSIAH GORGAS · *Born July 1, 1818*, in Running Pumps, Pennsylvania. He graduated from USMA in 1841. Early in 1847, while in Mexico, Gorgas had severe attacks of fever associated with weakness, prostration, and nonhealing ulcerations on his feet and legs. Unable to wear shoes or boots, he could not exercise. By July he was better, feeling that he had "sufficient fever to make him well." Having served in the Ordnance Department throughout his military service, he was appointed chief of Ordnance in the Confederate Army at the start of the Civil War. He was ill in January and July 1862; the July illness was compounded by the intolerable heat. Sluggishness of the liver, he stated, seemed to be inherent in his makeup, because he could not endure warm climates with impunity. He abstained from eating and thought he would feel better soon because, for him, a few days of fasting was worth all the medicine in the world. Whenever he felt ill he would diet. A half-grain of blue mass without anything else was another very good corrective for him in warm weather. Gorgas had facial neuralgia during the last of May 1864, but he was able to ride out to the battlefield on June 4. The neuralgia continued to cause him great suffering, although he took both opium and quinine, which gave him pleasant dreams or hallucinations all night. The pain left him on the twelfth, but he still felt unwell as a result of all the medication. He was promoted to brigadier general in November 1864. During January and October, and again in December 1865, Gorgas was confined to his bed with a cold and catarrh. He treated himself with a hot footbath and whiskey punch. After the war, Gorgas ran an ironworks in Alabama and in 1868 was made vice-chancellor of the University of the South at Sewanee, Tennessee. His attacks of facial neuralgia continued, and for the first few months of 1875 he was unable to sleep except when he took medication. Paroxysms of neuralgia recurred every few hours at night, and he had to get up to warm his painful arm. (His doctors reported he had atrophy of the muscles of his left arm.) Headaches that were made worse by sneezing or stooping bothered him in 1878. In February 1879, he seemed paralyzed, could hardly speak, and was intermittently confused. The pain in his arm also became more intense. Over his remaining years, his condition gradually deteriorated until he finally became helpless before his death on May 15, 1883, at Tuscaloosa, Alabama.[1] He was buried in Evergreen Cemetery in that city.

DEATH CERTIFICATE: NAD

1. OR, vol. 53:774; Josiah Gorgas to Ben Huger, June 7, 17, 26, July 10, 1847, Benjamin Huger Papers (no. 9942), UV; Vandiver, War Diary of Josiah Gorgas, 10, 167; Frank Everson Vandiver, Ploughshares into Swords: Josiah Gorgas and Confederate Ordnance, 118, 299, 308, 310–14; Josiah Gorgas Diaries, June 1, 4, 9, 13, 1864, Oct. 3, Dec. 17, 27, 1865, Alabama Department of Archives and History, Montgomery (hereafter cited as ADAH).

DANIEL CHEVILETTE GOVAN • Born July 4, 1829, in Northampton County, North Carolina. After graduation from the University of South Carolina, he went to California for the gold rush and spent time in Mississippi. He was in Arkansas engaged in farming when the war started. Govan raised a company that became part of the 2nd Arkansas Infantry, and he was made a lieutenant colonel. Sickness prevented him from participating in April 1862 in the Battle of Shiloh, and he had to take a leave. He was back in August and took part in the action at Murfreesborough in December 1862. His promotion to brigadier general ranked from February 1863. Outside of Nashville near the Granny White Pike on December 16, 1864, he was wounded in the throat. After recovering, he and his command left Augusta on March 18, 1865, for North Carolina.[1] Following the war he returned to farming in Arkansas until 1894, when he became an Indian agent in Washington state. He spent the last few years of his life living with one of his children, and he died March 12, 1911, in Memphis, Tennessee. He was buried in Hillcrest Cemetery at Holly Springs, Mississippi.

DEATH CERTIFICATE: Cause of death, primary, pulmonary edema; contributory, age.

1. CSR; OR, vol. 10, pt. 1:575, 577; vol. 20, pt. 1:860; vol. 45, pt. 1:740; vol. 47, pt. 3:742; CMH 10:200, Ark.; Buck, Cleburne and his Command, 300, 304.

ARCHIBALD GRACIE, JR. • Born December 1, 1832, in New York City. He graduated from USMA in 1854 and resigned from the U.S. Army two years afterward. He became a businessman in Mobile and joined a local militia company. After the Civil War began, Gracie was a member, sequentially, of the 3rd, 11th, and 43rd Alabama infantries, becoming the colonel of the last unit in 1862. His appointment to brigadier general ranked from November 1862. On December 14, 1863, near Bean's Station, Tennessee, his left arm was wounded by a rifle ball; that same day, after having it examined, he returned to the field. The surgeon could detect no lesion of the bones. Later examination revealed that the musket ball had struck his forearm posteriorly two inches below the elbow, passed deeply and transversely through the deep flexors, and had come out in front of the radius. Twenty days after the injury, the limb was markedly swollen, and the little and ring fingers were paralyzed. Abscesses formed, and at the end of six weeks, two exfoliations were removed. Rapid recovery followed. Gracie rejoined his brigade in April 1864, while it was located in the vicinity of Lick Creek. He was killed December 2, 1864, in the Petersburg trenches by the explosion of a Parrott shell. He was looking through a telescope at the time, the top of his head exposed. His neck was fractured, and he was struck three times in the shoulder. That very day Gracie had been granted a leave of absence to visit his wife and daughter. The child had been born the previous day, Gracie's birthday, in Richmond.[1] He was buried in Woodlawn Cemetery in New York City.

1. CSR; OR, vol. 31, pt. 1:534; MSHW, vol. 2, pt. 2:920; Lewellyn A. Shaver, *A History of the Sixtieth Alabama Regiment: Gracies Alabama Brigade*, 36, 42, 85; Josiah Gorgas Diaries, Dec. 7, 1864, ADAH; CV 5:429–32; CMH 12:412, Ala.

HIRAM BRONSON GRANBURY • *Born March 1, 1831,* in Copiah County, Mississippi. In his early twenties, Granbury moved to Texas, where he studied law and became a county chief justice. He entered the Civil War as part of the Waco Guards and was elected major and then colonel of the 7th Texas Infantry. Granbury was wounded at Chickamauga on September 19, 1863, but was back on duty by the end of the month. He was appointed brigadier general to rank from February 1864. In July 1864 he was absent for a short time due to illness. Granbury was one of the six Confederate general officers killed or mortally wounded at the Battle of Franklin, Tennessee, on November 30, 1864. On foot, he was struck in the face by a bullet, which hit just under the right eye and passed upward. He threw his hands up to his face and sank down on his knees, dead, and remained in that position until his body was taken off the field.[1] He was first buried at Franklin, but years later his remains were removed to Granbury, Texas.

1. CSR; OR, vol. 30, pt. 2:456; vol. 45, pt. 1:654, 685; CV 7:222; Purdue and Purdue, *Pat Cleburne*, 205, 252; Head, *Sixteenth Regiment, Tennessee Volunteers*, 377; James M. McCaffrey, *This Band of Heroes: Granbury's Texas Brigade, C.S.A.*, 120; Norman D. Brown, ed., *One of Cleburne's Command: The Civil War Reminiscence and Diary of Captain Samuel T. Foster*, 148.

HENRY GRAY • *Born January 19, 1816,* in the Laurens District, South Carolina. He was a county district attorney and legislator in Mississippi before moving to Louisiana. He enlisted as a private in a Mississippi regiment but then recruited the 28th Louisiana Infantry and was elected its colonel. Gray was wounded on April 14, 1863, in the battle on the Teche in western Louisiana. In command of Jean J. A. A. Mouton's brigade, he took part in the action on September 29, 1863, at the Fordoche Bridge. Gray was promoted brigadier general in March 1865. After the war he served a short period in the Louisiana state senate. In poor health for many years before his death, he lived in absolute retirement during the later days of his life.[1] He died December 11, 1892, at Coushatta, Louisiana, and was buried there in Springville Cemetery.

DEATH CERTIFICATE: NAD

1. OR, vol. 15:361; vol. 26, pt. 1:329–31; CMH 10:302; *New Orleans Daily Picayune*, Dec. 13, 1892.

JOHN BRECKINRIDGE GRAYSON • *Born October 18, 1806,* in Fayette County, Kentucky. He graduated from USMA in 1826. Served in the Florida and Mexican wars. He resigned from the U.S. Army and was appointed a brigadier general in the Confederacy in August 1861. The same month he was assigned to the military command of middle and eastern Florida. During early October 1861, he was confined to his bed with consumption. Because of poor health and inability to perform his duties, he was removed from command and died in Tallahassee on October 21, 1861.[1] He was buried in St. Louis Cemetery No. 1 in New Orleans, Louisiana.

1. CSR; *OR*, vol. 1:473; vol. 6:267, 287–89, 291, 341; vol. 53:182; *CMH* 9:237, Ky.

MARTIN EDWIN GREEN • *Born June 3, 1815,* in Fauquier County, Virginia. He had a sawmill in Missouri at the start of the war; he also organized a cavalry command. His appointment as brigadier general ranked from July 1862. Green was slightly wounded on June 25, 1863, at Vicksburg, and he was unable to visit the fortifications the next day. On the morning of the twenty-seventh, he was in the ditches, reconnoitering the positions of the enemy. While looking over the edge of the parapet, he was shot through the head by a sharpshooter and killed instantly. Warned not to look through the portholes until he had fired a few shots, he was supposed to have said that the bullet was not yet molded that would kill him.[1] He was first buried in the City Cemetery at Vicksburg, but the present location of his remains is unknown.

1. CSR; *OR*, vol. 24, pt. 2:329, 413, 420–21; *SHSP* 11:297; *CMH* 9:213, Mo.

THOMAS GREEN • *Born January 8, 1814,* in Amelia County, Virginia. Served in the Mexican War. Green studied law under his father; after moving to Texas he took part in the War for Texas Independence. He was a clerk of the Texas supreme court for the ten years prior to the Civil War and entered the Confederate Army as colonel of the 5th Texas Cavalry. His appointment as brigadier general ranked from May 1863. He had a "dumb chill" in October 1863, the first he had experienced since arriving in Louisiana. He thought he could break the chill in a minute with a little good brandy or whiskey or even rum (Louisiana lightning); however, there was nothing like that available in the wilderness of the Atchafalaya. Unless active operations occurred, Green had planned to try to obtain a furlough. During the Red River campaign at Blair's Landing, Louisiana, on April 12, 1864, a shell from one of the Federal gunboats took off the top of his head, killing him instantly.[1] He was buried in the Oakwood Cemetery in Austin, Texas.

1. CSR; *OR*, vol. 34, pt. 1:205, 453, 571, 610; *SHSP* 3:63; Taylor, *Destruction and Reconstruction,* 177; *CMH* 11:231, Tex.

ELKANAH BRACKIN GREER • *Born October 11, 1825,* in Paris, Tennessee. Following participation in the Mexican War, he became a farmer and merchant in Texas. In July 1861, he was appointed colonel of the 3rd Texas Cavalry. Greer was slightly wounded at Elkhorn in March 1862, yet remained on the field. In his report on the battle, he did not mention that he had been wounded.[1] Following his appointment as brigadier general in October 1862, he was made chief of the Bureau of Conscription in the Trans-Mississippi Department. After the war he lived in Marshall, Texas. He died March 25, 1877, while on a visit to DeVall's Bluff, Arkansas, and was buried in the Elmwood Cemetery in Memphis, Tennessee. Cause of death: Phthisis pulmonary.[2]

1. *OR*, vol. 8:293–94, 297–99; Warner, *Generals in Gray*, 118.
2. Burial record, 1877, 452, Elmwood Cemetery, Memphis, Tenn.

JOHN GREGG · *Born September 28, 1828,* in Lawrence County, Alabama. A lawyer, he was elected a Texas district judge in 1856 and was a member of the Provisional Confederate Congress in 1861. Resigning this position, he raised the 7th Texas Infantry and was elected its colonel. Gregg's assignment as brigadier general ranked from August 1862. At Chickamauga, on September 19, 1863, he rode out to reconnoiter the enemy lines and was halted by Federal skirmishers. Turning his mount to ride back, he was shot in the neck and fell from his horse. The Federal troops started to take his spurs and sword, but the Confederates charged forward and rescued him. He returned to the field January 1, 1864, and was assigned to duty with the Texas brigade. He was killed by a ball through the neck on October 7, 1864, on the Charles City Road in the vicinity of Richmond, Virginia.[1] Gregg was buried in the Odd Fellows Cemetery at Aberdeen, Mississippi.

1. CSR; *OR*, vol. 30, pt. 1:431, 436, pt. 2:454–55, 495; vol. 32, pt. 2:506, 517, 546; vol. 42, pt. 1:852, 876; *SHSP* 14:558; *CMH* 8:99.

MAXCY GREGG · *Born August 1, 1814,* in Columbia, South Carolina. Although he was in the Mexican War, he did not participate in any of the battles. He was a practicing lawyer at the outbreak of the Civil War and was made colonel of the 1st South Carolina Infantry. His promotion as brigadier general ranked from December 1861. Gregg was quite deaf and had trouble distinguishing sounds. At Sharpsburg on September 17, 1862, a bullet hit him near his right hip and almost knocked him out of the saddle. After he was lifted down and placed on the ground, examination revealed he had only been bruised. The next day he pulled his handkerchief out of his pocket, and when he opened it, out dropped a flat rifle ball! Gregg stated that this was the second time this had happened. Prior to the war he had been hit over his vest pocket while acting as a second in a duel at Charleston. At Fredericksburg on December 13, 1862, his command was in bivouac on the right of the Confederate line and in the rear of a gap between two brigades. Federal troops had penetrated the unprotected sector, and Gregg was shot from his horse by a minié ball that injured his spine and mortally wounded him. Later, some of the officers observed Gregg painfully pulling himself up by the side of a small tree and waving them on. Finally, he was carried off the field on a litter. When asked where he had been wounded, he pointed toward his back. He was given a cup of whiskey, and two blankets were put under him. He was taken in an ambulance about a mile to a house and placed in bed. Gregg said that when he was hit, he thought the wound was mortal because he was completely paralyzed, but by the time he was put in bed he had some sensation. The surgeons concluded his wound was mortal after they examined him. Dr. Hunter McGuire told Thomas J. Jackson that Gregg had been wounded. Jackson, who had a prior misunderstanding with Gregg, sent McGuire back to express his concern. Soon afterward, Jackson himself arrived and went in to see Gregg before he died on December 15, 1862.[1] He was buried in the Elmwood Cemetery in Columbia.

1. *OR*, vol. 19, pt. 1:981; vol. 21:547, 554, 632, 646; J. M. Anderson to Miss Gregg, Jan. 9, 1863, Maxcy Gregg Papers, SCL; Caldwell, *Brigade of South Carolinians*, 62; Freeman, *Lee's Lieutenants* 2:223–24, 357, 375; *SHSP* 13:16, 19:309; Oates, *War between the Union and the Confederacy*, 166.

RICHARD GRIFFITH • *Born January 11, 1814,* near Philadelphia, Pennsylvania. Prior to the Mexican War he taught in Vicksburg, Mississippi. On his return from Mexico, he became a banker in Jackson, Mississippi, and served two terms as state treasurer. He was made colonel of the 12th Mississippi on secession, and his promotion to brigadier general ranked from November 1861. At the Battle of Savage's Station, Virginia, on June 29, 1862, he fell from his horse, mortally wounded by a Federal artillery shell. A fragment of the shell struck Griffith on the inside of the thigh. In a slightly different version of the circumstances of his mortal wound, a shell struck the railroad section house just in front of the troops and exploded; a fragment was distinctly seen passing overhead before it struck Griffith. Borne off the field by members of his staff, he was transported to the home of W. Pierce, a banker in Richmond, where he died June 29, 1862.[1] He was buried in Greenwood Cemetery at Jackson.

1. CSR; J. F. H. Claiborne Papers, SHC; *OR*, vol. 11, pt. 2:664, 750; *CMH* 12:256, Miss.; *CV* 1:206; Dinkins, *By An Old Johnnie*, 44.

BRYAN GRIMES • *Born November 2, 1828,* in Pitt County, North Carolina. A prewar planter in North Carolina, he was a member of the state secession convention in 1861. He entered the Confederate Army as a major of the 4th North Carolina. A short time after his arrival at Manassas on July 29, 1861, he became ill with diarrhea and spent a few days in the Bull Run Mountains recuperating. His horse was killed at Seven Pines on May 31, 1862, and fell on Grimes's leg, but Grimes was not seriously injured. About the middle of July 1862, he had an attack of typhoid fever and went home to Raleigh to regain his health. He returned in time for the first invasion of Maryland. Crossing the Potomac River at White's Point near Edward's Ferry on September 5, 1862, Grimes was severely kicked on the leg by a horse. Because he could neither walk nor ride a horse, he was carried in an ambulance. On the fourteenth, he had to be lifted onto his horse, and he commanded his troops throughout the day—even on foot after his horse had been killed. That night four litter bearers carried him to the hospital. He was taken back to Virginia by wagon and then to Shepardstown, where he remained, as he was still unable to rejoin his command. Because of the serious nature of his leg injury, Grimes was sent to Winchester, and although an amputation was considered, it was not performed. He remained in Winchester or in camp until November, when he reported to duty, still not recovered. The indentation in the leg bone remained with him the rest of his life. At Chancellorsville on May 3, 1863, Grimes had his sword severed by a ball, his clothes perforated in many places, and his foot severely contused. He had only enough strength to climb over the earthwork from which they had started when he lost consciousness due to exhaustion and pain. He was awakened by having a canteen of water poured over his head and taken by litter to the hospital, where his foot was attended to. The next day he was able to ride over the battlefield. Owing to the injury to his foot, Grimes rode in an ambulance on the way to Gettysburg except when expecting an engagement. At Gettysburg on July 1, he led the 4th North Carolina Regiment. Later, on the retreat, he was ill after they had left Martinsburg, and he stayed with the wagons. At Spotsylvania on May 9, 1864, Grimes remained on duty despite his exhaustion and the slight wound to the instep of his left foot. His promotion as brigadier general ranked from May. Rheumatism and disordered bowels troubled him in May and June, and he was hospitalized in Lynchburg for a few days in July. Although he returned on August 6, he had a surgeon's certificate stating that he was still not fit for duty. He felt so bad on the thirteenth he was almost sorry that he had returned. At Strasburg, Virginia, on September 22, 1864, thinking they would fight on foot, Grimes left his horse behind and sprained his ankle while going down into a trench. His troops were almost surrounded when he ordered them to retreat; because of his crippled condition, he was in danger of being captured. Finding a horse from a disabled caisson, he was able to ride off and make his escape. A ball that had expended its force struck him on the leg without doing any damage at Cedar Creek, Virginia, on October 19, 1864. He did not even mention the incident in his official report. Grimes's appointment as major general ranked from February 1865. While at Petersburg on March 14, 1865, he suffered terribly from a sick, nervous headache. He attributed his problem to a glass of wine Robert E. Lee had recommended when Grimes had been looking pale and fatigued. Because this was an unusual suggestion for Lee, Grimes accepted and suffered as a consequence. Grimes was given division command and was paroled at Appomattox Court-House. After the war he returned to his plantation in North Carolina. On the evening of August 14, 1880, Grimes was shot from an ambush about two miles from his residence. He was hit with only one buckshot, which passed through his left arm and into his breast. Although there was no external evidence of bleeding, he died in a few minutes. His murderer had apparently been hired by individuals that Grimes, a leader of the community, was trying to have sent out of the country.[1] He was buried in a family cemetery on his plantation and has only a monument erected in his honor in the Trinity Churchyard in Pitt City.

DEATH CERTIFICATE: NAD

1. CSR; *OR*, vol. 11, pt. 1:956; vol. 19, pt. 1:1029; vol. 42, pt. 1:598; vol. 46, pt. 1:1277; John A. Young Diary, 1861, 4th N.C. Regiment, NCSA; Pulaski Cowper, comp., *Extracts of letters of Major-General Bryan Grimes to his Wife*, 11, 14–15, 18–21, 33, 51, 57–58, 70–71, 75–76, 97; Bryan Grimes to cousin, July 26, 1863, Bryan Grimes Papers, NCSA; Bryan Grimes to wife, May 26, 1864, Bryan Grimes Papers, SHC; CR, 145:120; *CMH* 4:314; Gallagher, *Letters of Bryan Grimes*, 6, 134; Clark, *Histories of Several Regiments* 1:253; *North State Press* (Washington, D.C.), Aug. 26, 1880; *Raleigh Farmer and Mechanic*, Aug. 19, 1880, in Bryan Grimes Papers, NCSA.

H

JOHNSON HAGOOD • *Born February 21, 1829*, in Barnwell, South Carolina. A graduate of the South Carolina Military Academy and a lawyer, he was a brigadier general in the militia before the war. He entered Confederate service as a colonel of the 1st South Carolina Volunteers in 1861 and was promoted brigadier general in July 1862. After the war he entered state politics and in 1880 was elected governor of South Carolina. He died January 4, 1898, at Barnwell and is buried there in the Episcopal Churchyard.

DEATH CERTIFICATE: NAD

WADE HAMPTON • *Born March 28, 1818*, in Charleston, South Carolina. He was a landowner and politician in South Carolina before the war. Hampton bore scars from having killed bears with a knife. At his own expense, he recruited and equipped the Hampton Legion, of which he became colonel. In June 1861, near Columbia, South Carolina, he was confined to his bed for two weeks because of illness. At the battle of First Manassas on July 21, 1861, a bullet grazed his scalp. The wound was slight and caused him no difficulty. He had the injury bandaged and resumed command. He was ill during the last of February 1862, but was back on duty in early March. On May 31, 1862, at Seven Pines, Hampton was severely wounded but refused to leave the field. While Hampton sat on his horse, and during heavy fire, a surgeon extracted a ball from his foot. A few minutes after removing the bullet, the surgeon was wounded in the right arm, which had to be amputated. Hampton's boot was put back on his wounded foot and he returned to the battle. The next day the boot had to be cut away because the foot had become so swollen and inflamed. Hampton was invalided to Columbia on crutches but returned in less than a month. On July 2, 1863, at Gettysburg, a bullet grazed his chest, and soon afterward he received a saber wound to the scalp. The gash was plastered shut, and he remained on duty. The next day he received two saber cuts on the lateral frontal area of his head, which opened the prior wound and left a four-inch-long gaping wound. His thick hair and felt cap prevented a more serious injury. A "courtsplaster" was put on the head wound, and he continued in the battle until a piece of shrapnel penetrated his right hip. Unable to ride, he was taken back, along with John B. Hood, in a carriage, wherein Hampton could not sit up and Hood could not lie down. He was too injured to help in the defense of the wagon train on July 5. By the middle of July, he was in Charlottesville and, optimistic about his improvement, expected to return soon. The outside of his head had healed, but the fragment in his right hip had not been removed. The surgeon who examined him in August reported he would not be fit for duty for at least a month. Although Hampton continued to improve, by late August he had still not been out of the house. He had a relapse, and it wasn't until October that he was on the mend again. He finally reported for duty early in November 1863. After the war he entered politics in South Carolina and became governor and United States senator. On November 7, 1878, he had a compound fracture below the right knee when he was thrown from a mule while hunting. He was found near twilight, and a road had to be cut to bring in a wagon to get him out. The next day he was taken to Columbia. The leg was set, but infection developed; although the area was lanced and drained, an amputation was required on December 9. His artificial leg was made of cork. Supposedly his son accidently shot him in the eye while hunting birds in November 1880, but he suffered only a minor injury. In December 1892, a boil on his leg caused him to use crutches. Dyspepsia and a "rapid heart" gave him difficulty in 1901. His health appeared improved that year until he caught a cold that bothered him considerably. Growing weaker, he was confined first to his chair and finally to the bed. He died April 11, 1902, of valvular heart disease complicated by his age at Columbia, South Carolina.[1] Hampton was buried at that city in the Trinity Episcopal Church Cemetery.

DEATH CERTIFICATE: NAD

1. CSR; *OR*, vol. 2:567; vol. 5:1082, 1090; vol. 11, pt. 1:991; vol. 27, pt. 2:298, 698, 725; vol. 29, pt. 2:817; John Bratton to wife, July 25, 1861, John Bratton Papers, SHC; Wade Hampton to Wigfall, July 15, Aug. 22, Oct. 2, 1863, Louis T. Wigfall Family Papers, Letters of Gen. Joseph Eggleston Johnston to Louis T. Wigfall, UTA; Manly Wade Wellman, *Giant in Gray: A Biography of Wade Hampton of South Carolina*, 44, 52, 64, 73–74, 76, 115–16, 120, 123, 127, 130, 301–4, 328, 330–32; Edward Cauthen, ed., *Family Letters of the Three Wade Hamptons*, 94; John Bell Hood, *Advance and Retreat*, 60; Garrett, *Obituaries from Tennessee Newspapers*, 151; *CMH* 1:697; *SHSP* 22:122–26; Chesnut, *Diary from Dixie*, 243, 252, 255, 257.

ROGER WEIGHTMAN HANSON • *Born August 27, 1827*, in Clark County, Kentucky. Served in the Mexican War. In January 1845, Hanson, a large, fat man, was wounded in a duel over a woman. The bullet shattered his right femur and left him with an abnormal gait for the rest of his life. He practiced law in Kentucky and served in the state legislature. When the Civil War started, he became a colonel in the Kentucky State Guard but was later given the same rank in the 2nd Kentucky Infantry. His promotion to brigadier general ranked from December 1862. During a charge at the Battle of Murfreesborough on January 2, 1863, he was wounded in the left thigh by the leaden strap of a shell. Gen. John C. Breckinridge held tightly to the artery of the leg to decrease bleeding. Hanson was promptly moved by ambulance to a house near the battlefield. Mary Breckinridge cut his boot off and tore strips of her own clothing for bandages. In spite of all his care, Hanson died on the morning of January 4. Dr. David Yandell, who examined the wound, stated that Hanson had lost too much blood to survive amputation of the leg.[1] He was buried in the City Cemetery in Lexington, Kentucky.

1. *OR*, vol. 20, pt. 1:670, 778, 787, 797, 825, 828; Davis, *Orphan Brigade*, 39, 157, 160–61; Duke, *Reminiscences*, 139; Liddell, *Record*, 105; *CV* 16:453–54.

WILLIAM JOSEPH HARDEE • *Born October 12, 1815,* in Camden County, Georgia. He graduated from USMA in 1838. Served in the Florida and Mexican wars. As a child, Hardee had dyspepsia. He was ill in November 1838 and was sent to the government hospital at St. Augustine where he remained until December 4. During May 1840, he was not able to perform his duties because of illness. He spent his sick leave in the hospital in St. Augustine and in a private home from June to October 1840. He met his future wife while staying in her family's home during this period. In Mexico during July and August 1846, Hardee had dysentery, which had previously bothered him in Florida, and was confined in the hospital at Carmargo. When he heard his regiment was going to have an engagement, he got up from his bed and reported back on September 3. Hardee was probably best known before the Civil War for his book *Rifle and Light Infantry Tactics*. He was appointed brigadier general in the Confederate Army in June 1861 and was promoted major general the following October. At Shiloh, on April 7, 1862, Hardee was slightly wounded in the arm and his coat was torn by multiple balls. Partly because of his injured arm and because he needed the opportunity to organize his troops, he was indisposed for a few weeks at Corinth. In July 1862 he was ordered to assume command at Tupelo. He spent a few days between the last of October and the middle of November 1862 in Chattanooga recuperating from a minor illness. In the middle of February 1865, Hardee was sick in bed in Charleston. He was sent away on the seventeenth by his surgeon but had returned by the twenty-eighth. On April 26, 1865, Hardee was paroled at Greensboro, North Carolina. Following the war, he became a planter in Alabama. He also owned land in Florida. As he grew older, he suffered more from dyspepsia. During a summer visit to White Sulphur Springs, West Virginia, in the early 1870s, he became critically ill. By 1872 it was known that he had cancer of the stomach. Suffering greatly, he tried changes in the climate and even tried the oranges from his Florida groves, which he thought made him more comfortable. Returning to White Sulphur Springs in the summer of 1873, he became ill and had difficulty in assimilating his food. After being confined to his bed all summer, he appeared to improve by the fall, but he still felt great pain. Because of his health, Hardee was taken back as far as Wytheville, Virginia, by train. He became too feeble to continue farther and was carried to the Buck Hotel near the station, where he died November 6, 1873.[1] He was buried at Selma, Alabama, in the Live Oak Cemetery.

DEATH CERTIFICATE: RNA

1. *OR*, vol. 10, pt. 1:389; vol. 24, pt. 3:1028; vol. 47, pt. 1:1044, 1066, pt. 2:1205, 1211, 1294; Nathaniel Cheairs Hughes, Jr., *General William J. Hardee: Old Reliable*, 15, 17–18, 30–31, 112, 115, 136, 312–13; T. B. Roy to Dr. E. L. Drake, Nov. 8, 1878, William Joseph Hardee Papers, ADAH.

WILLIAM POLK HARDEMAN • *Born November 4, 1816,* in Williamson County, Tennessee. A veteran of the War for Texas Independence and the Mexican War, Hardeman entered the Confederate Army as a captain of the 4th Texas Cavalry. He was absent sick on May 5, 1864.[1] His promotion to brigadier general ranked from March 1865. Following the war, he was a planter for a few years, then held a number of public positions. He died April 8, 1898, at Austin, Texas, and was buried in the State Cemetery in that city.

DEATH CERTIFICATE: NAD

1. *OR,* vol. 34, pt. 1:622.

NATHANIEL HARRISON HARRIS • *Born August 22, 1834,* in Natchez, Mississippi. Harris practiced law in Vicksburg and was mustered into the Confederate Army as captain of the 19th Mississippi Infantry. He was absent for ten days in October 1861 because of illness. Harris was slightly wounded on May 5, 1862, at Williamsburg, Virginia, but was back by the end of the month. Due to a wound received at Frayser's Farm on June 30, 1862, he was absent for another ten days in July. Harris was wounded during the battle of Second Manassas in August 1862, and was absent from September 15 to October 5. Because of enlargement of his spinal coccyx, he was absent in 1863, from August 23 to October 26. His appointment as brigadier general ranked from January 1864. Initially after the war he returned to his law practice in Mississippi, but later moved to South Dakota and California. Harris was an invalid for some time before his death.[1] He died at Malvern, England, on August 22, 1900.[2] His body was cremated and his remains were interred in the Green-Wood Cemetery, Brooklyn, New York.

DEATH CERTIFICATE: RNA (Passport Service, U. S. Department of State).

1. CSR; *OR,* vol. 27, pt. 2:288, 634; *The South,* n.i., in Nathaniel H. Harris subject file, MDAH.
2. Burial records and tombstone, The Green-Wood Cemetery, Brooklyn, N.Y.

JAMES EDWARD HARRISON • *Born April 24, 1815,* in Greenville District, South Carolina. After serving two terms in the Mississippi state senate, he moved to Texas and was a member of the Texas secession convention. Harrison entered the Confederate Army as a member of the 15th Texas Infantry, and his commission as brigadier general ranked from December 1864. Following the war he returned to Waco, Texas. In 1873, Harrison had what his physician brother called "rheumatic paralysis," which he thought was precipitated by long periods of overexertion. He had not been previously confined with rheumatism, as his habits were good; in fact, he had almost given up tobacco. The illness was accompanied by paralysis on the left side. By April 1874, he was able to walk with difficulty around the house, but at times his breathing was much affected. For treatment he was given mercury, quinine, strychnine, and iodide of potash.[1] He most likely had a cerebral vascular accident and some type of arthritis, but it is doubtful the two were related. He died February 23, 1875, at Waco and was buried there in the First Street Cemetery.

DEATH CERTIFICATE: NAD

1. Coke to J. E. Harrison, Dec. 9, 1873, Dec. 2, 1874, Dr. Richard Harrison to Dr. J. P. Fitlen, Apr. 5, 1874, Carter-Harrison Family Papers, Baylor University, The Texas Collection, Waco (hereafter cited as BU).

THOMAS HARRISON • *Born May 1, 1823*, in Jefferson County, Alabama. After studying law in Texas, he entered the Mexican War as a member of the 1st Mississippi Rifles. He was living in Waco, Texas, at the start of the Civil War and served at first in a militia company. Subsequently, he entered Confederate service in the 8th Texas Cavalry. For the first few months of 1862, Harrison was absent much of the time because of illness. On January 1, 1863, the second day of the Battle of Murfreesborough, he received a flesh wound of the hip but stayed in the fight all day. On April 27, he commanded a cavalry brigade at Smithville. His promotion to brigadier general ranked from January 1865. Harrison was disabled from a wound received March 10, 1865, while attacking Hugh H. Kilpatrick's camp near Fayetteville, North Carolina. He went to Greensboro to recover. At the time of the surrender of Joseph E. Johnston's army, he was on crutches.[1] Following the war he returned to Waco and was elected a district judge. He died in that city on July 14, 1891, and was buried there in Oakwood Cemetery.

DEATH CERTIFICATE: NAD

1. *OR*, vol. 33, pt. 2:798; vol. 47, pt. 1:1045, 1130, 1132; Paul Scott, "Eighth Texas Cavalry Regiment, CSA" (thesis), 64, 66, 84, 87; *Houston Tri-Weekly Telegraph*, Feb. 21, 1862; H. J. H. Rugeley, *Batchelor-Turner Letters*, 27; James K. P. Blackburn, *Terry's Texas Rangers: Reminiscences*, 38; Henry W. Graber, *The Life Record of H. W. Graber: A Terry Texas Ranger*, 245.

ROBERT HOPKINS HATTON • *Born November 2, 1826*, in either Steubenville or Youngstown, Ohio. At the age of fourteen, while living in middle Tennessee, he had a severe attack of fever. The oral mercury he received burned his lips and later caused him to froth when speaking. After being a teacher, he studied law and became a member of the state house of representatives and in 1859 was elected to Congress. He was made a colonel of the 7th Tennessee Infantry in May 1861. During November he had camp fever and was disabled for four days. Hatton's commission as brigadier general ranked from May 1862. In the last charge of the day at the Battle of Seven Pines on May 31, 1862, Hatton was killed by a minié ball just as his brigade reached the front lines.[1] He was buried in Cedar Grove Cemetery, Lebanon, Tennessee.

1. *OR*, vol. 11, pt. 1:991; Cummings, "Seven Ohio Confederate Generals," 214–15, 518, 523; Gustavus Smith, *The Battle of Seven Pines*, 100–101; Head, *Sixteenth Regiment, Tennessee Volunteers*, 354.

JAMES MORRISON HAWES • *Born January 7, 1824*, in Lexington, Kentucky. He graduated from USMA in 1845. Served in the Mexican War. He left the U.S. Army in 1861 to join the Confederacy. After resigning a commission as colonel of the 2nd Kentucky Cavalry, he became a major in the Regular Confederate Army. In December 1861 he had such difficulty with his rheumatism that he stated it would take months to get rid of it, particularly in the cold Tennessee climate. He stated that he preferred indoor work.[1] Hawes was commissioned brigadier general to rank from March 1862. After the war he entered business in Kentucky. He died November 22, 1889, at Covington, Kentucky, and was buried there in the Highland Cemetery.

DEATH CERTIFICATE: Cause of death, predisposing, age; immediate, cerebritis.

1. J. M. Hawes to W. W. Mahall, Dec. 26, 1861, Johnston Family Papers, The Filson Club, Manuscript Department, Louisville, Ky. (hereafter cited as FC).

ALEXANDER TRAVIS HAWTHORN • *Born January 10, 1825,* near Evergreen, Alabama. Hawthorn was practicing law in Arkansas when the war started, and he helped organize the 6th Arkansas Infantry. On May 29, 1863, he asked for a twenty-day leave of absence because of protracted illness. His surgeon reported that he needed a change of water and diet to recover his health. Hawthorn's commission as brigadier general ranked from February 1864. He was commanding troops in the field in April and took part in the action at Jenkins' Ferry on the thirtieth.[1] He went to Brazil following the war and returned to the United States in 1874, settling in Atlanta. He entered the Baptist ministry in 1880 and moved to Texas. He died May 31, 1899, at Dallas and was buried in the Greenwood Cemetery at Marshall, Texas.

DEATH CERTIFICATE: NAD

1. CSR; *OR*, vol. 34, pt. 1:783, 799.

HARRY THOMPSON HAYS • *Born April 14, 1820,* in Wilson County, Tennessee. Served in the Mexican War. Prior to the war he practiced law in New Orleans and took part in local and national politics. In 1861 he entered Confederate service as colonel of the 7th Louisiana Infantry. During the fight at Port Republic on June 9, 1862, Hays received a gunshot wound in the shoulder and a contusion. He recovered in the hospital and in private quarters. While at Liberty Mills in July, he was made a brigadier general, but as he still suffered from the effects of his wound, another had to take command of the brigade. Just before the Battle of Sharpsburg in September 1862, Hays rejoined his brigade. On May 9, 1864, at Spotsylvania Court-House, he was wounded again. Although other sources give the tenth as the date of his wound, the ninth is probably correct. In June he was in Lynchburg; in spite of his wound, on the seventeenth he helped with preparations for the impending battle. Hays returned to duty in Louisiana to recruit a brigade in August 1864 and remained assigned to recruiting service for the rest of the war. Following the war he returned to the practice of law in New Orleans and died at his residence on August 21, 1876.[1] He was buried at that city in the Washington Avenue Cemetery (Lafayette Cemetery no. 1).

DEATH CERTIFICATE: Cause of death, Bright's disease.

1. CSR; *OR*, vol. 12, pt. 1:741, 787; vol. 19, pt. 1:967; vol. 36, pt. 1:1029, 1072, 1074, pt. 2:983; *CMH* 10:304, La.; *SHSP* 22:295; Vandiver, *Diary of Josiah Gorgas*, 101; *New Orleans Daily Picayune*, Aug. 22, 1876.

LOUIS HEBERT · *Born March 13, 1820,* in Iberville Parish, Louisiana. Graduated from USMA in 1845 and resigned from the U.S. Army two years afterward. He had a varied career as a planter, politician, engineer, and militia officer. He entered Confederate service as colonel of the 3rd Louisiana Infantry. Hebert was slightly injured by a spent ball at the Battle of Elkhorn on March 7, 1862, and was captured. He was exchanged in fourteen days and soon resumed charge of his brigade. During the march from western Arkansas, he contracted a fever diagnosed as either typhoid or camp fever. When he reached the army at Summit, Mississippi, in May, the month he was promoted to brigadier, he was sent to the hospital in Canton, Mississippi, by the surgeon. He remained there for twenty days and then returned to the army. Preparation for the attack on Corinth was delayed on October 4, 1862, because Hebert was ill and had to be relieved of duty. He was transferred to Dabney H. Maury's division on October 22 and remained in the field the rest of the year. On the night of June 26, 1863, during the siege of Vicksburg, he was kept out of the trenches with a fever; at the time of the surrender of Vicksburg, he was still exhausted and ill.[1] After the war he edited a newspaper and taught school. Hebert died January 7, 1901, in St. Martin Parish and was buried in the family cemetery six miles north of Breaux Bridge, Louisiana.

DEATH CERTIFICATE: NAD

1. CSR; *OR,* vol. 8:231, 790; vol. 17, pt. 1:387, 389, pt. 2:736, 812; vol. 24, pt. 2:371; "An Autobiography of Louis Hebert," Louis Hebert Papers, SHC; Soldier's application for pension (no. 2663), filed June 27, 1899, St. Martin Parish, La.; William Watson, *Life in the Confederate Army,* 296, 303, 317.

PAUL OCTAVE HEBERT · *Born December 12, 1818,* in Iberville Parish, Louisiana. He graduated from USMA in 1840. Served in the Mexican War. Following nine years of service in the U.S. Army, he returned to Louisiana and was elected governor in 1852. Hebert was made a colonel of the 1st Louisiana Artillery at the start of the Civil War, and his commission as brigadier ranked from August 1861. During the Civil War he was frequently ill. On November 8, 1862, he sent a requisition from Houston for militia troops, but later in the month was unable to report because he was sick in San Antonio. In April 1863 he was in command at Monroe, Louisiana. Physical indisposition prevented him from reporting for duty as soon as expected in February 1864. He was present but ill in Houston in January 1865. Following the war he returned to Louisiana and was active in politics. He died on August 29, 1880, in New Orleans after a long and painful illness.[1] He was buried five miles north of Bayou Goula, Louisiana, at St. Raphaels.

DEATH CERTIFICATE: Cause of death, cancer of the tongue.

1. CSR; *OR,* vol. 15:925, 1057; *New Orleans Daily Picayune,* Aug. 30, 1880.

BENJAMIN HARDIN HELM · *Born June 2, 1831,* in Bardstown, Kentucky. He graduated from USMA in 1851, after which he served only a year in the cavalry before resigning due to poor health. He took an active part in Kentucky politics before the Civil War and helped recruit the 1st Kentucky (Confederate) Cavalry. He was made colonel in October 1861 and brigadier from March 1862. During May 1862 he was unable to perform any kind of duty because he could not sit except for a few hours at a time without pain. That month he had surgery for hemorrhoids and an anal fissure and received a leave of absence. He returned on July 8. On August 5, 1862, near Baton Rouge, Helm's horse fell with him and his right leg was broken. In November 1862, it appeared that Helm would not be able to return to active field duty for some months, so he was assigned as post commander at Chattanooga, Tennessee. He returned to his brigade in February 1863. At the Battle of Chickamauga, on September 20, 1863, Helm was mortally wounded by a bullet through his right side and fell from his horse. After his aides-de-camp did all they could for him on the field, he was carried back to the field hospital. His clothes were cut off and the wound was probed. In spite of all the attention he received, he died about midnight.[1] Helm was first buried in Atlanta, Georgia, but later his remains were moved to the Helm family cemetery at Elizabethtown, Kentucky.

1. CSR; *OR*, vol. 15:77, 90; vol. 20, pt. 2:417, 508; vol. 30, pt. 2:24, 35, 146, 206; Davis, *Orphan Brigade*, 34, 166, 191; Thompson, *History of the Orphan Brigade*, 385; *CMH* 9:243, Ky.

HENRY HETH · *Born December 16, 1825,* in Chesterfield County, Virginia. He graduated from USMA in 1847. During his third-year class encampment at West Point, Heth was struck in the thigh by a bayonet, which a plebe had thrown into the crowd. It passed through the leg, just missing the femoral artery. He was hospitalized flat on his back for weeks. During the summer of that same year, he was hospitalized with swelling of his submaxillary glands. While in Mexico he had yellow fever, or what his doctor called "acclimating fever." He was delirious, but in about two weeks he had improved. Heth also contracted diarrhea while there, which continued after his return to the States in 1848. The diarrhea, along with a milk and rice diet, made him so sick that he was sent home. While on the trip, he had a relapse and had to remain in Cleveland for a while. Later, in Philadelphia, Heth consulted a physician who told him to stop taking medicine and return home. He was told to eat small pieces of rare beefsteak or mutton chops and get some exercise when he felt like it. He also recommended that Heth's mother make him calf's foot jelly. Following all of these instructions, Heth recovered slowly; he did not return to duty until March 1850. While hunting rabbits in 1851, he was thrown from his horse and injured his left arm. For eighteen months he had only partial use of the limb. Heth resigned from the U.S. Army in 1861 and entered Confederate service as colonel of the 45th Virginia Infantry. His promotion as brigadier general ranked from January 1862. He was slightly wounded at Chancellorsville on May 3, 1863, but remained on the field. Outside of Gettysburg on July 1, 1863, he was knocked unconscious by a minié ball that hit his hatband. The ball broke the outer table of the skull, supposedly cracked the inner table, but did not penetrate the brain. How a diagnosis of a crack of the inner table was made without an X-ray was not stated. Heth thought he had been saved because of the thickness of the paper placed under his sweatband. On July 2, he insisted on coming to the field, where he was present during a consultation between Robert E. Lee and other officers, and he was back in command on the seventh. After the war he was involved in the insurance business in Richmond. In poor health, he had a stroke several months before he died on September 27, 1899, in Washington, D.C.[1] He was buried in Hollywood Cemetery, Richmond.

DEATH CERTIFICATE: Cause of death, primary, chronic interstitial nephritis and cardiac hypertrophy and dilatation; immediate, uremic coma (duration, 8 months).

1. OR, vol. 25, pt. 1:803, 889, 905, pt. 2:768; vol. 27, pt. 2:298–99, 317, 607, 650; Morrison, *Memoirs of Henry Heth*, 14, 18–19, 51, 53, 70–73, 77, 81, 104–5, 174–77; Walter Lord, ed., *The Fremantle Diary*, 206.

EDWARD HIGGINS · *Born in 1821* at Norfolk, Virginia. Appointed a midshipman at an early age, he had mostly sea duty until he resigned from the navy in 1854. When the war started, he was made a captain of the 1st Louisiana Artillery and rose through grades. Although on sick leave in November 1862, he planned to proceed to Vicksburg with the consent of his surgeon by the end of the month. While at Vicksburg, he had leave on surgeon's certificate of disability during March and April 1863. His promotion to brigadier ranked from October 1863. He was absent again because of illness in March 1864, and it was feared he would not be able to resume his post. He was listed as in command of his brigade on June 30, 1864. After the war, he lived in Norfolk and San Francisco. He died as the result of a heart attack on January 31, 1875, in San Francisco.[1] He is buried in the Calvary Cemetery in that city.

DEATH CERTIFICATE: RNA

1. CSR; OR, vol. 32, pt. 1:403; vol. 39, pt. 2:678; *San Francisco Alta*, Feb. 1, 2, 1875.

AMBROSE POWELL HILL · *Born November 9, 1825*, in Culpeper, Virginia. He graduated from USMA in 1847. Served in Florida and Mexican wars. As a cadet at the U.S. Military Academy he contracted gonorrhea during the summer of 1844. He was admitted to the Academy Hospital in September 1845 with a urethral stricture and a fistula, and he required catheterization. At the time of his discharge from the hospital in October he was still ill and went home on sick leave. He was under the care of the post surgeon in February 1846 because of catarrh. The following May he was back in the hospital for a week with difficulty urinating. Because of his illness, he graduated one year later than his class. Typhoid fever, contracted while in Mexico City in November 1847, caused Hill to be sick for six weeks. Twice while in Florida, in 1850 and again in 1855, he was very ill with what was diagnosed as possible yellow fever. Because this viral disease should confer immunity, at least one episode must have been due to some other condition. After he left the U.S. Army in March 1861, he was made colonel of the 13th Virginia Infantry and was promoted to brigadier general in February 1862. Hill was incapacitated due to sickness before the war from December 1860 to January 1861, after the start of the war in August and September 1861, and again in September 1862. He had an unusual swelling of one arm in November 1862, which rendered the limb useless. At Chancellorsville on May 2, 1863, soon after the command had been turned over to Hill, a projectile (minié ball or shell fragment) hit him in the calves of his legs. He hobbled back to the lines but was unable to walk or ride a horse. Still paralyzed below the knees the next day, he was able to resume command on the fifth. During the Gettysburg battle on July 1, 1863, he was sick. Throughout 1864 and 1865, he was frequently ill and on leave. Good evidence suggests that Hill's frequent illness were due to the earlier gonorrhea with resulting prostatitis and stricture formation. These problems lead ultimately to chronic infection, impaired renal function, and uremia. Hill was killed by a Federal trooper on the Petersburg line on April 2, 1865. He was attempting to capture some Federal soldiers and had his pistol in his hand when the fatal ball cut off the thumb of his left hand, passed directly through his heart, and came out his back. At the time he was killed, he had sick leave he had not used.[1] Hill was buried under his monument at the intersection of Laburnum and Hermitage avenues in Richmond, Virginia.

1. OR, vol. 25, pt. 1:799, 855, 887, pt. 2:768, 775, 782; vol. 36, pt. 1:1042, pt. 2:974, pt. 3:814; vol. 46, pt. 1:1272; Paul E. Steiner, "Medical-Military Studies on the Civil War. 1. Lieutenant General Ambrose Powell Hill, C.S.A.," Military Medicine 130:225–28; Hassler, A. P. Hill, 11, 139–40, 184, 193, 236, 238; Robertson, A. P. Hill, 11–12, 17, 22, 25, 33, 43–45, 134, 157, 206, 249–50, 258, 263, 268, 270, 272–73, 299, 310, 312–13; Von Borcke, Memoirs of the Confederate War 2:252; Lord, Fremantle Diary, 230; CV 1:235–36, 12:493–94; Clark, Histories of Several Regiments 4:195; SHSP 11:564–69, 19:184–85.

BENJAMIN JEFFERSON HILL • Born June 13, 1825, near McMinnville, Tennessee. A businessman, he was elected to the Tennessee state senate in 1855. When the war started he was made a colonel in a state unit, which later became the 35th Tennessee Volunteer Infantry. At Richmond, Kentucky, on August 30, 1862, Hill was struck by three bullets and had two horses shot from under him. In spite of his injuries, he led his brigade without apparent interruption. He was provost marshal of the Army of Tennessee from late 1863 until August 1864. In November 1864 he was made a brigadier general. Following the war he returned to his business in Tennessee. It was not long before the hardships and exposure of four years in the field started taking their toll on his nervous system and his health began to fail.[1] He died January 5, 1880, at McMinnville and was buried there in the Old City Cemetery.

DEATH CERTIFICATE: NAD

1. OR, vol. 16, pt. 1:948; Head, Sixteenth Regiment, Tennessee Volunteers, 234.

DANIEL HARVEY HILL • Born July 12, 1821, in the York District, South Carolina. He graduated from USMA in 1842. Served in the Mexican War. He was in poor health while at the military academy, and his back was slightly bent from a spinal problem. In 1849 he resigned from the army and held faculty positions at a number of colleges until the start of the war. He joined the C.S.A. as a colonel of the 1st North Carolina Infantry. At the Battle of Big Bethel on June 10, 1861, Hill received a slight contusion of the knee but did not have to leave the field. He was promoted the next month to brigadier general. After being absent for five to six weeks in an attempt to recover from a severe sickness made worse by his constant duties at Yorktown, he returned on September 3, 1861, looking feeble. On November 16, Hill was relieved of command in North Carolina and was assigned to command of the North Carolina Brigade in the Potomac District. In March 1862 he was appointed major general. That same month he had an attack similar to the one he had at Yorktown. Although there are no details concerning this illness, one of the soldiers said that Hill had "brain fever." Hill felt it was unfortunate that he had been in command of a post, as the sedentary life was injurious to his spinal disease. In May 1862 Hill suffered from chills and dysentery complicated by piles, which caused great difficulty. He was listed as in command of his division during the Seven Days' battles in June 1862. Hill was writing a letter in an exposed position at Malvern Hill on July 1 when a shell exploded in front of him, rolling him over the ground. He sustained no real injury. During the winter of 1862, Hill experienced more trouble with his spine because of the cold weather. He was chilled at night and could not get warm. At home in North Carolina in January 1863, he talked of resigning because of continued poor health, saying that there had not been a moment he had been free from pain since he had been in the service. He was assigned command of the troops in the state of North Carolina in February 1863. At New Bern on March 16, Hill started out with his throat in a terrible condition, and he thought it might cost him his life. James Longstreet was not sure that Hill's health would permit him to carry out his duties. However, Hill wrote him that although he had a frail, good-for-nothing body, he had more heart for the work than some of the big fellows. He was ordered to report for duty to Braxton Bragg in July 1863. At his own request he was relieved of division command on May 21, 1864. In October he was home unemployed, but he spent the winter of 1864 in the Petersburg trenches. On January 9, 1865, Hill was at Montgomery ready for duty. Ordered to report to Augusta on the nineteenth, he was placed in command of the area from Branchville to Millen, Georgia, the following day. Following the war Hill returned to teaching, but his poor health continued. In addition to his arthritic problems, he had piles, which incapacitated him for six months in 1870. In 1889 he developed a "stinging rash," and his skin would become cold with distended veins. He used a hairbrush to scratch his skin to obtain relief, but the continued irritation made it impossible for him to sleep.[1] He died September 24, 1889, at Charlotte, North Carolina, and was buried in the Davidson College Cemetery, Davidson, North Carolina.

DEATH CERTIFICATE: NAD

1. CSR; *OR*, vol. 4:662, 700; vol. 12, pt. 2:484; vol. 18:189, 851, 938; vol. 23, pt. 2:189, 909; vol. 36, pt. 3:821, 1163; vol. 47, pt. 2:1001, 1023, 1030; vol. 51, pt. 2:513; Leonard Hal Bridges, *Lee's Maverick General, Daniel Harvey Hill,* 15, 18, 29, 147, 162, 268–69, 276–79; Freeman, *Lee's Lieutenants* 1:20–21; *SHSP* 19:240; Moore, *Life for the Confederacy,* 110; D. H. Hill to James Longstreet, Mar. 17, 1863, Daniel Harvey Hill Papers, *CWTI* Coll., USAMHI; D. H. Hill to Ewell, Aug. 11, 1870, in Brown-Ewell Papers, TSLA; Gordon, *Reminiscences,* 67–68.

THOMAS CARMICHAEL HINDMAN · *Born January 28, 1828,* in Knoxville, Tennessee. Served in the Mexican War. Along with Patrick R. Cleburne, he was wounded in a street fight on May 24, 1856. A bullet hit his rib and lodged under the pectoral muscles. Hindman refused an anesthetic, and the projectile was cut out while he calmly smoked a cigar. When he and Cleburne could travel, they were taken to the home of a Dr. Ellis in Booneville, Mississippi, until they had recovered. During a storm in 1858, a tree blew over on top of Hindman's buggy and fractured his leg. When the fracture healed, one leg was shorter than the other, and he had to wear a boot with a higher heel. He was elected to Congress from Arkansas in 1858 and was a factor in that state leaving the Union. Commissioned a colonel of the 2nd Arkansas Infantry, he was promoted to brigadier general in September 1861. At Shiloh on April 6, 1862, Hindman's horse was shot from under him and his thigh was broken by the fall. He had to be carried off the field and could not return. That month he was promoted to major general. On May 9, still lame, he dined with nurse Kate Cumming. The following day he reported back to duty and was assigned to the command of Daniel Ruggles's division. While at McLemore's Cove, Tennessee, following the skirmish on September 11, 1863, Hindman became sick and had to give up his command. He resumed it at Chickamauga on the afternoon of September 19. The following day he received a contusion of the neck from a shell fragment. Although he remained in the saddle, he turned over his command that evening. He was in Newnan, Georgia, on September 26. On December 15, Hindman arrived at Dalton, Georgia, and took command of the corps. While riding his horse in the Atlanta campaign on the night of July 3, 1864, he was struck across the face by a tree branch. His eyes became inflamed and his sight was impaired for several months. In late July it was reported that he probably would not return to command due to illness. President Jefferson Davis wrote that Hindman's physical disability for immediate service would justify a leave of absence. Hindman requested a transfer to the Trans-Mississippi Department, in part because of his physical condition. In Kirby Smith's reorganization of January 30, 1865, Hindman was assigned command of a division. When the war ended, Hindman moved to Mexico but in 1868 returned to Arkansas and his law practice. Soon afterward, on September 28, 1868, he was assassinated in his home at Helena, Arkansas. While at his mother's bedside, giving her medicine, he was shot in the jaw and upper part of the throat. There was severe hemorrhage, but he was able to tell a group outside that he forgave his killer. He sank into a chair and died from the blood loss.[1] Hindman was buried in the Maple Hill Cemetery at Helena.
DEATH CERTIFICATE: NAD

1. *OR,* vol. 10, pt. 1:389–90, 466, 569, 574, pt. 2:510, 538; vol. 30, pt. 2:35, 302, 305, 319, 416; vol. 31, pt. 3:833; vol. 38, pt. 5:904, 926; vol. 41, pt. 2:1031; vol. 48, pt. 1:1352; Nash, *Biographical Sketches,* 66–70, 75, 217–18, 263; *CV* 1:172; Cumming, *Kate,* 34, 145; *SHSP* 13:367, 24:69, 31:164–65; Manigault, *Carolinian Goes to War,* 195; *CMH* 10:293, Ark.

GEORGE BAIRD HODGE · *Born April 8, 1828,* in Fleming County, Kentucky. He graduated from the U.S. Naval Academy in 1845, but after five years of service, he resigned and took up law and politics. When the war started, he enlisted as a private but was soon elected to the Confederate Congress. In addition to holding this position, he was on Gen. John C. Breckinridge's staff and was promoted to colonel through ranks. Although his two promotions to brigadier general were rejected by the Senate, he was paroled at the end of the war as a brigadier. He returned to his law practice in Kentucky and later moved to Florida. Hodge died August 1, 1892, in Longwood, Florida, and was buried in the Evergreen Cemetery in Southgate, Kentucky.

DEATH CERTIFICATE: RNA

JOSEPH LEWIS HOGG • *Born September 13, 1806, in Morgan County, Georgia.* Served in the Mexican War. Planter, lawyer, and politician, he cast his vote in the secession convention for Texas to leave the Union. He helped raise troops for the Confederacy and was appointed brigadier general in February 1862. Hogg and his command were ordered to Corinth, Mississippi, in April 1862. Conditions at Corinth were bad, with many of the troops sick with diarrhea and transportation of patients poor. Hogg contracted dysentery after his arrival. He was removed, along with his Negro body servant, to a private house a few miles from the camp. A doctor was with him almost all of the time, and although he received the best care, he died May 16, 1862.[1] He was buried near the Mount Holly School House; later his remains were moved to the Confederate Cemetery at Corinth.

1. CSR; *OR,* vol. 10, pt. 2:434; *CMH* 11:267, Tex.; *CV* 14:494, 15:379; Manigault, *Carolinian Goes to War,* 20.

ROBERT FREDERICK HOKE • *Born May 27, 1837, in Lincolnton, North Carolina.* Hoke was educated at the Kentucky Military Institute and was in charge of his family's business when the Civil War started. He entered Confederate service as a second lieutenant of the 1st North Carolina Volunteers. During the Battle of Mechanicsville on June 26, 1862, Hoke was wounded and had to leave the field. He was listed as in command on July 23 and fought at Manassas in August. On December 13 during the first battle at Fredericksburg, a shell struck his horse on the head, causing it to fall to its knees. Hoke fell off and caught one foot in the stirrup. When the horse ran, it dragged him by his leg. Although addled for a while, he recovered and remained in command. After passing through ranks, he was promoted brigadier general in January 1863. He was severely wounded in the action near Fredericksburg on May 4, 1863. A minié ball entered the lateral portion of the left clavicle, passed through the shoulder joint, and smashed the head of the humerus and acromion process of the scapula. The ball exited in the area of the scapula. Surgery was performed the same day, with resection of the head of the humerus and acromion process. He returned in December 1863 and, although not fully recovered from his wounds, fought at New Bern on January 30. In April 1864 he was promoted to major general. In late January 1865, Hoke was unable to get around much because of a carbuncle on his face. In February he was in the general hospital no. 4 at Wilmington, North Carolina. It is not clear when after the war Hoke first had a diagnosis of diabetes mellitus, but it manifested itself for some years prior to his death. The disease became worse the last few weeks of his life, and he finally alternated between stupor and consciousness before he died July 3, 1912, at Raleigh, North Carolina.[1] He was buried there in Oakwood Cemetery.

DEATH CERTIFICATE: NAD

1. CSR; *OR*, vol. 11, pt. 2:836, 839, 899; vol. 12, pt. 2:676, pt. 3:649; vol. 25, pt. 1:803; vol. 27, pt. 2:439, 473; vol. 46, pt. 2:1139; Summary of the sick and wounded of the 21st North Carolina Regiment, Apr. 1, 1862–June 20, 1863, 183, Museum of the Confederacy, Eleanor S. Brockenbrough Library, Richmond, Va. (hereafter cited as MC); *CMH* 4:317; Clark, *Histories of Several Regiments* 3:273; Oates, *War between the Union and the Confederacy,* 166–67; *Baltimore Sun,* July 4, 1912; *Raleigh News and Observer,* July 4, 1912.

THEOPHILUS HUNTER HOLMES • *Born November 13, 1804,* in Sampson County, North Carolina. He graduated from USMA in 1829. Served in Florida and Mexican wars. He resigned from the U.S. Army in April 1861, and after joining the Confederate service was appointed brigadier general in June 1861, major general in October 1861, and lieutenant general in October 1862. Holmes was apparently quite deaf and at times was totally unaware of extremely loud gunfire. On July 14, 1863, he returned from an expedition against Helena, Arkansas. Soon thereafter, he was confined to his bed by a severe headache and was unable to attend to business of any kind or have visitors. In late July, Gen. Sterling Price was ordered, as a consequence of Holmes's illness, to assume command of the District of Arkansas. Holmes continued on sick leave from July to September 25, when he took command of the district. By November 1863, his health had improved. In January, Kirby Smith reported that Holmes's memory was failing and that he should be replaced by a younger man. At his own request in March 1864, Holmes was relieved from command of the District of Arkansas and was told to report to Richmond. In May he was ordered to take command of the reserve forces of the state of North Carolina. He was admitted to the general hospital in Wilmington on September 16, 1864, but no diagnosis was recorded. In December 1864 he volunteered his services and assumed command of Wilmington.[1] Following the war he settled on a small farm near Fayetteville, North Carolina. He died June 21, 1880, in that city and is buried there in the MacPherson Presbyterian Church Cemetery.

DEATH CERTIFICATE: NAD

1. CSR; *OR*, vol. 22, pt. 1:520, pt. 2:936, 938, 942, 1097; vol. 36, pt. 3:778, 844; vol. 42, pt. 3:1303; vol. 53:915; *Battles and Leaders* 2:390; T. H. Holmes to Jefferson Davis, July 14, 1863, and Special Order, Little Rock, Aug. 9, 1863, both in Theophilus H. Holmes Papers, DU; William M. McPheeters Civil War Diary—June 1, 1863 to June 20, 1865, Sept. 24, 1863, William M. McPheeters Papers, MHS; Robert E. Shalhope, *Sterling Price: Portrait of a Southerner,* 241–45.

JAMES THADEUS HOLTZCLAW • *Born December 17, 1833,* in McDonough, Georgia. Although he had an appointment to West Point, he entered the law profession instead. He joined the Confederacy as a lieutenant of the Montgomery True Blues in 1861. At Shiloh on April 6, 1862, he was wounded by a minié ball through the right lung. The wound was considered to be fatal; however, within three months he rejoined his regiment. At Chickamauga on September 19, 1863, he was injured when he was thrown from his horse; nevertheless, he remained on the field. After having been a major and colonel, he was promoted to brigadier general in July 1864. Holtzclaw was sick and had leave on a surgeon's certificate during August and September. While trying to rearrange his line near Franklin on December 17, 1864, he received a severe contusion of the ankle and required medical help. In April 1865 he was back on the field.[1] Holtzclaw returned to Alabama after the war and took an active roll in politics. He died July 19, 1893, at Montgomery, Alabama, and was buried there in the Oakwood Cemetery.

DEATH CERTIFICATE: NAD

1. CSR; *OR*, vol. 10, pt. 1:557; vol. 30, pt. 2:405; vol. 39, pt. 2:833; vol. 45, pt. 1:707; vol. 49, pt. 2:1184; *CMH* 12:417, Ala.; *Battles and Leaders* 3:675.

JOHN BELL HOOD • *Born June 1, 1831,* in Owingsville, Kentucky. He graduated from USMA in 1853. On July 20, 1857, an arrow pinned his left hand to his bridle during a fight with Indians at Devil's River, Texas. He broke off the projectile head and tried to pull the arrow out, but the feathers would not pass through the wound. Finally he freed himself by pulling on the feathered end and continued in the fight. He left the U.S. Army in April 1861 and was subsequently promoted to brigadier general in March 1862, major general in October 1862, and full general in July 1864. Hood spent several days in October 1861 at the Spotswood Hotel, recovering from the flux. On September 19, 1862, during the retreat from Sharpsburg, Hood was not well. He was wounded in the left arm by shrapnel at Gettysburg on July 2, 1863. He fell from his horse, utterly prostrated, and almost fainted. Although the wound did not appear serious, he sent for his surgeon. He was so dazed when he reached the field hospital, probably at the J. E. Plank farm on a litter, that he scarcely observed the bursting of a shell almost in his face. The division surgeon found that Hood had been shot through the hand, forearm, elbow, and biceps. At first it was feared that he would lose his arm. He was taken two hundred miles back to Staunton in a carriage with Gen. Wade Hampton, who had also been wounded. Hampton was unable to sit up, and Hood could not lie down. Hood was confined for more than two months and lost the full use of his arm. He remained for a period of one month under medical treatment, first at Staunton and then at Charlottesville, before proceeding to Richmond. About the middle of September 1863, when his division passed through the capital, he rejoined them with his arm still in a sling. A few days later, on September 20 at the Battle of Chickamauga, a minié ball struck Hood in the right thigh and fractured the femur. He was carried to a nearby house with his leg dangling off the side of the litter. At the field hospital, he underwent a primary amputation at the junction of the upper and middle thirds of the femur. On the next day, he was carried on a litter some fifteen miles to a private residence, where he remained for about one month under the care of a doctor and the family who owned the residence. In mid-October he was sitting up for short periods and was moved to

Dalton. He was then transferred to Atlanta. In early November he went to Richmond where he spent the winter of 1863–64 recovering from the amputation. In December he still had to be lifted from a carriage and helped into the house. His stump healed promptly but remained painful because it was so short that an artificial limb was hard to fit. The men of his old brigade contributed money and presented it to him for the purchase of an artificial limb. By mid-January he was able to stand without his crutches, walk very slowly, and ride a horse. In February 1864 he was ordered to proceed to Dalton, Georgia, to command a corps. He wrote to President Jefferson Davis in March that his health had never been so good. He wore a boot and spur on his artificial limb and could ride up to fifteen miles a day without difficulty. However, by July 1864, the pain in Hood's stump was aggravated by long hard rides. His poor health and an episode of rheumatism in November delayed the preparation of his reports. In Columbus, South Carolina, in January 1865, he could stand well without his crutches. As a businessman after the war, he wore a glove on the injured hand, presumably because it was unsightly. He became ill and delirious on August 27, 1879, while in New Orleans, and died in three days.[1] He was buried in that city's Metaire Cemetery.

DEATH CERTIFICATE: Cause of death, Yellow fever.

1. *OR*, vol. 19, pt. 1:833; vol. 27, pt. 2:298–320, 359, 362; vol. 30, pt. 2:24, 35, 288, 512; vol. 32, pt. 2:699, 804, pt. 3:607; vol. 39, pt. 3:880; Heitman, *Historical Register and Dictionary* 2:25; Richard M. McMurry, *John Bell Hood and the War for Southern Independence*, 19–20, 31, 79–80, 99; Wade Hampton to Wigfall, July 15, 1863, in Louis T. Wigfall Family Papers, Letters of Gen. Joseph Eggleston Johnston to Louis T. Wigfall, UTA; *CV* 5:552; *MSHW*, vol. 2, pt. 3:218, Case 108; Hood, *Advance and Retreat*, 12, 59–61, 64–65; Freeman, *Lee's Lieutenants* 3:231–32; Coco, *Sea of Misery*, 144; Maury, *Recollections of a Virginian*, 92; Steiner, *Medical-Military Portraits*, 221–22, 228; Chesnut, *Diary from Dixie*, 332, 355, 368, 473–74; *New Orleans Daily Picayune*, Aug. 3, 1879.

BENJAMIN HUGER · *Born November 22, 1805*, in Charleston, South Carolina. He graduated from USMA in 1825. Served in the Mexican War. In late 1847 he had a bad cold with a sore throat and vertigo. The cold continued into January 1848 and was associated with a bout of rheumatism. During March and April, he experienced considerable pain in his leg, which limited his activities. It is difficult to determine the exact problem with Huger's leg. He was too ill to do his duty in mid-April and obtained a three-month leave of absence on surgeon's certificate. With the start of the Civil War, he resigned his United States Army commission and was appointed a Confederate brigadier general in June 1861 and major general in October. In May 1861, Huger went to Richmond but was delayed by sickness on the way. On the morning of May 8, 1862, he was unable to attend a conference because of an illness that lasted for only a few days. Following the war he settled on a farm in Virginia. A year or two before he died, he had an attack of apoplexy, and from that time on his health slowly deteriorated. He returned to Charleston, and just prior to his death, he intermittently vomited blood, had pain all over his body, and slept most of the time.[1] He died December 7, 1877, at Charleston and was buried in Green Mount Cemetery at Baltimore, Maryland. Cause of death: Paralysis.[2]

1. *OR*, vol. 2:863; Huger Journal from Mexico, Apr. 16, 17, Oct. 15, 16, 22, 1847, Jan. 13, 19, 20, 23, Mar. 18, 20, 21, 25, Apr. 4, 10, 12, 16, 22, 1848, Ben Huger Papers (no. 9942), UV; Jeffrey L. Rhoades, *Scapegoat General: The Story of Major General Benjamin Huger, C.S.A.*, 43–44, 120.

2. Registers of Charleston County deaths compiled by the Charleston County Health Department, Charleston County Library, Charleston, S.C.

WILLIAM YOUNG CONN HUMES • *Born May 1, 1830*, in Abingdon, Virginia. A prewar lawyer, in 1861 he joined the Confederacy as a lieutenant of artillery. He was wounded in the foot during a fight at Farmington, Tennessee, on October 7, 1863. Later he was promoted to brigadier general and was ordered to proceed to Dalton on November 19 for assignment. On March 10, 1865, while charging Kilpatrick's camp near Fayetteville, North Carolina, Humes was wounded in the leg.[1] Returning to Memphis after the war, he resumed the practice of law. He died September 11, 1883, in Huntsville, Alabama, and was buried in the Elmwood Cemetery in Memphis.[2]

DEATH CERTIFICATE: NAD

1. *OR*, vol. 30, pt. 2:725; vol. 31, pt. 3:721; vol. 47, pt. 1:1045, 1130, 1132.

2. *Memphis Daily*, Sept. 14, 1883.

BENJAMIN GRUBB HUMPHREYS • *Born on either August 24 or 26, 1808*, in Claiborne County, Mississippi. Dismissed from West Point in 1827, he studied the law and became a politician and planter. He raised a company for the Confederate Army, then was made a captain in the 21st Mississippi Infantry in May 1861 and colonel in November. He was sick in March 1862. His old enemy, the flux, returned June 30, 1862, the night of the Battle of Frayser's Farm, and he turned over his command to William L. Brandon. Following a stay in a Richmond hospital, Humphreys went home to Mississippi but returned in time for the battle at Sharpsburg in September. At Fredericksburg on May 3, 1863, he was blinded in his left eye for a time when a minié ball drove the vizor of his cap back into the eye. In August he was promoted to brigadier general. He was admitted again to a general hospital in Richmond on May 24, 1864, with recurrence of the flux and returned to duty June 15. Four miles from Berryville on September 3, 1864, Humphreys was wounded. A minié ball entered at the right nipple, passed around the front of the chest, and came out at the left nipple. He was admitted to the hospital in Charlottesville on September 13, 1864. This was followed by a transfer to a hospital in Richmond, and he spent the winter of 1864–65 at home. In February 1865 he was prevented from returning to the army by Federal cavalry. He was assigned to command of the Subdistrict of Homochitto in April. After the war he was an insurance agent and planter. When more than sixty years of age, he still stood six feet tall and weighed two hundred pounds. Purportedly, his severe wound undermined his health and hastened his death.[1] He died December 20, 1882, at his plantation in Leflore County, Mississippi, and was buried in the Winter Green Cemetery at Port Gibson, Mississippi.

DEATH CERTIFICATE: NAD

1. CSR; *OR*, vol. 42, pt. 1:875; vol. 49, pt. 2:1243; J. F. H. Claiborne Papers, SHC; James B. Blackwell to Sis. Priss (Mrs. A. G. Duncan), Sept. 29, 1864, in Lionel Baxter Coll. Letters, *CWTI* Coll., USAMHI; *CV* 2:242; D. A. Humphreys to Dr. Dunbar Rowland, May 28, 1907, Benjamin G. Humphreys subject file, MDAH; *SHSP* 11:246, 14:422.

EPPA HUNTON • *Born September 22, 1822*, in Fauquier County, Virginia. Hunton studied the law and was admitted to the bar in 1843. He rose to brigadier general of the Virginia militia and was a member of the secession convention. On entering Confederate service, he was appointed colonel of the 8th Virginia Infantry in May 1861. After the First Battle of Manassas in July 1861, he had great difficulty with an anal fistula. He was laid up in Leesburg until October 10, when he went to his brother's home in a spring wagon fitted with a camp bed. By the nineteenth he had rejoined his troops. On the twenty-second, following the Battle of Leesburg, Virginia, he left the field in a wagon and spent the night in town. Hunton left his command on sick leave on November 24, 1861, and had surgery on the fistula in Richmond. This probably consisted of opening up the fistula tract through the overlying skin and muscle with a knife or cautery and allowing it to heal from within. Following the surgery, however, the site did not heal properly. Twice he reported to Centreville but was judged unfit for duty both times and was sent home. He returned to Richmond, and although he received cautery treatments on a regular basis, he did not heal. Again he reported to Centreville but had to return home. He finally returned to his troops on March 20, 1862, although still unfit for duty. Following the Battle of Williamsburg in May, Hunton was so ill he almost fell off his horse. He had a leave in Lynchburg in May and June. Against the advice of his physician, he left his sick bed and rejoined his regiment on June 26. Throughout the Seven Days' battles he fell frequently due to pain and exhaustion. At one time he became separated from his command because he was too exhausted to keep up. Hunton's continuing ill health prompted James Longstreet to send him back to Lynchburg on July 15, 1862. At Gettysburg on July 3, 1863, he was too sick to go into battle on foot as ordered and rode his horse. He was wounded in the right leg just below the knee by a bullet during the charge at Cemetery Heights. His courier led his horse to the rear, where the wounded horse collapsed. Hunton half walked and was half carried back to an ambulance and transported to a field hospital. His wound was dressed, but it was not possible for him to return to the field because of blood loss. During the retreat he rode in a conveyance taken from the Gettysburg Carriage Works and made it back to Virginia. He was promoted to brigadier in August, and following a six-week leave in Virginia, he returned to the field. Late in January 1865 he had a short medical leave. In the last of March, Hunton united his command with George E. Pickett's division and, although sick, remained with his men. On the thirty-first of March at Hatcher's Run, his clothing was ripped by a shell fragment and his sword scabbard bent by a minié ball. At Sayler's Creek, Virginia, on April 6, 1865, he was captured. He was suffering so severely with his chronic diarrhea and fistula that he had to be put on a horse and taken to the rear. He was cared for at Federal general George A. Custer's headquarters, where Custer's physician gave him a bottle of imported brandy and a hair mattress to sleep on. At Fort Warren, with the change in climate and diet, the diarrhea decreased and he gained weight. After the war, President Jefferson Davis told him that his poor health had impeded his promotion during the war. Hunton resumed his law practice and became a politician. When he returned to Richmond, he had attacks of vertigo two to three times a week. He could neither sit nor attempt to lie down without falling. His attacks continued until early 1902. He was blind and deaf for several months before his death.[1] Hunton died October 11, 1908, at Richmond and was buried there in the Hollywood Cemetery. Cause of death: Natural causes.[2]

1. CSR; *OR*, vol. 11, pt. 2:767, 769; Eppa Hunton, *Autobiography of Eppa Hunton*, 45–46, 53, 62–64, 66, 68, 74, 81–82, 90–92, 101–2, 123–24, 128–29, 138, 233–34; John E. Divine, *8th Virginia Infantry*, 9, 22, 25–26, 34; *SHSP* 34:268; *CV* 7:223–24, 16:589; *CMH* 3:603–8; Hunter H. McGuire, Jr., M.D., to author, Jan. 10, 1984.
2. Burial register, Hollywood Cemetery, Richmond, Va.

I

JOHN DANIEL IMBODEN • *Born February 16, 1823,* near Staunton, Virginia. A teacher, lawyer, and politician, he went into Confederate service in 1861 as a captain of the Staunton Artillery. At the battle of First Manassas on July 21, 1861, while firing an artillery piece, he perforated his left eardrum. Subsequently he was totally deaf in that ear. He also received multiple superficial wounds from shell fragments. Later, when he was trying to stop some of his men from running away, one of them raked the skin of Imboden's left arm from wrist to shoulder with his bayonet and knocked him to the ground. Imboden's promotion to brigadier general ranked from January 1863. In the summer and fall of 1864, his health was so impaired from an almost fatal attack of typhoid fever that he was not capable of performing his duties in the field. He was posted to Aiken, South Carolina, in December 1864 to command all the prisons west of the Savannah River.[1] After the Civil War he returned to Richmond and resumed his law practice. He died August 15, 1895, in Damascus, Virginia, and was buried in the Hollywood Cemetery in Richmond. Cause of death: Cholera.[2]

1. CSR; *OR*, vol. 43, pt. 2:937; CR, 145:143; *SHSP* 1:187–88; *Battles and Leaders* 1:235–36.
2. Burial register, Hollywood Cemetery, Richmond, Va.

ALFRED IVERSON, JR. • *Born February 14, 1829,* in Clinton, Georgia. Served in the Mexican War. Directly commissioned into the regular army in 1855, he served as a first lieutenant until he resigned and joined the Confederacy in 1861. He was elected colonel of the 20th North Carolina Infantry. At Cold Harbor on June 27,

1862, he was seriously wounded while leading his regiment. After recovering he took part in the Maryland campaign and fought at South Mountain in September. He was promoted to brigadier the following November. During the Chancellorsville campaign on May 3, 1863, Iverson received a contusion in the groin from a spent shell, which made walking very painful. At Gettysburg he was able to be back in command. In the fighting at Sunshine Church, Georgia, on July 31, 1864, Iverson was sick and not on duty.[1] He initially returned to Georgia after the war, but in 1877 he went to Florida and grew oranges. His death occurred on March 31, 1911, at Atlanta, Georgia, and he was buried there in the Oakland Cemetery. DEATH CERTIFICATE: Cause of death, chronic nephritis.

1. *OR*, vol. 11, pt. 2:554, 625, 644; vol. 19, pt. 1:1029; vol. 25, pt. 1:987; vol. 32, pt. 2:287, 578, 818; Lewis A. Lawson, *Wheeler's Last Raid*, 79.

J

ALFRED EUGENE JACKSON · *Born January 11, 1807*, in Davidson County, Tennessee. Prior to the Civil War he was an active trader all over the South with a variety of holdings. He joined the Confederate service in 1861 as a major in the Quartermaster Corps and was appointed brigadier general in February 1863. On November 23, 1864, because he was physically unfit for active duty in the field, Jackson was ordered to report to John C. Breckinridge for such light duty as he could perform.[1] Later, Jackson undertook farming, having lost everything as a result of the war. His previous holdings were finally restored to him through a special pardon by President Johnson. He died October 30, 1889, at Jonesborough, Tennessee, and was buried there in the Old Jonesborough Cemetery.
DEATH CERTIFICATE: NAD

1. *OR*, vol. 45, pt. 1:1240.

HENRY ROOTES JACKSON · *Born June 24, 1820*, in Athens, Georgia. Served in the Mexican War. Jackson had an extensive and productive career prior to the war. He was a lawyer, newspaper editor, judge, and member of the Georgia secession convention. Appointed as a brigadier general in the Confederate service in June 1861, he resigned in December 1861 to accept the command of Georgia state troops. With changes in the laws, the Georgia troops were turned over to the Confederacy and Jackson was again appointed brigadier in the Confederate Army in September 1863. Following the war he resumed the practice of the law in Georgia, and for almost two dozen years he was president of the Georgia Historical Society. He died May 23, 1898, at Savannah and was buried there in Bonaventure Cemetery. Cause of death: Paralysis.[1]

1. Department of Cemeteries, City of Savannah, Ga.

JOHN KING JACKSON • *Born February 8, 1828,* in Augusta, Georgia. Jackson was practicing law when the war started, and he was elected colonel of the 5th Georgia Infantry in May 1861. He was promoted to brigadier general in January 1862. He returned to his law practice after the war, and within a few months he died on February 27, 1866, at Milledgeville, Georgia. He was buried in the City Cemetery (Magnolia) at Augusta. Cause of death: Pneumonia.[1]

1. Burial records, Magnolia Cemetery, Augusta, Ga.; *Milledgeville (Ga.) Southern Recorder,* Mar. 6, 1866, in Special Collections, Library, Georgia College, Milledgeville, Ga.

THOMAS JONATHAN JACKSON • *Born January 21, 1824,* at Clarksburg, [West] Virginia. He graduated from USMA in 1846. Served in Florida and Mexican wars. Jackson had malaria at age twelve. After the Mexican War, while on a visit to West Point, he was convinced that one of his legs was bigger than the other and that one of his arms was heavier than the other. In December 1857 he had an inflamed throat and trouble with his right eustachian tube. This episode eventually led to permanent impairment of his hearing in both ears, but was more marked in the right. An operation on his throat in 1858 did not alter his condition. He had various symptoms referable to his digestive system and problems with his arms, eyes, legs, and other areas of his body. The weakness of his eyes was a particular problem because it made reading by artificial light difficult. He never ate pepper because it supposedly produced weakness of his left leg, and chronic constipation caused him to ingest large amounts of water. For a time he ate only while standing as an effort to improve his digestion by "straightening the digestive tract." Also, he rigidly limited his diet because of dyspeptic symptoms, a problem that caused him so much suffering that in later years he said he could never forget it. If a man could be driven to suicide, he said, it might be from dyspepsia. Considering his gastrointestinal symptom complex and proclivity to sleeping upright, he most certainly had reflux esophagitis. In July 1860 he had a bilious attack with high fever and spent the summer in New England to improve his health. During the war he was frequently seen sucking lemons, although no one knew how he obtained them. His various systemic complaints virtually ceased once active field duty started. At First Manassas on July 21, 1861, he was wounded in the left hand. The wound was so painful that he carried the arm upright and stopped at the first hospital he reached. The surgeon proposed amputation of the finger, but when he turned his back, Jackson mounted his horse and rode off until he located Dr. Hunter McGuire. The ball had hit one side of the middle finger of the left hand just below the articulation between the first and second phalanges and had carried off a small piece of bone. The upper fragment had been split longitudinally and the articulation was exposed. McGuire placed a splint along the palmar surface of the finger to support the fragments and held it in place with adhesive plaster. A lint-and-water dressing was applied, and McGuire told him to keep it wet with cold water. Later, Jackson was seen pouring cup after cup of water over his hand for several hours at a time. McGuire had him keep the extremity in a sling and elevated. Passive motion was started the twentieth day after the injury and was continued so that there was little resulting deformity. Jackson had been noted to have a mannerism of holding his arm up prior to this injury, and McGuire thought this was why he continued the habit later. On September 6, 1862, when his new horse did not move, Jackson touched her with his spur. She reared instantly, lost her balance, and went over backward. Jackson was stunned for half an hour and was compelled to lie where he had fallen. The pain was so severe that he turned over his command and remained in an ambulance for the remainder of the day. On the following Sunday, he rode to church in an ambulance. While at Moss Neck in January 1863, he developed a severe earache and had to move from his cold tent into a small office building for three months. At Chancellorsville on the evening of May 2, 1863, Jackson, along with other members of his staff, rode down the pike. When they were fired on by Federal troops, the group wheeled about to escape and rode toward their own lines. Confederate troops, not realizing who they were, fired on them by mistake. Jackson was struck in three places and was almost knocked from his horse by the bough of a tree. Before he could dismount, he fell slumping into his companions' arms and was in such a condition that they had to disengage his feet from the stirrups. He was carried a few yards into the woods, where an attempt was made to bind the wound and a sling was rigged to support his arm, which had been mangled. Within a short time, the enemy's battery began to fire on them again, and Jackson was moved back variously by walking and being carried on a litter. When a stretcher-bearer fell, Jackson was dropped on his wounded side and received a contusion of the chest. Replaced on the litter, he was hurried toward the field hospital near Wilderness Run and placed in an ambulance. He was given whiskey and morphine, and after his sleeve was cut away, a handkerchief was tied around his left arm as a makeshift tourniquet to stop the bleeding. There is some confusion as to whether one handkerchief was tied above the wound or whether two handkerchiefs, one above and one below, were applied. When Dr. McGuire met him with an ambulance and examined him by candlelight, Jackson was cold, clammy, and in obvious shock. McGuire compressed the artery with his finger and readjusted the handkerchief, which had slipped and allowed the wound to bleed. After being given more morphia and whiskey, and while McGuire kept his finger resting on the vessel in case bleeding recurred, Jackson was taken back to a field hospital. Placed in a tent on a camp bed, he was covered with blankets and given more whiskey with water. About two and a half hours later he was examined under chloroform anesthesia, having given permission to amputate if necessary. A round ball under the skin of the back of the right hand was removed first. The ball had penetrated the palm of his hand, fractured the second and third metacarpals, and lodged under the skin on the dorsum. A simple lint-and-water dressing was applied, and the hand was splinted to immobilize the bone fragments. The left arm had two wounds, the more serious about three inches below the shoulder. One ball had fractured the humerus and severed the brachial artery, and the other had struck the forearm an inch below the elbow and exited on the opposite side just below the wrist. The arm was amputated two inches below the shoulder with an ordinary circular operation. Superficial skin wounds on the face were dressed with isinglass plaster. Afterward, talking about the chloroform, Jackson said it was the most delightful physical sensation he had ever experienced. The early postoperative course was favorable, and it was thought he would recover. On the third day following surgery, he was moved by ambulance some twenty-five miles to a safer location. When he arrived at Fairfield, they learned that there had been a number of cases of erysipelas in the main house, and so Jackson was placed in a small building in the yard. By the fourth day his amputation was healing, partially by first intention and by healthy granulation. The hand wound gave him little pain, and the discharge appeared healthy. During the following night he became nauseated, and on the morning of May 7, examination suggested a right pleural pneumonia. It was stated he might have a pulmonary contusion with a secondary hemothorax as a result of having been dropped. Others suggested it developed because he already had a cold, or that Jackson himself had brought on the pneumonia because he wrapped himself in wet sheets. However, Dr. McGuire reported the wet cloths could not be implicated because of the short time interval between their application and the development of symptoms. Cups were applied, and mercury with antimony and opium was administered. On the sixth day, the discharge from the wounds had decreased and healing continued. Although the pain in his side had disappeared, he still had trouble breathing and was exhausted. A blister was applied. Consultants from Richmond and Lexington came, but Jackson weakened and expired of pneumonia on May 10, 1863.[1] He was buried in the Jackson Memorial Cemetery at Lexington, Virginia. There was also a "grave" for his amputated arm outside of Chancellorsville.

1. CSR; *OR*, vol. 2:478, 500; vol. 19, pt. 1:1019; vol. 25, pt. 1:799, 885, pt. 2:791–92; Steiner, *Medical-Military Portraits*, 262–64; Douglas, *I Rode with Stonewall*, 126, 149–50, 225; McHenry Howard, *Recollections of a Maryland Confederate Soldier and Staff Officer Under Johnston, Jackson, and Lee*, 102; James L. Mathis, "Building of the Wall—Thomas Jonathan Jackson," *Military Medicine* 129:449–56; Robert L. Dabney, *Life and Campaigns of Lieut.-Gen. Thomas J. Jackson*, 65, 73–74, 145, 686–96, 711–18; McGuire, "Clinical Reports on Gun-Shot Wounds of Joints," 147–50; Hunter McGuire, "Last Wound of the Late Gen. Jackson," *Richmond Medical Journal* 1:402–12; *MSHW*, vol. 2, pt. 2:719, Case no. 88; W. N. Pendleton to wife, Nov. 9, 1863, W. N. Pendleton Papers, SHC; *CV* 1:112, 4:308–9, 13:229–32; Freeman, *Lee's Lieutenants* 2:641; *SHSP* 6:268–72, 14:154–62, 19:304, 43:38; *Battles and Leaders* 1:236, 238, 2:620; Maury, *Recollections of a Virginian*, 71; Lord, *Fremantle Diary*, 105.

WILLIAM HICKS JACKSON • *Born October 1, 1835*, in Paris, Tennessee. He graduated from USMA in 1856. Jackson resigned his commission in May 1861 and joined the Confederate service as a captain of artillery. In the Battle of Belmont, Missouri, on November 7, 1861, he was wounded by a minié ball, which remained in his side even after the war. His father came to take care of him and to help him get home. Jackson rested well the night of the tenth, and on the eleventh smoked a cigar and took soup and milk. The following day he ate foot jelly with milk, wine, and sugar.

Arrangements were made to transport him home in an ambulance. He was back on the field in early 1862. In December 1862 he was promoted to brigadier general. He was ill on July 19, 1863, and unable to take the field. However, he returned the following day.[1] Following the war he raised and developed thoroughbred horses. He died March 30, 1903, at "Belle Meade" near Nashville, Tennessee, and was buried in Mount Olivet Cemetery at Nashville.

DEATH CERTIFICATE: RNA

1. *OR*, vol. 3:828–29, 355; vol. 10, pt. 1:652; vol. 24, pt. 2:659, pt. 3:1019, 1021, 1027; *CMH* 8:316; *CV* 4:235; Alexander Jackson to wife, Nov. 11, 12, 1861, and R. P. Neely to W. H. Jackson, Nov. 21, 1861, William Hicks Jackson Papers, TSLA.

WILLIAM LOWTHER JACKSON • *Born February 3, 1825,* in Clarksburg, [West] Virginia. A prominent lawyer and politician in Virginia, he enlisted in the Confederate service as a private. He soon became colonel of the 31st Virginia Infantry and was promoted to brigadier general in December 1864. Unable to practice law in West Virginia after the war because he was a former Confederate, he moved to Kentucky. In a few years he became a judge. Jackson died March 24, 1890, at Louisville, Kentucky, and was buried there in Cave Hill Cemetery.

DEATH CERTIFICATE: Cause of death, acute nephritis.

ALBERT GALLATIN JENKINS • *Born November 10, 1830,* in Cabell County, [West] Virginia. A lawyer and member of the Federal Congress, he resigned his seat in April 1861. He recruited a company of men and soon was made colonel of the 8th Virginia Cavalry. At Scary Creek in Kanawha County on July 16, 1861, he was seen with his hat off and blood coming down his hair and neck. There are no other details, and it is not known for sure if he had been injured. During a skirmish near Piggot's Mill, West Virginia, on August 25, 1861, Jenkins's arm was slightly injured when his horse fell. In February 1862 he resigned because he had been elected to represent the Fourteenth Virginia Congressional District in the first Confederate Congress. He was promoted to brigadier general in August and was ordered to report for duty. In December there was concern about him being able to join his men at Bristol because of poor health. Jenkins was wounded on the head by an exploding shell on July 2, 1863, while at Gettysburg. Three days later, when the army was retreating, he was able to ride up on a hill near the wagons and observe the Federal troops. After taking leave and recuperating in Lexington, Virginia, he returned in the fall to the Department of West Virginia. On May 9, 1864, while collecting a force at Cloyd's Mountain near Dublin, Virginia, a musket ball shattered his left arm and he was captured. He was taken along with two other wounded Confederate officers to the nearby John Guthrie home, which had been established by the Federal troops for wounded officers. The next day he gave his parole to the Federal troops to report as soon as he was able to travel. The remaining wounded officers were left with five Federal surgeons, and all of them were taken by Confederate troops on the twelfth. On the thirteenth, a Federal surgeon with Confederate surgeons in attendance amputated Jenkins's arm near the shoulder using chloroform. A son of the Guthrie family and a Negro boy took the arm wrapped in a sheet and buried it in the orchard. Cared for by his wife and the Guthrie daughters, Jenkins seemed to improve. However, he subsequently developed pneumonia and rapidly bled to death from secondary hemorrhage on May 21, 1864.[1] He was buried in the Dublin Chapel Cemetery but was moved in 1866 to the family cemetery at Greenbottom. Later he was finally interred in Spring Hill Cemetery, Huntington, West Virginia.

1. CSR; OR, vol. 5:115, 816; vol. 20, pt. 2:474; vol. 27, pt. 2:310–11, 698; vol. 30, pt. 4:740; vol. 37, pt. 1:11, 44, 45, 47; Southern Commanders and Staff Officers folders, RLB Coll., USAMHI; SHSP 24:344–46; CMH 2:133, W.Va.; CV 9:229, 17:599; Jack L. Dickinson, Jenkins of Greenbottom: A Civil War Saga, 44, 49–50, 64–67, 69–75.

MICAH JENKINS • *Born December 1, 1835,* on Edisto Island, South Carolina. As a young child, Jenkins promised his mother he would not drink alcohol. When he was twelve years of age, he refused an offer of whiskey when a doctor cut a fishhook out of his wrist without anesthesia. Following his graduation from the South Carolina Military Academy in 1854, he assisted in the establishment of a military school at Yorkville, South Carolina. Still associated with the school in 1861, he was elected colonel of the 5th South Carolina. At Seven Pines on May 31, 1862, he was struck on the knee. Although the injury drew blood, it did little more than ruin his trousers. Grapeshot struck his shoulder and a shell fragment hit him on the breast during the June 30 fight at Frayser's Farm. Other shell fragments hit his sword, clothes, and horse's bridle, but Jenkins sustained only minor wounds and continued on duty. He was promoted to brigadier general in July and was assigned to a brigade in early August 1862. At Second Manassas on August 30, he was severely wounded. Jenkins rejoined his unit on October 29, when it passed through Front Royal, and he was placed in command the next day. On Sunday, May 1, 1864, he was sick in his tent. On the fifth, he looked unwell, was evidently in pain, and had been riding in an ambulance. To reach the battle, he had to leave his ambulance and continue on horseback. On May 6, 1864, the second day of the Wilderness fight, he was riding at the side of James Longstreet when they were accidentally fired on by Confederate troops. Both were wounded. A bullet struck Jenkins's forehead and paralyzed one side of his body. Although unconscious, he repeatedly lifted his nonparalyzed hand to his head and continued to talk. Most observers agree that he died about five hours later.[1] He was buried at Charleston, South Carolina, in the Magnolia Cemetery.

1. CSR; OR, vol. 12, pt. 2:567; vol. 19, pt. 1:842; vol. 36, pt. 1:1028, 1055; John P. Thomas, Career and Character of General Micah Jenkins, C.S.A., 8–10, 14–17, 20–21, 23; SHSP 1:68; Haskell, Memoirs, 66.

ADAM RANKIN JOHNSON • *Born February 2, 1834,* in Henderson, Kentucky.[1] In the years prior to the war, he was a surveyor and Overland Mail station contractor in West Texas. First serving as a scout for Bedford Forrest, he was appointed a colonel in August 1862 and a brigadier general in June 1864. On August 21, 1864, while attacking a Federal encampment at Grubb's Crossroads, Kentucky, Johnson was accidentally shot in the head by his own men. An ambulance took him to the rear, and he was nursed in a private home. Treatment consisted of bathing the wound in water. Totally blind, he was captured and sent to Fort Warren. Examination by a Federal surgeon revealed that the ball had entered his right eye at the external angle, passed beneath the bridge of the nose, and had come out his left eye, cutting out both eyes. During the time he was a prisoner at Fort Warren, he fell into the basement and was injured. Because Johnson needed help at all times, he was paroled to a private house until the Federal authorities could decide on his case. After being exchanged in February, he refused to retire and returned in March 1865 to the Invalid Corps on a medical certificate. Following the war, despite his blindness, he was very active and established the town of Marble Falls in Texas.[2] He died on October 20, 1922, at Burnet, Texas, and was buried at Austin.

DEATH CERTIFICATE: Cause of death, heart failure and senility.

1. Death certificate.
2. CSR; *CV* 8:117–18, 12:595; Adam R. Johnson, *Partisan Rangers of the Confederate States Army,* 174, 197, 199–201.

BRADLEY TYLER JOHNSON • *Born September 29, 1829,* in Frederick, Maryland. After his admission to the Maryland bar, he was active in politics until the start of the Civil War. Initially, he served as major and colonel with the 1st Maryland (Confederate) Infantry and was promoted to brigadier general in June 1864. He returned to his law practice and politics in Virginia after the war but spent the last few years of his life in Baltimore, Maryland, as an author. He died October 5, 1903, at Amelia, Virginia, and was buried in Loudon Park Cemetery at Baltimore. Cause of death: Bright's disease.[1]

1. Burial records, Loudon Park Cemetery, Baltimore, Md.

BUSHROD RUST JOHNSON • *Born October 7, 1817,* in Belmont County, Ohio. He graduated from USMA in 1840. Served in the Florida and Mexican wars. During February and March 1843, Johnson was unfit for duty because of "Florida Swamp Fever," which was probably malaria. His regiment went to St. Louis in April, and he had a relapse of the fever in November. During a sixty-day leave to Cambridge City, Indiana, in October 1845, he had another episode of the fever. After an extended leave on certificate of ill health, he returned to his company in Corpus Christi, Texas, on February 28, 1846. The army moved in March to the Rio Grande opposite Matamoros. Johnson swam in the river on June 5, 1846, and was sick the next day. In July he had a leave to New Orleans. He reported himself sick at Pass Christian, Mississippi, on August 8 and did not rejoin his company until September 12. Between leaves and illness, he was absent for over six months during a nine-month period in 1846. While in Mexico in May 1847, Johnson contracted yellow fever. He had the "black vomit" and was prostrated in body and mind. The illness and "violent treatment" disabled him for six weeks. After Johnson resigned his army commission in 1847, he taught and was active in local militia groups until

1861. He joined the Confederacy as a colonel of engineers and was promoted to brigadier general on January 24, 1862. On April 6, 1862, at Shiloh, the explosion of a shell knocked Johnson to the ground, and he had to be carried to the rear. He was in Columbus, Mississippi, on April 21, reportedly improving as rapidly as could be expected and hoping to be ready soon for duty. On May 22, Johnson returned sick to his quarters. After recovery, he went into the Kentucky campaign. After the war his health was broken and he never returned to full vigor. For a while he was Chancellor of the University of Nashville, but because of poor health, he returned to his farm. In 1880, a cerebral vascular accident left him with residual paralysis.[1] He died September 12, 1880, near Brighton, Illinois, and was originally buried there in the Miles Station Cemetery. His remains were moved in 1975 to the Old City Cemetery in Nashville, Tennessee. Cause of death: Heart failure and stroke.[2]

1. CSR; *OR*, vol. 10, pt. 1:408, 437, 444–45, pt. 2:431, 537; Charles M. Cummings, *Yankee Quaker, Confederate General: The Curious Career of Bushrod Rust Johnson*, 16, 19–20, 81–82, 92, 100, 219, 374; Cummings, "Seven Ohio Confederate Generals," 9–15, 26–27, 104–5, 109–13, 117–20, 134.

2. State of Illinois, Permit for Disposition of Dead Human Body, Permit no. 12.

EDWARD JOHNSON · *Born April 16, 1816,* in Salisbury, Virginia. He graduated from USMA in 1838. Served in the Florida and Mexican wars. In Mexico he received a wound near the eye that subsequently caused him to twitch, so Johnson appeared to be continuously winking. He left the U.S. Army in June 1861 and joined the Confederate service as a colonel of the 12th Georgia Infantry. In July 1861 he was sick at Camp Monterey. Johnson was promoted to brigadier general in December 1861. On May 8, 1862, at the Battle of McDowell, he was severely wounded. Although some reports say he was hit in the leg, most later reports refer to the ankle as the main site of injury. Robert E. Lee stated that because Johnson could not take the field in September 1862, he might be able to take command of a depot at Winchester. In October he was still unable to perform his duties because the bone in the ankle had not healed properly. Johnson was disabled for a year, and while recuperating in Richmond during the winter of 1862–63, he went around on crutches. When sitting, he would support the ankle and hold his leg as straight as a ramrod. In February 1863 he was promoted to major general and was assigned command in May. At Gettysburg on July 3, his horse was killed and he was wounded. He took part in the action of Payne's Farm on November 27. At Spotsylvania Court-House on May 12, 1864, Johnson hobbled about using a stick and was captured along with Gen. George H. Stewart. He was among the officers taken from Fort Delaware in June to be sent to Hilton Head, South Carolina. After his exchange, Johnson reported to John B. Hood in Atlanta on August 22. On foot and unable to move very well, he was captured again on December 16, 1864, during the Battle of Nashville. Following his release in July 1865, he returned to farming in Virginia.[1] He died March 1, 1873, in Richmond and was buried there in the Hollywood Cemetery.[2]

DEATH CERTIFICATE: Cause of death, apoplexy of lungs.

1. CSR; *OR*, vol. 12, pt. 1:472, 481, 483; vol. 19, pt. 1:139, pt. 2:683–84; vol. 25, pt. 2:762, 787; vol. 29, pt. 1:846; vol. 35, pt. 2:147–48; vol. 36, pt. 1:68, 335, 410, 1072; vol. 38, pt. 5:983; vol. 45, pt. 1:81, 660, 690, 699; vol. 51, pt. 2:181; John H. Worshaw, *One of Jackson's Foot Cavalry*, 79; Freeman, *R. E. Lee* 3:317; Chesnut, *Diary from Dixie*, 299.

2. Death certificate.

ALBERT SIDNEY JOHNSTON • *Born February 2, 1803*, in Washington, Kentucky. He graduated from USMA in 1826. Served in the Mexican War. When he had cholera in August 1832, his treatment consisted of being wrapped in heavy blankets, drenched with vinegar and salt, and then dosed with brandy and cayenne pepper. During August and September of 1836, while in the Texas Army, Johnston had "the fever of the county," which was probably malaria. In a duel with Gen. Felix Houston on February 5, 1837, using horse pistols, Johnston was hit on the sixth shot. The ball passed through the orifices of the pelvis, injured the sciatic nerve, but missed the bones. The examining surgeon did not think he would recover, and he was moved to Texana, where he lay for weeks. By April he tried to exercise but experienced considerable pain and was unable to ride his horse. He turned over command of the army on May 7 and went to New Orleans, where consultants recommended complete rest. On June 27 he tendered his resignation from the Army of the Republic of Texas, which was declined. In December, when his health had improved sufficiently, he returned to Texas. For the remainder of his life he had a limp and was bothered by some loss of muscle mass and numbness, associated with occasional pain in one foot. From 1847 to 1850 he was in poor health from recurring malaria and had to ask for leave in April 1850. He took his family to Kentucky, and in September he went to New Orleans. Returning on shipboard, he had an attack of yellow fever. He apparently treated himself and was able to return to duty in November. At Fort Mason in January 1856, Johnston had remittent bilious fever. On arrival at San Antonio in April, he had a relapse and did not completely recover until the winter of 1856 while in Utah. He was commanding the Department of the Pacific when he resigned his commission in May 1861 and was appointed full general in the Regular Army of the Confederacy.[1] At Shiloh on April 6, 1862, Johnston was riding along the front with Dr. David Yandell and Governor Harris. When they came upon wounded Federal prisoners, Johnston ordered Dr. Yandell to care for them. Soon afterward, Johnston was dead. Exactly how this occurred, the sequence of his wounds, the final minutes of his life, and why he died are all in some dispute and demonstrate observer differences. However, later that night Dr. Yandell examined the body and discerned that the fatal wound had been made by a spent minié ball that had struck Johnston just below the knee and had penetrated as far as midway in the leg. In its course it had torn, without severing, the right popliteal artery, where it divided into the anterior and posterior tibial arteries. This description of the fatal wound was recorded by the only medical observer and should be the most accurate. The ball was removed by Dr. Samuel Choppin of Gen. P. G. T. Beauregard's staff. Besides the fatal wound,

Johnston had been struck three times. One wound was from a spent ball that hit him about the middle of the right thigh on the outside. The second was from a shell fragment just above and to the rear of the right hip, and the third was a minié ball that cut the left boot sole. Supposedly blood was welling over the top of the boot, but if the amount of blood lost was adequate by itself to account for Johnston's death, or if other factors such as underlying coronary artery disease played a role, it is only speculative. It is possible that the altered sensation in his leg from the nerves damaged by his 1837 dueling wound prevented him from realizing in the excitement of battle how badly he had been wounded. In an unusual move, Dr. Yandell had issued tourniquets to all of Johnston's staff officers; one was in Johnston's pocket at the time he died. Dr. Yandell later wrote that if the tourniquet had been applied or if he had been present to tie the vessel, Johnston's life could have been saved.[2] He was buried in the Texas State Cemetery, Austin, Texas.

1. Wm. Preston Johnston, *The Life of Gen. Albert Sidney Johnston*, 47, 74–85, 165, 189; *SHSP* 11:263.

2. *OR*, vol. 10, pt. 1:387, 390, 404–5; *Battles and Leaders* 1:565; *CV* 5:609–13, 6:66, 314, 16:629; William Preston to wife, Apr. 19, 1862, Johnston Family Papers, FC; D. W. Yandell to William, Nov. 11, 1877, 14–17, Mrs. Mason Barret Collection of Albert Sidney and William Preston Johnston Papers (box 17, folder 32), Tulane University Libraries, Howard-Tilton Memorial Library, Tulane University, New Orleans, La.

GEORGE DOHERTY JOHNSTON • *Born May 30, 1832,* at Hillsboro, North Carolina. He was active in Alabama politics before the war. Johnston entered Confederate service as a second lieutenant of the 4th Alabama Infantry and was commissioned major of the 25th Alabama in January 1862. At Murfreesborough, on December 31, 1862, he was wounded on the thigh by a shell fragment. He was listed as in command April 1, 1863. He was made a colonel in September and was promoted to brigadier general in July 1864. One of the bones in Johnston's leg was fractured by a bullet on July 28, 1864, at Ezra Church. He supported the wounded limb on his bridle rein and continued in command of the brigade until exhausted. During the Tennessee campaign, he was on crutches most of the time.[1] After the war he returned to politics in Alabama and died December 8, 1910, at Tuscaloosa, where he was buried in Greenwood Cemetery.

DEATH CERTIFICATE: Cause of death, epilepsy; duration of illness six days.

1. Confederate States Army Casualties, roll 4; *OR*, vol. 23, pt. 2:735; vol. 38, pt. 3:688, 767, 780; vol. 47, pt. 3:698; *CMH* 12:419, Ala.

JOSEPH EGGLESTON JOHNSTON • *Born February 3, 1807,* at Farmville, Virginia. He graduated from USMA in 1829. Served in the Florida and Mexican wars. As a boy, he was kicked on the leg by a horse as they rode over the mountains. He sustained a compound fracture and had to be carried down the mountain on his companions' shoulders. In 1838, during the Seminole War, Johnston was severely wounded in a fight near Jupiter Inlet, Florida. While with a small detachment, he was ambushed; a bullet struck his forehead and passed around his skull. Initially he thought he would die, but after putting his finger into the wound and finding no bones broken, he got up and continued. Years later he said that he had been running toward the Indians when shot, and it had felt like his whole head had been blown off. Johnston was confined to the house during the winter of 1841 and suffered inflammation of an eye the following summer. He was severely wounded twice by musket fire on April 12, 1847, at Cerro Gordo during the Mexican War. While recuperating, he shared a reed house with Dabney H. Maury for about ten days and was then taken to Jalapa and to Benjamin Huger's quarters. His nephew, Preston Johnston, helped take care of him, and he recovered in time to return to the field. At the Battle of Chapultepec on September 13, 1847, Johnston was wounded again. He resigned from the U.S. Army in April 1861 and was commissioned a brigadier in the Regular Army of the Confederacy. In May 1861 Johnston was sick, and his debility compelled him to stop at Abington, Virginia. He wrote from Winchester on July 9, 1861, that he had been so sick the preceding day that he had been unable to write. His promotion to full general ranked from that month. About dusk on May 31, 1862, at Seven Pines, a musket ball hit his right shoulder; a moment later a shell fragment struck him in the chest. Wounded and unconscious, he fell from his horse. When Dr. Gaillard was dressing Johnston's arm, he himself was wounded and lost an arm. Johnston was carried about a quarter of a mile away from the Federal fire and was placed on a stretcher. Examination revealed that his shoulder blade and two ribs were broken. He was next moved several miles in an ambulance to a house where a surgeon dressed his wounds. The following day, with his wife in attendance, he was taken to Richmond to recover. The prescribed treatments were bleeding, blistering, and depletion of his system. When he was finally able to make his report on the battle in late June 1862, he was still feeble and weak. During October he had a lot of pain and difficulty with his side. By November 1862 he was taking some exercise on horseback, and he reported for duty on the thirteenth. The wound caused him continued pleuretic pain due to adhesions between the lung and the chest wall. In January 1863 Johnston was unfit for duty and put himself in the care of a surgeon. On the twenty-second, he was well enough to inspect the defenses of Mobile. The next month he spent three weeks in Tennessee before returning to Mobile. Ordered back to Tennessee, he arrived at Tullahoma on March 18. Too feeble to command, he became seriously ill in a few days. His poor health continued throughout April, and though still unfit for field duty, he left Tullahoma on May 10 and arrived in Jackson on the thirteenth to take command. Johnston helped collect wood for the train on May 23, and the exertion caused pain in the sites of the wounds received at Seven Pines. Following the war he had an acute episode of rheumatism in January 1873, which continued to bother him for a couple of months. Sickness interfered with his correspondence in December 1874. He sustained a severe sprain in 1880 but felt lucky that he had found a physician who understood such cases. Treatment consisted of keeping the joint under a jet of water, which removed the pain and inflammation within twenty-four hours. The use of the limb was limited until its strength returned. He died March 21, 1891, in Washington, D.C., supposedly as the result of a cold contracted while marching bareheaded in the funeral procession of his old adversary, William T. Sherman.[1] However, his death certificate does not support this diagnosis. He was buried in Green Mount Cemetery, Baltimore, Maryland.

DEATH CERTIFICATE: Cause of death, immediate, heart failure; primary, fatty degeneration of the heart of unknown duration. Duration of last sickness, three weeks.

1. CSR; OR, vol. 2:856, 969; vol. 11, pt. 1:934–35; vol. 17, pt. 2:727, 757; vol. 24, pt. 1:238; vol. 51, pt. 2:69; "Military Reminiscences of Major Campbell Brown, 1861–1863," 22, in Campbell Brown-Ewell Papers, TSLA; J. E. Johnston to Pres. (J. Preston Johnston), May 13, 1842, Joseph E. Johnston to grandniece, Sally, Mar. 9, 1873, and Joseph E. Johnston to T. T. Gantt, Aug. 25, 1880, all in Joseph E. Johnston Papers, CWM; B. Huger to wife, April 28, May 13, 1847, both in Benjamin Huger Papers (no. 9942), UV; Mrs. Wigfall to son, Oct. 9, 22, 1862, and Lou to brother, Nov. 14, 1862, all in Louis T. Wigfall Family Papers, UTA; J. E. Johnston to Wigfall, Nov. 12, Dec. 3, 1863 and J. E. Johnston to S. Cooper, Nov. 1, 1863, all in Louis T. Wigfall Family Papers, Letters of Gen. Joseph Eggleston Johnston to Louis T. Wigfall, UTA; Heitman, Historical Register and Dictionary 2:26; Gilbert Eaton Govan, A Different Valor: The Story of General Joseph E. Johnston, C.S.A., 156–58; Joseph E. Johnston, Narrative of Military Operation, Directed during the Late War Between the States, 138–39, 147, 161–64, 167–68, 173–74, 506; Haskell, Memoirs, 27; Lord, Fremantle Diary, 99; Lloyd Lewis, Sherman, Fighting Prophet, 652; Maury, Recollections of a Virginian, 38–40, 145, 153; Chesnut, Diary from Dixie, 248; SHSP 1:412, 18:185–88, 19:338–39; CMH 1:644; Battles and Leaders 3:473–78.

ROBERT DANIEL JOHNSTON • Born March 19, 1837, in Lincoln County, North Carolina. An attorney, he joined the Confederacy as a captain in the 23rd North Carolina Infantry. At Seven Pines on May 31, 1862, he was wounded in the arm, face, and neck and had his horse killed under him. By September he was able to return to the field. Johnston was slightly wounded at Gettysburg on July 1, 1863. While being taken on the retreat through South Mountain on Sunday night, he was captured by Hugh J. Kilpatrick's cavalry near Monterey Springs. However, he was rescued by Confederate cavalry and carried to Williamsport. In September 1863 he was promoted to brigadier and was ordered to report to Richard S. Ewell for assignment to brigade command. At Spotsylvania on May 12, 1864, after planting the regimental flag on the enemy's works, he was shot in the head and fell from his horse. He was hospitalized at the general hospital in Charlotte, North Carolina. During the Valley campaign under Jubal A. Early he was again in command. As he climbed the Federal works at Hare's Hill on March 25, 1865, he severely sprained his ankle. Unable to either walk or mount a horse, he accompanied the retreat in an ambulance. When Federal cavalry were about to capture the group, he collected a few stragglers and fought them off. Later, when the wagon train was captured, he mounted a mule and retook the line with the help of a group of soldiers.[1] He practiced law in Alabama for a number of years following the war and then moved to Birmingham, where he became president of a bank. He died February 1, 1919, at Winchester, Virginia, and was buried there.

DEATH CERTIFICATE: Cause of death, pneumonia; contributory, a deep cold for fifteen days.

1. CSR; *OR*, vol. 11, pt. 1:963–64; vol. 27, pt. 2:287, 559, 563; vol. 29, pt. 2:706; vol. 36, pt. 1:1072, 1074, 1079; *SHSP* 25:175; Clark, *Histories of Several Regiments* 2:205, 223, 238, 244, 264, 266; *CMH* 4:320.

DAVID RUMPH JONES • *Born April 5, 1825*, in Orangeburg District, South Carolina. He graduated from USMA in 1846. Served in the Mexican War. He resigned from the U.S. Army to join P. G. T. Beauregard as chief of staff when the war started. In June 1861, Jones was promoted to brigadier general but was unwell the next month. Appointed to major general in March 1862, he became ill that spring; although his health did not improve, he returned to duty in June. Soon after the Battle of Sharpsburg in September, Jones was pronounced unfit for duty because of a heart condition that had been present for some time. He was relieved from duty on November 6. His report on the Maryland campaign was delayed until December 8, 1863, because of his illness and absence from the field. Jones's poor health continued, and he died in Richmond the next month. Although the date of his death has been reported to be the fifteenth or the seventeenth, the nineteenth was probably correct.[1] He was buried in Hollywood Cemetery, Richmond, Virginia.

1. CSR; *OR*, vol. 19, pt. 1:149, 885; Freeman, *Lee's Lieutenants* 1:272; *CMH* 5:406; Warner, *Generals in Gray*, 164; *CV* 15:236.

JOHN MARSHALL JONES • *Born July 26, 1820*, in Charlottesville, Virginia. He graduated from USMA in 1841. Jones was an instructor at the military academy and did not participate in the Mexican War. He left the U.S. Army as a captain and joined the Confederacy with the same rank. In January 1862, Jones was relieved from duty because of continuous ill health and went to Charlottesville to recuperate. On Richard S. Ewell's staff during the summer of 1862, he was on the field at Cold Harbor in June. His promotion to brigadier ranked from May 1863. At Gettysburg on July 2, 1863, during the assault on the first line of the Federal entrenchment, Jones received a flesh wound of the thigh. Because of excessive bleeding, he gave up his command and had to be carried off the field. He was admitted to the receiving hospital at Gordonsville, Virginia, on July 27 and left the hospital to return to duty in September. Jones led his division on November 27, 1863, to Payne's Farm, where he received a serious wound to the head. However, he reported back within a few days, before he had fully recovered. On May 5, 1864, his brigade opened the fight in the Wilderness. He sustained the first attack by Gouverneur K. Warren's corps, but his men were driven back in confusion. While attempting to rally his brigade, he and his aide-de-camp were killed.[1] He was buried in Maplewood Cemetery at Charlottesville, Virginia.

1. CSR; *OR*, vol. 11, pt. 2:568; vol. 12, pt. 1:780; vol. 27, pt. 2:299, 310–11, 320, 447, 504, 532; vol. 29, pt. 1:848, 856, pt. 2:727; vol. 36, pt. 1:1028, 1070, 1074; Register Book, Receiving Hospital, Gordonsville, Va., June 1, 1863–May 5, 1864, 141, Eleanor S. Brockenbrough Library, MC; *CMH* 3:612.

JOHN ROBERT JONES • *Born March 12, 1827,* at Harrisonburg, Virginia. Before the war he was a teacher at a number of institutions and entered the Confederacy as captain of a company of the 33rd Virginia. Jones was at home on sick leave in August 1861. His promotion to brigadier general ranked from June 1862. He had a contusion of the knee from a shell fragment on the night of July 1, 1862, at the Battle of Malvern Hill, yet the next day he returned and assumed command. Later that month, he left on sick leave and did not return to brigade command until September 6. On September 17 at Sharpsburg, he was disabled by the explosion of a shell above his head and retired from the field. However, he was at Winchester, Virginia, on October 1. On the second day at Chancellorsville, May 2, 1863, owing to the ulcerated condition of one of his legs, he was compelled to leave the field. He was captured July 4, 1863, and admitted to the Federal hospital at Frederick, Maryland, because of a contusion to his leg. He spent the remainder of the war as a prisoner. After returning to Virginia, he was engaged in business.[1] He died April 1, 1901, in the town of his birth and was buried there in Woodbine Cemetery. DEATH CERTIFICATE: RNA

1. CSR; *OR*, vol. 11, pt. 2:587, 591; vol. 18:751; vol. 19, pt. 1:149, 1008, 1012; vol. 25, pt. 1:1005; *CMH* 3:614; John D. Chapla, *42nd Virginia Infantry*, 16–17, 25, 34.

SAMUEL JONES • *Born December 17, 1819,* in Powhatan County, Virginia. He graduated from USMA in 1841. Served in the Florida wars. On his resignation from the United States Army in April 1861, he was appointed a major of artillery in the Confederate Regular Army. He was promoted to brigadier general to rank from July 1861 and to major general from March 1862. His Confederate service was punctuated by a series of illness. His arrival to take command of the army at Pensacola, Florida, in January 1862 was delayed because he was sick en route; instead he assumed command in February. Jones was detained in Brooksville, Mississippi, in June 1862 for a week because of illness. On June 24, 1863, he was in Salt Sulphur Springs with an attack of chills and fever. He was delayed at Abingdon for five or six days in September by an illness diagnosed as diphtheria. Jones was ill again in December. In April 1864 he arrived in Charleston, South Carolina, and on May 4 was temporarily confined to his house because of illness. In November 1864 he was again absent because he was sick. There is not enough information available to determine why Jones was sick so much of the time.[1] He farmed in Virginia after the war until 1880, when he became a clerk in the War Department. Jones died July 31, 1887, at Bedford Springs, Virginia, and he was buried in the Hollywood Cemetery at Richmond. Cause of death: Jaundice.[2]

1. CSR; *OR*, vol. 6:816, 819, 820, 890; vol. 27, pt. 3:929; vol. 30, pt. 2:604; vol. 31, pt. 3:792; vol. 35, pt. 2:471, 647, 650; J. F. Gilmer to wife, Apr. 19, 1864, in J. F. Gilmer Papers, SHC.

2. Burial records, Hollywood Cemetery, Richmond, Va.

WILLIAM EDMONDSON JONES • *Born May 9, 1824,* in Washington County, Virginia. He graduated from USMA in 1848 and served on the frontier until his resignation in 1857. When Virginia left the Union, he became captain of a company he had organized. He later was colonel of the 1st and then the 7th Virginia Cavalry. On August 2, 1862, he received a saber wound while leading a charge at Orange Court-House, but he was back on the field by August 9. From August 23 to August 30 Jones was under medical care in private quarters. His promotion to brigadier general ranked from September 1862, and he was assigned to the command of a cavalry brigade in November. At the battle of Piedmont on June 5, 1864, while encouraging his men in the front line, he was struck in the head by a ball and fell dead from his horse. His body was captured by Federal troops.[1] He was buried in the yard of the Old Glade Spring Presbyterian Church in Washington County, Virginia.

1. CSR; *OR*, vol. 12, pt. 2:182, 184; vol. 19, pt. 2:705; vol. 37, pt. 1:95, 118, 150.

THOMAS JORDAN • *Born September 30, 1819*, in Luray, Virginia. He graduated from USMA in 1840. Served in the Florida and Mexican wars. He resigned from the U.S. Army in May 1861 and assumed staff positions in the Confederate Army during the Civil War. His promotion to brigadier general ranked from April 1862. Jordan was absent with typhoid fever from the middle of May to mid-June 1862. He had been too ill and weak to withstand the slightest exertion, so he had stayed with his brother a few days in June to recover his strength. He was made adjutant and inspector general and chief of staff of the department under P. G. T. Beauregard in September 1862. For the rest of the war, he mainly had staff duties with Beauregard.[1] After a varied postwar career as an author and editor, he suffered poor health in 1892. He died November 27, 1895, at New York City and was buried near Hastings-on-Hudson in Mount Hope Cemetery.

DEATH CERTIFICATE: Cause of death, tubercular lymphadenitis.

1. CSR; *OR*, vol. 10, pt. 2:602; vol. 14:609.

K

JOHN HERBERT KELLY • *Born March 31, 1840*, at Carrollton, Alabama. He resigned from West Point in December 1860 and was shortly thereafter commissioned a second lieutenant of artillery in the Confederate Army. He was slightly wounded in the arm at Murfreesborough on December 31, 1862, but was listed as present the next month. After passing through grades, he was promoted to brigadier general to rank from November 1863. In the course of Joseph Wheeler's raid on Federal communications at Franklin on September 2, 1864, he was shot through the chest by a sharpshooter and fell from his horse. He was placed on a blanket and his coat cut off. Afterward, he was moved to a brick house about half a mile down the road and placed in the care of a nurse. Later, he was moved again and was left with the Harrison family five miles south of town, where he died September 4, 1864.[1] He was buried first in the yard of the Harrison home but was later removed to the Magnolia Cemetery at Mobile, Alabama.

1. CSR; *OR*, vol. 20, pt. 1:776, 847, 859, 869; vol. 38, pt. 3:961; Warner, *Generals in Gray*, 168; Lawson, *Wheeler's Last Raid*, 202.

JAMES LAWSON KEMPER · *Born June 11, 1823*, in Madison County, Virginia. He returned to his law practice following the Mexican War and served five terms in the Virginia House of Delegates. Starting in the 1850s, Kemper had occasional episodes of poor health but on the whole was a strong and healthy man. He went into Confederate service as colonel of the 7th Virginia Infantry in 1861 and was promoted to brigadier general in June 1862. The last of May 1861 he was very sick and was unable to work. On July 3, 1863, at Gettysburg, Kemper was one of the general officers too sick to go on foot and led his brigade on horseback. As the division concentrated on making the final assault, he was seriously wounded and fell off of his horse. He had been struck by a minié ball on the inside of the left thigh near the femoral artery. The ball glanced up the femur, passed through the cavity of the body, and lodged near the base of his spine. At first the lower half of his body was paralyzed. A Federal officer with some of his men placed him on a blanket and started to take him to the rear. Soon afterward, he was recaptured by Confederate troops. Kemper, while being borne back to Bream's Mill on a litter, told Robert E. Lee that he was mortally wounded. He was placed in an ambulance but was thrown to the ground when it was hit by a Federal shell. He was picked up and moved to a farmer's house where he bled profusely. During the retreat he was captured again by Federal troops. Three weeks after the battle, while still among the Federals, Kemper was taken to the Lutheran Theological Seminary in Gettysburg, which was being used as a hospital. Gen. Isaac R. Trimble was brought into the same hospital on August 3. Later, Kemper was transferred to a hospital in Baltimore. After three months' imprisonment, he was exchanged in late September. He served on a court of inquiry from October through November 1863. Although the wound he received at Gettysburg healed rapidly, the ball remained where it had lodged. His pain continued, and his left leg was practically useless. His injuries prevented service in the field, and he was given command of the reserve forces of the state of Virginia for the rest of the war. His poorly healed wound prevented him from traveling on horseback, and he surrendered to Federal troops at Danville. Kemper's condition continued to improve slowly until the late 1860s, but he never regained full use of the leg. Later, even when his general health was good, he felt pain whenever traveling by carriage, stage, train, or horse. During Kemper's 1873 campaign for governor of Virginia, he was exhausted and in pain from standing for long periods during his speeches. Although a brief illness in October prevented one appearance, he traveled four thousand miles and made sixty speeches during a two-month period. After his election as governor, he suffered daily with pain and experienced increasing difficulty with locomotion.

Kemper was frequently confined to bed during his term of office, and although he performed his duties, he was difficult to deal with on occasion. With advancing age, his ability to get around decreased even with the aid of crutches, and he had a number of serious falls. Service buildings were built around his main house, including one with a pool, which was used for its therapeutic effects on his old wound. Also, large quantities of whiskey were purchased, which probably helped alleviate his pain. By 1891 his condition was further complicated by heart disease, and he was barely able to move from room to room. In 1894 he could not stand any motion of his left hip and leg because of excruciating pain. Swelling of his abdomen, day and night bronchitis, and asthma bothered him continuously during the last year of his life.[1] He died April 7, 1895, at his plantation in Orange County, Virginia, and was buried in the family cemetery (Walnut Hill Cemetery) beside his plantation.

DEATH CERTIFICATE: RNA

1. CSR; *OR*, vol. 27, pt. 1:80, pt. 2:298, 321, 362, 386; vol. 36, pt. 2:1012; vol. 51, pt. 2:881; Robert Rivers Jones, "Conservative Virginian: The Postwar Career of Governor James Lawson Kemper" (diss.), 8, 10–11, 207, 211, 305, 331, 354–55, 381, 388, 390–92; *CMH* 3:620; *SHSP* 31:234; Coco, *Sea of Misery*, 148.

JOHN DOBY KENNEDY • *Born January 5, 1840*, in Camden, South Carolina. He was admitted to the bar a short time before the start of the Civil War and was elected captain of a company in the 2nd South Carolina Infantry in April 1861. On July 21, 1861, during the battle of First Manassas, Kennedy was bruised on the side by a ball. He was made colonel of his regiment in January 1862. Following the battle of Savage's Station on June 29, he was disabled by fever. He was wounded during the first charge at Sharpsburg on September 17, 1862, but three months later he was able to participate in the Battle of Fredericksburg. He was absent on a surgeon's certificate for thirty days starting February 24, 1863. Kennedy was wounded at Gettysburg on July 2 but was listed as in command on August 31. He was wounded again outside of Knoxville, Tennessee, on November 18. He was promoted to brigadier in December and on the thirty-first was listed as in command. At the Wilderness on May 6, 1864, Kennedy was severely wounded and carried to the rear. He was in private quarters on the nineteenth and requested medical leave. Still absent in October because of this wound, he recovered sufficiently to be listed as in command in December 1864. Besides the multiple wounds during his service, Kennedy was hit fifteen times by spent balls! After the war he was prominent in South Carolina politics. His death occurred suddenly from a stroke on April 14, 1896, at Camden, South Carolina.[1] He was buried in the Quaker Cemetery in that city.

DEATH CERTIFICATE: NAD

1. CSR, *OR*, vol. 2:526; vol. 11, pt. 2:733; vol. 19, pt. 1:865; vol. 21:592; vol. 27, pt. 2:369; vol. 29, pt. 2:682; vol. 31, pt. 1:495, 508, pt. 3:890; vol. 42, pt. 3:1364; CR, 145:88; *CMH* 5:408; Warner, *Generals in Gray*, 171.

JOSEPH BREVARD KERSHAW • *Born January 5, 1822*, in Camden, South Carolina. Served in the Mexican War. He was a lawyer and politician and served in the South Carolina secession convention in 1860. He was made colonel of the 2nd South Carolina when the war started and was promoted brigadier to rank from February 1862 and major general from May 1864. Following the war he returned to the practice of law and again entered politics. He was elected circuit court judge in 1877 and served in that position until 1893, when he resigned because of poor health.[1] He died April 12, 1894, at Camden and was buried there in the Quaker Cemetery.[2]

DEATH CERTIFICATE: NAD

1. *CMH* 5:409–11.
2. Tombstone, Quaker Cemetery Association, Camden, S.C.

WILLIAM WHEDBEE KIRKLAND • *Born February 13, 1833*, at Hillsboro, North Carolina. He entered West Point in 1852 but resigned and was commissioned in the U.S. Marine Corps in 1855. He left the corps in August 1860 and was appointed a captain in the Confederate Army in March 1861. The following June he was elected colonel of the 21st North Carolina Infantry. In the First Battle of Winchester on May 25, 1862, Kirkland was shot through both thighs and was carried off the field on a litter. While recuperating, he acted as chief of staff to Patrick R. Cleburne at the Battle of Murfreesborough. He rejoined his regiment during the invasion of Pennsylvania and fought at Gettysburg. His promotion to brigadier general ranked from August 1863. The ulnar bone of his left arm was fractured by a bullet at Bristoe Station, Virginia, on October 14, 1863. Kirkland remained a few days at the receiving hospital in Gordonsville, Virginia, before going on to a general hospital in Richmond where he had some type of surgery on the day of his arrival. He went to Savannah, Georgia, to recuperate and in December requested a sixty-day extension of his leave on a surgeon's certificate. Upon recovery, he returned to command on February 20, 1864. He was badly wounded at Cold Harbor on June 2 when a rifle ball struck him in the right thigh muscles. He was admitted to the Jackson Hospital in Richmond on June 14. In August he was able to take command of a brigade in Robert F. Hoke's division.[1] At the end of hostilities he went to Savannah but later moved to New York, where he worked in the post office. Kirkland became an invalid and spent the last years of his life in a soldiers' home in Washington, D.C., where he died May 12, 1915. He was buried at Shepherdstown, West Virginia, in Elmwood Cemetery.

DEATH CERTIFICATE: Cause of death, primary, general arteriosclerosis; immediate, uremic poisoning.

1. CSR; *OR*, vol. 12, pt. 1:780, 795; vol. 29, pt. 1:427, 432; vol. 42, pt. 2:1190, 1207; CR, 178:74, 588; Register Book, Receiving Hospital, Gordonsville, Va., June 1, 1863–May 5, 1864, 289, Eleanor S. Brockenbrough Library, MC; *CMH* 4:321; Oates, *War between the Union and the Confederacy*, 98; Buck, *Cleburne and his Command*, 22 n.22; Clark, *Histories of Several Regiments* 3:244, 246; Morrison, *Memoirs of Henry Heth*, 189.

L

JAMES HENRY LANE • *Born July 28, 1833,* at Mathews Court House, Virginia. Following his graduation from the Virginia Military Institute and the University of Virginia, he became a teacher. When the war started, he was elected major of the 1st North Carolina Volunteers. On June 27, 1862, at First Cold Harbor, he received a slight head wound. Three days later, while at Frayser's Farm, Lane suffered a flesh wound of the right cheek; however, he refused to leave the field. His promotion to brigadier ranked from November 1862. He was injured when his horse was shot from under him at Gettysburg on July 3, 1863, but remained in command. During the advance on Turkey Ridge on June 2, 1864, Lane was wounded in the groin by a sharpshooter. In early August he was at the post headquarters in Richmond on a surgeon's certificate. He resumed command August 29, 1864, but, as he was not fully recovered, he took a sick leave October 30. On February 28, 1865, Lane was listed as in command, and he took part in the actions with his brigade in April. He returned to teaching after the war and was professor of civil engineering at the Alabama Polytechnic Institute when he died.[1] He died on September 21, 1907, at Auburn, Alabama, and was buried there in the Pine Hill Cemetery.

DEATH CERTIFICATE: RNA

1. CSR; *OR,* vol. 11, pt. 2:839, 893; vol. 27, pt. 2:664; vol. 42, pt. 2:1207, 1218; vol. 46, pt. 1:1285, pt. 2:1272; *SHSP* 9:241–46; *CMH* 4:323; *CV* 2:150; Clark, *Histories of Several Regiments* 3:91.

WALTER PAYE LANE • *Born February 18, 1817,* in County Cork, Ireland. On April 21, 1836, during the Texas Revolution, a Mexican soldier pierced Lane's shoulder with a lance, throwing him off his horse. His head struck the ground and he was knocked senseless. The lance nearly went through his shoulder blade. A little over three months after the battle of San Jacinto, he was ill and obtained his discharge from the Texas Army. Later, while going by horseback from Houston to San Augustine, he had an illness characterized by chills and fever that lasted for six months. While Lane was working with a surveying crew near Richland Creek in Texas's eastern Navarro County on October 8, 1838, he was wounded in a fight with the Kickapoo Indians. He was shot through the calf of the leg, and the bullet splintered the bone and cut the tendons. Walking on his heel, he hobbled to cover in a ravine. There was rather severe bleeding, and the wound was bandaged as soon as possible. To escape he had to travel almost ninety miles. He was laid up for two months while the splintered bone fragments worked themselves out of his leg. During the American occupation of Mexico, Lane was shot in the leg in one of the engagements with Indians and guerrillas. He was involved in mining at the start of the Civil War and was elected lieutenant colonel of the 3rd Texas Cavalry in 1861. In the spring of 1863 he became ill while en route to Van Buren, Arkansas. He developed a rising or boil on his head as well as fever. He was left at a farmhouse in the Indian Nation for three weeks, but instead of improving, his condition worsened. Because there was no drainage of the infection, his physician made an incision below the ear. Unfit for duty, Lane went to Marshall, Texas, and did not return for two months. Prior to the attack on the fort at Donaldsonville in June 1863, Lane's artillery fought on the Mississippi with Federal gunboats. A 140-pound shell struck the bank just below him and exploded, turning over the planks he was standing on and covering him with dirt. His only injury was a cut on the forehead from a plank. At the Battle of Mansfield, Louisiana, on April 8, 1864, Lane was shot through the thigh and had six bullets pass through his coat, two of which drew blood from him. He was taken back to Marshall in an ambulance. Although he returned and his promotion to brigadier general ranked from March 1865, this was his last major combat. He returned to Texas after the war and was prominent in local affairs and various veterans' organizations. He had been in poor health for more than a year before his death and was quite ill for a few days before dying on January 27, 1892, at Marshall.[1] He was buried in that town in the Old Marshall Cemetery. Cause of death: Cirrhosis of the liver.[2]

1. Walter P. Lane, *The Adventures and Recollections of General Walter P. Lane*, 12–13, 19, 29, 30–38, 40, 69, 105, 107, 110, 115–16, 118, 162; newspaper clipping, n.i., n.p., n.d., in Walter P. Lane biography file, Library of the Alamo, San Antonio, Tex.

2. Register of Death and Burials of the City of Marshall, Rains and Herndon Funeral Home, Marshall, Tex.

EVANDER MCIVER LAW • *Born August 7, 1836*, at Darlington, South Carolina. He graduated from the South Carolina Military Academy in 1856 and spent the years before the war teaching. He recruited a company of Alabama state troops and was later elected lieutenant colonel of the 4th Alabama. Law was severely wounded in the left arm at First Manassas on July 21, 1861, and was absent through October. He was listed as in command during the summer of 1862, and his promotion to brigadier general ranked from October. At Second Cold Harbor on June 3, 1864, while standing on the Confederate works, he was wounded in the head. The ball fractured the orbit procep, os frontis, and hemicrania and injured the left eye. He applied for a furlough in August from general hospital no. 4 in Richmond. Law did not return to his brigade, as he was relieved at his own request and desired cavalry service. In October 1864 he was back on the field. He was relieved from duty with the Army of Northern Virginia on January 7, 1865, and was instructed to report to Gen. Braxton Bragg at Wilmington, North Carolina. In March he was on duty. Following the war he was a major factor in the establishment of public education in Florida. A pension examination in 1917 revealed that Law's left arm was shrunken and practically useless. The elbow was stiff, and the rotary motion of the forearm was gone. The head wound had severed the supraorbital nerves of the left eye and paralyzed the left frontal quarter of his scalp.[1] He died October 31, 1920, at Bartow, Florida, and was buried there in Oakhill Cemetery.

DEATH CERTIFICATE: Cause of death, primary, paralysis for seven days; contributing factor, senility.

1. CSR; *OR*, vol. 12, pt. 2:483; vol. 36, pt. 1:1059; vol. 42, pt. 1:876; vol. 46, pt. 2:1179; vol. 47, pt. 1:1123, pt. 2:998, 1204; CR, 145:134; *CV* 20:511; *CMH* 12:422, Ala.; Pension application of Evander McIver Law, filed Apr. 24, 1917, Florida Department of State, Division of Archives, History and Records Management, the Capitol, Tallahassee, Fla.

ALEXANDER ROBERT LAWTON • *Born November 4, 1818,* in Beaufort District, South Carolina. He graduated from USMA in 1839 and resigned from the U.S. Army two years later to study law. He moved to Savannah, Georgia; besides practicing the law, he was a railroad president and a member of the Georgia legislature. His commission as brigadier general was confirmed in August 1861. At the Battle of Sharpsburg on September 17, 1862, Lawton was severely wounded in the leg and had to be borne off the field. He was taken to Henry Kyd Douglas's father's home for care and then to Staunton, where his wife joined him. During the first part of October he was moved to Jeremy F. Gilmer's quarters in Richmond. Although the bone was injured, it was not broken, and the wound appeared to heal well. However, he also suffered from nervous prostration and a disordered condition of his stomach and bowels. The large amounts of morphine he required made him nervous and restless, causing his wife to decide that he needed a physician more than a surgeon. In addition, the wound was complicated by a fever that was variously diagnosed as camp fever, typhoid, or intermittent fever because it returned every four days. By the nineteenth of October, the inflammation from Lawton's wound had extended down his leg almost to the ankle. Under chloroform, the area was examined by a probe and a searching needle. It was confirmed that no bones were broken but that the inflammation below the wound was caused by a sinus tract that extended downward. A lance was used at the lowest point to provide a vent for the accumulated pus, and a "tent" or "seton" was inserted to keep it open. Within a few days, after drainage of the area, Lawton improved and suffered mainly from the restlessness and confusion produced by the opiates he was given. All of the family helped with his care, and he ate oysters and beefsteak and drank eggnogs. He continued to have an elevated temperature, which Jeremy F. Gilmer blamed on his diet. In December, Lawton and his wife left Richmond for Savannah. By the end of the month, he still could not use the leg or foot and was on crutches. In May 1863 he thought his health was sufficiently restored to return to duty. He sat in on the examinations at Virginia Military Institute, and his increased efforts to walk produced some lameness. In July he stopped at Rockbridge Bath, Virginia, for the benefit of the hot water on his legs. He was placed in command of the Quartermaster General's Department in the fall of 1863. Following the end of hostilities he returned to Georgia and had a major role in state and national politics. In March 1875, because of illness and duties with the legislature, he was unable to keep up with his correspondence.[1] He died July 2, 1896, at Clifton Springs, New York, and was buried at Savannah in Bonaventure Cemetery.

DEATH CERTIFICATE: Cause of death, apoplectic paralysis.[2]

    1. CSR; *OR*, vol. 19, pt. 1:147, 923, 956, 968, pt. 2:683–84; A. Porter to J. F. Gilmer, Sept. 27, 1862, Sally (Mrs. A. W. Lawton) to J. F. Gilmer, Oct. 2, 1862, J. F. Gilmer to Mrs. J. F. Gilmer, Oct. 16, 19, 22, Dec. 25, 1862, and Mrs. J. F. Gilmer to J. F. Gilmer, Dec. 31, 1862, all in Jeremy F. Gilmer Papers, SHC; William W. Mackall to wife, Oct. 2, 1862, in W. W. Mackall Papers, SHC; Alexander R. Lawton to Jos. E. Johnston, Mar. 11, 1875, in Joseph E. Johnston Papers, CWM; Douglas, *I Rode with Stonewall*, 168; Warner, *Generals in Gray*, 175–76.

    2. Village Clerk, Clifton Springs, N.Y.

DANVILLE LEADBETTER · *Born August 26, 1811,* at Leeds, Maine. He graduated from USMA in 1836. He was sick in August 1850, but no details are available. He resigned from the U.S. Army in December 1857 and was appointed chief engineer of the state of Alabama. He was commissioned a major of engineers in March 1861. In late November 1861, while in East Tennessee, he was ill from the "weather and water" and turned over his command, but he was back on duty by December 3. He spent his time in service as an engineer, and he was promoted to brigadier general from February 1862. When he arrived in Mobile on November 4, 1862, Leadbetter was in very bad health, cold and jaundiced. By the end of the month he was actively engaged in his duties.[1] He went to Mexico after the close of the war and then moved to Canada, where he died at Clifton on September 26, 1866. Leadbetter was buried in Magnolia Cemetery, Mobile.

DEATH CERTIFICATE: RNA (Passport Service, U.S. Department of State).

    1. *OR*, vol. 7:712, 747; vol. 15:867; vol. 20, pt. 2:405, 443; Th. L. Smith to Danville Leadbetter, Aug. 31, 1850, in Danville Leadbetter Papers, ADAH.

EDWIN GRAY LEE · *Born May 27, 1836,* at "Leeland," Virginia. Lee was never in the best of health, and his lassitude and coughing spells were diagnosed as tuberculosis by a physician in New York in October 1860. Although it was recommended that he have exercise and fresh air in a cold, dry climate, he was unable to leave Shepherdstown, where he was just starting a law practice. He entered the Confederate Army as a second lieutenant of the 2nd Virginia. He felt well in June 1861 while at a camp near Winchester. However, the cold, rainy weather of the following autumn affected his lungs, and he had to leave his unit. He stayed in a private home near Forest Depot in Bedford County, and he returned to winter quarters at Winchester. In June 1862 he obtained a twelve-day leave on surgeon's certificate to rest at Lexington, not because of anything specific, but because the uninterrupted exposure had exhausted him and weakened his lungs. He left camp in August on surgeon's orders. By September his health was still bad, and assignment to post duty during the winter was considered. However, Lee, who had risen through grades to colonel, resigned on the advice of Dr. Hunter McGuire in December 1862 because of his lung disease. He was recommissioned a colonel in 1863. In the summer of 1864, he was assigned to temporary command at Staunton, Virginia, and took part in the operations near there in June and near Waynesboro in September. His appointment as brigadier general ranked from September. In

November 1864 he received six-months' leave of absence for his health. He and his wife ran the blockade in December and went to Montreal, Canada. During the winter of 1865, he had a cold that became worse, and his doctor recommended a diet of oysters, milk, and "gamy" partridges. In the spring of 1866 the Lees returned to Shepherdstown. However, his lungs could not withstand the cold winter weather, so he and his wife went to Texas. He returned home in May 1867, still very sick. Despite his poor health, he went to Washington in July to testify at the trial of John H. Surratt. The rest of the summer he remained in Shepherdstown trying to regain his strength. The winter of 1867–68 was spent at Aiken, South Carolina, where the climate was recommended for those with lung disease. His health visibly worsened during the summer of 1869. After returning to Lexington, his greatest problem was his inability to walk, and he was unable to exert himself with anything more strenuous than office work. He died supposedly from tuberculosis on August 24, 1870, while trying the waters at Yellow Sulphur Springs.[1] He was buried at Lexington, Virginia, in Jackson Memorial Cemetery.

DEATH CERTIFICATE: RNA

1. CSR; *OR*, vol. 36, pt. 1:151–52, pt. 2:1017; vol. 43, pt. 1:615, pt. 2:926; Edwin G. Lee to W. N. Pendleton, June 14, 1862, in W. N. Pendleton Papers, SHC; Alexandra Lee Levin, *"This Awful Drama": General Edwin Gray Lee, C.S.A., and His Family*, 22, 27, 33–34, 40–41, 43, 55–56, 176, 183–87, 190, 192–93; CMH 3:621–22; Bean, *Stonewall's Man Sandie Pendleton*, 64.

FITZHUGH LEE · *Born November 19, 1835*, in Fairfax County, Virginia. Graduated from USMA in 1856. On May 13, 1859, in a fight with Comanche Indians in the Nescutunga Valley, Texas, he was shot through the lungs with an arrow. Blood came from his mouth but not from the wound entrance. He was taken almost two hundred miles across the plains using a mule litter. At one point the animal began running wildly; due to the jostling, Lee's wound reopened. Lee recovered in three months and was able to write by June 3. In January 1860 he was back fighting the Indians, and after home leave in the summer was assigned to West Point in December. He left the U.S. Army in May 1861 and entered the Confederacy as a first lieutenant. He was made a lieutenant colonel of the 1st Virginia Cavalry in August 1861 and a brigadier general in July 1862. Toward the end of September 1862 he was kicked on the leg by a mule and was unable to return to duty until November. In May and early June 1863, Lee was incapacitated with inflammatory rheumatism but returned to command his brigade on June 24, even though he was still suffering from the disease. His promotion to major general ranked from August 1863. In January 1864 he left Moorefield with his feet frozen to such an extent that the surgeon considered amputation. On August 29 and 30, 1864, he was sick with an intermittent fever and was confined to bed. At the Third Battle of Winchester on September 19, 1864, in the midst of an artillery barrage, Lee's horse was shot, and Lee himself received a minié ball in the left thigh. He spent November recovering in Richmond, but in December the wound was complicated by infection and abscesses. He rejoined his troops at Staunton and in March 1865 was appointed to command the cavalry corps of the Army of Northern Virginia.

Following the war he became a farmer in Virginia. He developed an eye infection in the fall of 1869 and had treatment in Washington and Alexandria. In 1885 he was elected governor of Virginia. Overweight in 1895, he had difficulty breathing with exertion. On April 28, 1905, while on the train to Washington, D.C., he had a stroke involving his left side. The doctor who traveled with him from New York administered strychnine. On arrival at Washington, Lee was taken by ambulance to a hospital, where he remained conscious until just before his death on April 28, 1905.[1] He was buried in Hollywood Cemetery in Richmond, Virginia. Cause of death: Apoplexy.[2]

1. CSR; *OR*, vol. 19, pt. 2:141, 669, 712; vol. 27, pt. 2:692, pt. 3:7–8; vol. 43, pt. 1:1009; Fitzhugh Lee to Mrs. E. V. D. Miller, May 28, 1886, in Earl Van Doran Papers, ADAH; Heitman, *Historical Register and Dictionary* 2:28; Francis Dawson, *Reminiscences of Confederate Service, 1861–1865*, 132, 138; James L. Nichols, *General Fitzhugh Lee: A Biography*, 10–13, 54, 78–79, 97, 146, 173, 177; Von Borcke, *Memoirs of the Confederate War* 1:273; CMH 3:622; CV 13:280; SHSP 35:143.

2. Burial register. Hollywood Cemetery, Richmond, Va.

GEORGE WASHINGTON CUSTIS LEE • *Born September 16, 1832*, at Fortress Monroe, Virginia. The son of Robert E. Lee, he graduated from USMA in 1854. In May 1861 he resigned from the army and became a captain of engineers in the Confederate service. In June 1861, while in Richmond, he became ill. During the first part of July he was ordered to North Carolina to inspect the forts and works. William D. Pender visited him in Richmond on May 22, 1862, and found him ill from typhoid and looking as though he would not recover for some time. Lee was still quite weak in August. His promotion to brigadier general ranked from June 1863. In July 1864, Lee supposedly had typhoid fever again but had almost recovered by August 8. However, President Jefferson Davis did not think that Lee was physically equal to duty in the Shenandoah Valley. He improved and, promoted to major general, was ordered to resume his command in October 1864. By the end of the month, however, he was bothered by boils. In January 1865 he was assigned to command a division.[1] Following the war in July 1865, he was ill and planned to stay near Centreville for the next one to two months. After his father's death in 1870, Lee succeeded him as president of what is now Washington and Lee University. His tenure in office was marked by a series of illnesses, long absences because of his health, and frequent attempts to resign. When he tried to resign in 1893, he was too ill to submit a written statement. Unfortunately, there are few descriptions of his symptoms, and his students and colleagues who later wrote about him did not detail his illness. Lee did spend time at White Sulphur Springs and had difficulty with rheumatism, particularly of his hands. This condition confined him to his house except on warm days, but he inferred that there were other problems with his health without being specific. Some authors have attributed his illness to psychosomatic causes due to frustration and because he was overshadowed by his father. About six weeks before his death, he slipped on the staircase and fractured his hip. He never left his bed after this accident. He had lived the life of a recluse and had guarded his seclusion so persistently in his later years that few of the general public outside his native state knew that he was still alive.[2] He died February 18, 1913, at his residence at "Ravensworth" near Alexandria, Virginia, and was buried in Lexington, Virginia, in the Lee Chapel on the grounds of the Washington and Lee University.

DEATH CERTIFICATE: Cause of death, chronic parenchymatous nephritis of one year's duration; contributory, hydrostatic pneumonia of five days' duration.

1. OR, vol. 42, pt. 3:1141; vol. 43, pt. 1:992; vol. 46, pt. 2:1025; Jeremy F. Gilmer to Mrs. J. F. Gilmer, Aug. 8, 1862, in Jeremy F. Gilmer Papers, SHC; Hassler, General to His Lady, 145; Robert E. Lee, The Wartime Papers of R. E. Lee, 46, 54, 56, 251, 851, 865.

2. James Lewis Howe, Annals of Washington and Lee University, Washington and Lee University, the University Library, Lexington, Va. (hereafter cited as WLU); Charles Bracelan Flood, Lee: The Last Years, 70; Olinger Crenshaw, General Lee's College: The Rise and Growth of Washington and Lee University, 178–81; G. W. C. Lee to Dear "Mrs. Nowell," Aug. 20, 1895, G. W. C. Lee to My Dear Cousin, Apr. 28, 1896, July 16, 1903, all in Robert Edward Lee Papers, WLU; Dr. George Bolling Lee to Dear Professor (James L. Howe), Feb. 8, 1940, in James Lewis Howe Papers, WLU; SHSP 39:167.

ROBERT EDWARD LEE · Born January 19, 1807, in Westmoreland County, Virginia. He graduated from USMA in 1829. Preparing for the September 13, 1847, attack on Chapultepec, Mexico, he was almost paralyzed by the strain. He was slightly wounded during this assault and had to leave the field because of loss of blood. While supervising construction of Fort Carroll in Baltimore Harbor in 1849, he had a febrile illness, probably malaria. When Virginia left the Union, he resigned his commission in the United States Army and accepted a position as commander in chief of Virginia forces. He was appointed brigadier general in the Regular Confederate States Army in May 1861. The next month he was appointed general. Lee contracted a cold in the hot weather of June 1862, he thought from being too heavily clad. During the first part of July, he was tired and not well. On August 31, at Stewart's farm, Virginia, Lee had both hands injured by a fall. One hand was badly sprained and the other had several bones broken. Water was poured on them until the pain subsided, and both hands were put into splints. He had to carry one of his hands in a sling for some time and was unable to ride his horse for almost two weeks. Lee suffered with a bad cold the first week in April 1863, which was aggravated by living in a tent. The doctors moved him into the home of the Yerby family because they thought he had developed pericarditis. Although he did not feel very sick, he had paroxysms of sharp pains in the chest, back, and arms associated with some fever. He thought that it was similar to the illness others had when he was in Richmond, and that he had caught it from them. His treatment consisted of quinine and the frequent attention of physicians, who he said tapped him all over like an old steam boiler before they condemned it. One visitor thought that if she made him an all-cotton shirt to wear, it would extract the pain. His doctors and Lee had little faith in the idea, so it was not tested. Although confined to his room, he was still able to do his daily paperwork. By the eleventh of April, he was able to ride, although his legs were weak and his pulse was about ninety per minute. The next day his cough was better and he was free of pain. He returned to camp on the sixteenth but was still feeble and could do little. During the battle at Gettysburg, Lee had diarrhea and possibly a recurrence of malaria. On August 8, 1863, he suffered with a rheumatic malady. He experienced increasing failure of strength; in addition, it appeared that he had not fully recovered from the illness he had the previous spring. Becoming less capable of exertion and unable to perform his duties, he asked to be relieved of his command. Following a trip to Richmond in September, Lee had another severe cold, which exacerbated the rheumatism in his back. The intense pain when riding his horse prompted him to use a spring wagon that on rough roads was almost as painful as horseback riding. The doctors gave him a lotion that he applied to his back for a week with little benefit, although he almost excoriated himself. The violent back pains were attributed variously to lumbago, sciatica, or rheumatism. Attributing these symptoms to angina, as has been done by later writers, does not seem to be correct. By October 1863, Lee's rheumatism became so severe that he was confined to his tent. He could not mount a horse, and when he did, every motion gave him pain. During mid-November he rode a great deal but still had twinges of pain and general stiffness. In December he seemed to be aging hourly, and his hair and beard turned white. There was continuation of the sharp paroxysmal pain intermittently in his left side. He became very sick on the night of May 23–24, 1864, with violent intestinal complaints that one observer said was bilious dysentery. He was worse on the twenty-fifth and was confined to his tent. On the twenty-ninth, Lee was so sick he could hardly leave headquarters. He had improved enough after two days to get about in a carriage, and he was taking some brandy that had been sent to him. There was a continuation of the vague sciatica, lumbago, or rheumatism during the last months of the war.[1] In the fall of 1867, Lee had a severe cold complicated by rheumatism and was confined to bed for two weeks. He was able to ride his horse back to Lexington and arrived there in the middle of September. His health had worsened by the summer of 1868, and he could no longer make long trips by horseback. His physicians recommended that he drink large amounts of the mineral waters at White Sulphur Springs. He had occasional episodes of subacute or chronic rheumatism. In October 1869 he had an attack of subacute pericarditis with muscular pain of the back and right side, which later extended to his arms. There was never any evidence of pericardial effusion. During the first part of 1870, he could not walk much farther than 150 yards without stopping to rest. Early in March 1870, he became more feeble, his rheumatism more bothersome, and he was continually sad and depressed. By April, when he attempted to walk faster than a very slow gait, the pain or stricture in his chest was always there. Although these episodes have been diagnosed in retrospect as angina due to arteriosclerotic heart disease, the recurrent rheumatism and pericarditis diagnosed by his doctors at the time are more suggestive of rheumatic heart disease. On his return to his home in Lexington on September 28, he lost his ability to speak, his consciousness became impaired, and there was a disposition to doze. His pulse was slightly rapid and weak, but his respirations and skin temperature were normal. His attending physicians made a diagnosis of venous congestion induced by fatigue. He was given hot footbaths, and cold compresses were applied to his head. Afterward, his consciousness improved enough so that he assisted the doctors as they removed his clothes, and, pointing to his shoulders, said, "You hurt my right shoulder." He had slight diarrhea. His consciousness improved again on September 29; he was easily awakened and responded intelligently to questions. His symptoms were thought to indicate sluggish capillary circulation of the brain. A blister was applied behind each ear and on the back of his neck. That evening he was given a purgative enema and was able to raise himself and take nourishment. On the thirtieth he was quite conscious. His physicians took six or eight ounces of blood, and he was given ten grains of calomel at bedtime. Although he seemed to be improving during the first part of October, his condition deteriorated on the eleventh. He became less observant, respirations were fast, and his pulse was 120 per minute. Stimulants were given, but his decline was rapid, and he died soon after 9:00 A.M. on October 12, 1870. His physicians thought that he "died of a broken heart and its strings were snapped at Appomattox." In reference to the cause of Lee's death, his physicians were of the opinion that it was due to passive congestion of the brain, not proceeding far enough to produce apoplexy or effusion. There was no paralysis of motion or sensation, but marked debility from the first. His symptoms, in many respects, they thought, resembled concussion without its attending syncope. All his symptoms were compatible with a stroke. Recently, based on the same information, it has been proposed that his stroke involved one or both frontal lobes of the brain, which would account for his lack of paralysis and the syndrome of abulia or "absence of will."[2] Lee had heart disease, an ischemic stroke before he died, and probably had aspiration pneumonia as a terminal event. Abulia is certainly a distinct possibility, but without better observations, a partial, nonfluent expressive aphasia cannot be ruled out. He was buried at Lexington in the Lee Chapel on the grounds of the Washington and Lee University.

DEATH CERTIFICATE: Cause of death, congestion of the brain.

1. *OR,* vol. 19, pt. 2:588; Harris D. Riley, Jr., "Robert E. Lee's Battle with Disease," *CWTI* 18:12–22; Ben Huger to Wife, Sept. 16, 1847, in Benjamin Huger Papers (no. 9942), UV; R. E. Lee to Mary Stuart, Apr. 5, 1863 (typed copy), WLU; W. D. Pender to Fanny Pender, Apr. 1, 3, 8, 1863, all in W. D. Pender letters, SHC; Heitman, *Historical Register and Dictionary* 2:28; Freeman, *Lee's Lieutenants* 1:589, 2:340, 502–3, 3:170–71, 172, 185, 189, 214, 356–58, 364; Lee, *Papers,* 190, 431–32, 438, 589–90, 595, 611, 614, 619, 624, 756; Josiah Gorgas Diaries, June 1, 1864, ADAH; *CMH* 1:633; Douglas, *I Rode with Stonewall,* 145; Snow, *Lee and his Generals,* 29; Sorrel, *Confederate Staff Officer,* 102–3, 256; McDonald, *Stonewall Jackson's Topographer,* 124.

2. R. L. Madison and H. T. Barton, "Letter," *Richmond and Louisville Medical Journal* 10:516–23; Marvin P. Rozear et al., "R. E. Lee's Stroke," *Virginia Magazine of History and Biography* 98:291–308; Flood, *Last Years,* 168, 194, 214–15, 225, 241.

STEPHEN DILL LEE • *Born September 22, 1833,* in Charleston, South Carolina. He graduated from USMA in 1854. Served in the Florida wars. In 1854 he had intermittent fever but reported to duty in Texas in December. He resigned his commission from the United States Army in February 1861 and became a captain and aide-de-camp to Gen. P. G. T. Beauregard. Having passed through ranks, he was appointed brigadier general in November 1862. He was slightly wounded in the shoulder on May 16, 1863, at Baker's Creek. The arm was painful and later turned black from the shoulder to the elbow. He was promoted to major general in August 1863 and to lieutenant general the following June. After the Battle of Nashville and during the retreat at Spring Hill on December 17, 1864, Lee was severely wounded in the foot and had to leave the field. A shell fragment had taken off his spur and shattered a few bones in his heel. He traveled as far as Florence, Alabama, where he was hospitalized for several days. Lee was on leave in January 1865. Using crutches to walk, he was married on February 8, 1865. In March, Richard Taylor thought that if Lee's wounds would permit, he should rejoin his corps. On recovery, Lee took command and on March 18, 1865, led his troops from Augusta to North Carolina. Following the war he moved to Mississippi, where he was a farmer, state senator, president of Mississippi State College, and a major figure in the United Confederate Veterans. In 1900 he was bothered by severe colds, insomnia, rheumatism, and carbuncles. During March 1903, he was at Hot Springs, Arkansas; the water helped decrease the soreness in his arm, chest, and back. He had pneumonia in 1905, and his sight was impaired by cataracts. The next year he had a diagnosis of diabetes mellitus, which improved with treatment. Lee gave a speech at the National Military Park at Vicksburg on May 22, 1908. Later, he returned to the Carroll Hotel and ate a heavy supper. He suffered with indigestion that night but had improved by the next day. Afterward he was moved to the home of W. T. Rigby, where he continued to improve until the night of the twenty-fifth, when he had a stroke. He was unconscious for the last twelve hours of his life and died May 28, 1908. The cause of death was reported as an apoplectic stroke affecting his left side.[1] He was buried at Columbus, Mississippi, in Friendship Cemetery.

DEATH CERTIFICATE: NAD

1. CSR; *OR*, vol. 45, pt. 1:655, 661, 673, 686, 706; vol. 49, pt. 1:1027; Hattaway, *General Stephen D. Lee*, 87, 146–48, 228; Herman Hattaway, "Stephen Dill Lee: A Biography" (diss.), 33–34, 242–43, 246–49; S. D. Lee to J. F. H. Claiborne, June 12, 1878, in J. F. H. Claiborne Papers, SHC; S. D. Lee to Capt. Rigby, Mar. 19, 1903, in Stephen D. Lee Letters, MDAH; *CV* 12:51, 271, 350; *CMH* 1:688; *Vicksburg (Miss.) Herald*, May 29, 1908.

WILLIAM HENRY FITZHUGH LEE ("ROONEY") • *Born May 31, 1837,* at the Custis home, "Arlington," in Virginia. He was the second son of Robert E. Lee. In 1857 he was commissioned directly into the United States Army. He only stayed in the service for two years and then started farming. After entering the Confederate service as a captain of cavalry in May 1861, he was made lieutenant colonel and then colonel of the 9th Virginia Cavalry. At Boonsboro, on September 15, 1862, he was unhorsed and run over while crossing a bridge. Bruised and initially unconscious, he lay by the road for some time. When Henry Kyd Douglas returned home on September 16, he found that Lee was being cared for by Douglas's family. Lee's promotion to brigadier general ranked from that September. On November 18, Lee was ordered to go with his brigade to Fredericksburg to assume command of the cavalry and other forces there. At the Battle of Brandy Station on June 9, 1863, Lee had a flesh wound of the thigh. Neither the bone nor the artery of the leg was injured. Because of this wound, R. E. Lee sent Rooney to his mother's home on June 17. On the twenty-sixth of June, Rooney was captured at Hickory Hill by a Federal raiding party and put in the hospital at Fort Monroe. The Federal surgeon who examined him reported that the ball had passed entirely through Rooney's thigh when he was wounded at Brandy Station. By August 1, Lee was able to walk on crutches. He was not exchanged until March 1864, and reached J. E. B. Stuart's camp on the twenty-ninth. His promotion to major general was from the next month. He was absent sick on August 25, 1864, and missed the action at Reams' Station. Following the war he had an active life. He farmed, served as a state senator, and was a member of Congress.[1] He died October 15, 1891, near Alexandria, Virginia, and was buried there. His remains were later moved to the Lee Chapel on the grounds of Washington and Lee University at Lexington, Virginia.

DEATH CERTIFICATE: RNA

1. CSR; *OR*, vol. 21:1020; vol. 27, pt. 2:683, 771, 794, 796; R. T. L. Beale to wife, June 10, 1863, in Beale Family Papers (no. 7754), UV; R. E. Lee to G. W. C. Lee, Mar. 29, 1864, Dr. Hunter McGuire Collection, VSL; Lee, *Wartime Papers*, 511–12, 542, 567, 597; *CMH* 3:625–26; Clark, *Histories of Several Regiments* 1:435, 470; Douglas, *I Rode with Stonewall*, 166.

COLLETT LEVENTHORPE • *Born May 15, 1815*, at Exmouth, England. He served in the British Army before coming to the United States. He was elected colonel of the 34th North Carolina at the start of the Civil War. On July 1, 1863, at Gettysburg, he was wounded, and one bone of his left arm was broken. The Confederate wagons carrying Leventhorpe and the other wounded men south left Gettysburg on July 4. They were captured by Federal cavalry, and Leventhorpe, along with the others, was put in the Theological Seminary at Mercersburg, Pennsylvania. His wound was cauterized with nitric acid without benefit of anesthesia. Supported by the chaplain, he was able to walk to the ambulance when they were moved on the twenty-first. In October, Leventhorpe was in the hospital at Fort McHenry. The wound had broken down and the remaining bone fragments had come out, so healing improved. By February 1864 his health was good, but his arm had not completely healed. In April 1864 his surgeon stated that chronic inflammation or subacute ophthalmia of Leventhorpe's eyes was making sight difficult, particularly from the left eye, and that there had been recent deterioration of his vision. He described thickening of the conjunctiva with chronic engorgement of the blood vessels and said that the condition, the result of an accident, was one he had been treating for two years. The surgeon thought continued service in the field would aggravate the problem, and the situation was particularly precarious if Leventhorpe lost the sight in his left eye. Leventhorpe was assigned to command of the three Home Guard Regiments that were assembled at Kinston in September 1864. He was appointed brigadier general in February 1865.[1] After the war he entered into a number of business enterprises and traveled. He died

December 1, 1889, in Wilkes County, North Carolina, and was buried in the Episcopal Cemetery at Happy Valley near Lenoir, North Carolina.

DEATH CERTIFICATE: NAD

1. CSR; *OR*, vol. 27, pt. 2:638, 643, 645, 1016; Philip Schoff, D.D., "The Gettysburg Week," *Scribner's Magazine* 16:21–30; Leventhorpe to wife, Oct. 5, 1863, Feb. 8, 1864, both in Collett Leventhorpe Papers, NCSA; *CMH* 4:326; Clark, *Histories of Several Regiments* 5:7.

JOSEPH HORACE LEWIS • *Born October 29, 1824*, near Glasgow, Kentucky. After being admitted to the bar, he served in the Kentucky legislature. In September 1861 he was commissioned a colonel of the 6th Kentucky Infantry. Although his health began to seriously decline while at Corinth in May 1862, he remained with his troops until after they reached Vicksburg. About July 20, Lewis became so ill he sought medical attention in the country, and another was in command of his troops during the fighting at Baton Rouge on August 5. Lewis took part in the action at Murfreesborough in December 1862 but was absent on sick leave in February and March 1863. His promotion to brigadier general ranked from September 1863. He was bruised on the left breast by shrapnel at Jonesborough on August 31, 1864, but was able to continue in command.[1] When he returned home he practiced law, served in the state legislature, and was elected to Congress. His last years were spent on his farm. He died July 6, 1904, in Scott County, Kentucky, and was buried in the City Cemetery in Glasgow, Kentucky.

DEATH CERTIFICATE: NAD

1. CSR; *OR*, vol. 20, pt. 1:831; Thompson, *History of the Orphan Brigade*, 390, 392; Davis, *Orphan Brigade*, 117; *CV* 4:329, 12:403.

WILLIAM GASTON LEWIS • *Born September 3, 1835*, in Rocky Mount, North Carolina. His prewar career was varied, having been a teacher and a surveyor. When the war started, he served in the Bethel Regiment and was elected major of the 33rd North Carolina. Having been made lieutenant colonel of the 43rd North Carolina, he was promoted to brigadier general from May 1864. On July 20, 1864, at Stephenson's Depot during a clash between Stephen D. Ramseur's and William W. Averell's cavalry, Lewis was wounded. His wife helped nurse him back to recovery. He was back on the field in October but still had tenderness and some suppuration of his wound. In a rear guard fight at Farmville, Virginia, on April 7, 1865, he was seriously wounded by a minié ball through the thigh and was taken prisoner. After the war he resumed the profession of engineering. On May 10, 1894, because of illness, Lewis was not able to present an address on William Dorsey Pender. His death occurred at Goldsboro, North Carolina, on January 8, 1901, and he was buried in Willow Dale Cemetery in that city. He died reportedly of pneumonia.[1]

DEATH CERTIFICATE: NAD

1. CSR; H. Battle to Gaston (W. G. Lewis), July 29, 1864, W. G. Lewis to wife, Oct. 31, Nov. 16, 20, 1864, and J. B. Gordon to W. G. Lewis, Aug. 21, 1886, all in W. G. Lewis Papers, SHC; *SHSP* 18:245, 22:301;

Clark, *Histories of Several Regiments* 3:284, 400; *CV* 9:32; *Raleigh News and Observer Company,* May 11, 1894, in William Dorsey Pender Papers, SHC; *Washington (N.C.) Times,* Jan. 10, 1901, in CSR.

ST. JOHN RICHARDSON LIDDELL • *Born September 6, 1815,* near Woodville, Mississippi. In 1851, while trying to save a small black child, he was badly burned and almost lost his life. As part of a feud, he killed two men in 1852. Arrested for murder, he was finally acquitted in 1854. He joined the Confederacy as aide-de-camp to Gen. William J. Hardee and soon was given the rank of colonel. On January 16, 1862, he left Richmond for Bowling Green in a crowded, cold, railroad car. By the third day, when the train reached Chattanooga, Tennessee, Liddell had developed a bronchial condition with a painful cough. To restore his health he obtained a thirty-day leave to go home. He rejoined the army near Murfreesborough about the twentieth of February. Returning to Richmond in May 1862, he again became ill. On the trip back to the army, he was reported to have typhoid by the time he reached Huntsville, Alabama, and when he arrived at Tuscumbia he was completely prostrated. General Hardee's surgeon considered Liddell's condition critical, and a telegram was sent to his wife in Louisiana. During this period, Hardee stayed with him when possible and nursed him himself. On Hardee's departure, Liddell was placed under the care of a local doctor in Tuscumbia and Mrs. J. B. Barton, who had to force his parched mouth open to pour in the "necessary acids" and food to sustain his system. Finally, when he could walk, he took an open train to Corinth. Constant exercise helped him to regain his strength, and he left Corinth with the troops on May 28. His promotion as brigadier general ranked from July 1862. After the war he returned to Louisiana. Liddell was killed February 14, 1870, as a result of a feud that went back to the 1852 duel. He was eating dinner on a steamer going down the Black River when Col. Charles Jones and his two sons came on board. When Liddell stood up, Jones fired at him twice while Liddell's bullet went wild. After he fell, several more shots were fired at him. A doctor who later examined him found that he had been hit seven times, three of which could have been fatal. Two bullets had entered his chest near the left nipple and another had hit him in the neck.[1] He was buried in a private family cemetery on his plantation outside of Jonesville, Louisiana.

DEATH CERTIFICATE: NAD

1. Liddell, *Liddell's Record,* 19, 25, 46–49, 52, 62–67, 205; *New Orleans Daily Picayune,* Feb. 16, 1870.

ROBERT DOAK LILLEY • *Born January 28, 1836,* near Greenville, Virginia. Prior to the Civil War he sold surveying instruments invented by his father. In May 1861 he recruited a company of troops in Virginia and was chosen their captain. He was promoted to major in January 1863 and to lieutenant colonel later that summer. He had a twenty-day sick leave in early 1864. His promotion to brigadier was from May. During a reconnaissance near Winchester on July 20, 1864, Lilley was wounded three times: first he was hit in the left thigh by a shell fragment; then his right arm was shattered near the shoulder by a minié ball; finally, a minié ball went through the already injured thigh. Disabled after the second wound, he dismounted. His horse was running to the rear when Lilley received the third wound. Almost ready to collapse, he lay down under a tree and was captured. His arm was amputated at the shoulder the next day and the wounded thigh was treated by a Federal surgeon. Left in Winchester by the Federal troops, Lilley was found by the Confederates four days later. By November 1864, although his stump still had not healed completely, he was assigned to command the reserve forces of the Valley District.[1] After the war he devoted most of his time to obtaining funds for Washington and Lee University. He died in Richmond, Virginia, on November 12, 1886, and was buried at Staunton, Virginia, in the Thornrose Cemetery.

DEATH CERTIFICATE: Cause of death, paralysis.

1. CSR; *OR*, vol. 43, pt. 2:926; Jos. A. Waddell, *Annals of Augusta County, Virginia with Reminiscences*, 332; *CMH* 3:627.

LEWIS HENRY LITTLE · *Born March 19, 1817*, in Baltimore, Maryland. Served in the Mexican War. Little was commissioned directly into the U.S. Army in 1839 and served until he resigned in May 1861. He joined the Confederacy as a major of artillery. In May 1862 he was promoted to brigadier general, but he was ill most of the month with chills, weakness, fever, and diarrhea. The quinine, opium, and blue mass he took made him feel worse. Little was too ill to participate in the fight on May 6 and developed piles during the middle of the month. Although still feverish, he assumed command of a division on June 12. On the fifteenth, he suffered from the effects of multiple flea bites. He was so sick and the swelling so severe that he thought he had erysipelas, but the doctor assured him he did not. He did well until July 22, when a boil developed on his buttocks and made it agony to ride a horse. After the boil spontaneously drained on August 1, he felt better. Little had diarrhea throughout the month of August and had to ride in an ambulance to Tupelo on the seventh. During the first week of September, the diarrhea and weakness continued. He developed a fever on the ninth and took quinine, but he thought there was something wrong with it because he felt stuporous and his stomach was upset. He left for Iuka, Mississippi, in an ambulance on the twelfth and on the fourteenth could hardly ride his horse. On the day of his death, September 19, 1862, he went to take command of the left wing and was just behind the Confederate lines conferring with Gen. Sterling Price. A minié ball struck him on the line of scalp over the left eye, passed through his head and stopped under the skin on the occiput. He died instantly.[1] He was initially buried at Iuka, but his remains were later removed to Green Mount Cemetery, Baltimore, Maryland.

1. CSR; *OR*, vol. 17, pt. 1:122–23; Sul Ross to Lizzie Ross, Sept. 24, 1862, in Ross Family Papers, BU; Lewis Henry Little Civil War Diary in *CWTI* Coll., USAMHI; Note by Rev. J. Bannon in Lewis Henry Little Civil War Diary in *CWTI* Coll., USAMHI; *CMH* 9:89, Mo.; *SHSP* 29:212–15.

THOMAS MULDRUP LOGAN • *Born November 3, 1840,* in Charleston, South Carolina. At the beginning of the Civil War, he served as a volunteer but was promoted to captain in the summer of 1861. He received a severe flesh wound of the top of his foot from a shell fragment at the battle of Cold Harbor on June 27, 1862. He rode from the battlefield to Richmond in the front seat of an ambulance with the driver. He was disabled for two months. His promotion to brigadier general ranked from July 1863. Logan was wounded again in the fight at Riddell's Shop on June 13, 1864. On July 9 he requested a furlough but was back by September. An adept businessman and developer, he made and lost fortunes after the war. Logan died August 11, 1914, in his apartment in New York City, suffering from a "complication of diseases." He had recently had a nervous breakdown, and the summer heat aggravated his condition.[1] He was buried in Hollywood Cemetery at Richmond, Virginia.

DEATH CERTIFICATE: Cause of death, Pott's disease, nephritis with pus; contributory, edema of lungs.

1. CSR; *Richmond Times Dispatch,* Aug. 12, 1914, and (Edgefield, S.C.) newspaper clipping, n.i., Jan. 30, 1879, all in Thomas Muldrup Logan Papers, SHC; *CMH* 5:411; Haskell, *Memoirs,* 36.

LUNSFORD LINDSAY LOMAX • *Born November 4, 1835,* in Newport, Rhode Island. He graduated from USMA in 1856. Serving on the frontier at the beginning of the war, he resigned his commission and joined the Virginia state forces as a captain. He held a number of staff positions and in February 1863 was promoted to colonel of the 11th Virginia Cavalry. In July 1863 he was promoted to brigadier general and in August 1864 appointed major general. Following the war he returned to Virginia, where he farmed until 1885, when he was elected president of Virginia Polytechnic Institute. He resigned this position in 1899 and spent the next few years helping compile the *Official Records.* Lomax died May 28, 1913, at Washington, D.C., and was buried at Warrenton, Virginia, in the City Cemetery.

DEATH CERTIFICATE: RNA

ARMISTEAD LINDSAY LONG • *Born September 3, 1825,* in Campbell County, Virginia. He graduated from USMA in 1850. Long resigned from the United States Army in June 1861 and accepted the rank of major of artillery in the Confederate Army. He served primarily as a staff officer and was commissioned brigadier general of artillery in September 1863. During the winter of 1863–64, his health failed, and although he had facial paralysis and disability, he continued in active service. Long was ill in May 1864. He turned over his command in August and was on medical furlough through November. In March 1865, he was in command of the artillery of the central line, Army of Northern Virginia. Long surrendered with the army at Appomattox, his appearance much changed because of neuralgia of the face. He worked as an engineer after the war. In 1870 he became blind, supposedly from exposure during the war. Using a slate, he wrote a biography of Robert E. Lee. Long's health was poor for three years prior to his death; however, his demise was unexpected. The day of his death, April 29, 1891, at Charlottesville, Virginia, he awoke and asked for a fire to be built in his room, but later, when his daughter brought him a cup of coffee, he was unable to answer her. He did not recover consciousness, and his family and doctor were at his side when he expired.[1] He was buried at Charlottesville in Maplewood Cemetery.

DEATH CERTIFICATE: RNA

1. CSR; *OR*, vol. 36, pt. 1:1048; vol. 42, pt. 1:859, 862, 866; vol. 46, pt. 1:516, 1279, pt. 3:1316; CR, 145:148; *SHSP* 13:247; Armistead Lindsay Long, *Memoirs of Robert E. Lee*, 426; three newspaper clippings, n.i., n.d., from Mrs. Pauline Long Dunn, great-niece of General Long.

JAMES LONGSTREET • *Born January 8, 1821*, in Edgefield District, South Carolina. He graduated from USMA in 1842. While carrying the regimental flag on September 13, 1847, at Chapultepec in Mexico, Longstreet was wounded in the thigh. He was cared for in a private home in Mexico City. Able to travel by the first of December, he returned home for a month's leave. In the autumn of 1848, he returned to duty at Jefferson Barracks. Longstreet resigned from the United States Army in June 1861 and was appointed brigadier general in the Confederate Army that same month. He was promoted to major general in October 1861. Early in September 1862, a boot chafed his heel and the skin did not heal, causing him to wear a slipper and ride sidesaddle at Sharpsburg. He was promoted to lieutenant general from October 1862. During the Battle of Fredericksburg on December 13, 1862, Longstreet came close to having an accident similar to the one that had disabled Leonidas Polk in November of the previous year. A large Parrott cannon, having been fired for some hours, burst on about the thirty-ninth discharge. Although Longstreet and others were standing close by, no one was hurt. In late February 1863, he was sick with a sore throat that kept him in his quarters at Petersburg. On May 6, 1864, at the Wilderness, Longstreet was accidently wounded by Confederate troops. Because of his large size, it took three men to lift him from his horse. He was placed by the roadside with bloody foam coming from his mouth and blood pouring over his breast. A minié ball had entered near his throat and passed into the right shoulder. The bloody foam suggested a pulmonary injury. Hemorrhage was severe, though a surgeon was soon there to stop it. Longstreet was promptly carried to the rear, placed in an ambulance, and taken as far as Parker's Store in tolerable comfort. Four doctors made a partial examination of the wound and determined it was not necessarily fatal. He was taken to his old quartermaster's house, where his wound was treated for a few days. He then went by train to Lynchburg and was cared for by a relative, the widow of Gen. Samuel Garland. When Longstreet was finally able to ride, he was transported in a carriage to a home at Campbell Court-House. His wound appeared to be healing, but his right arm was paralyzed. Because of the threat of Federal raiders, he went first to Augusta, Georgia, and then to Union Point. By July he was just able to sit up but still unable to write, and he preferred to convalesce until his arm improved, if his services were not essential. In early October 1864, Longstreet reported that he would not regain use of his arm for at least a year, and he therefore wanted either duty he could perform or an extended leave. However, he returned October 19 and assumed command of the troops on the north side of the James River. When Longstreet returned to the army, his right arm was still paralyzed and useless, but he had taught himself to write with his left hand. Following the advice of his doctor, he continually pulled on the disabled arm, and its use was partially restored in later life. After the war he settled in New Orleans and joined the Republican party. His actions and writing made him a controversial figure. For many years before his death he was partially deaf. In 1902 he suffered severely from rheumatism, and pain in his feet made it impossible for him to stand for more than a few minutes at a time. His usual weight of two hundred pounds had decreased to 135 pounds by January 1903. Cancer developed in his right eye, and in December he had X-ray therapy in Chicago to combat the disease. While visiting his daughter in Gainesville, Georgia, he contracted pneumonia; large amounts of blood came from his mouth. He lost consciousness and died soon afterward on January 2, 1904.[1] He was buried at Gainesville in the Alta Vista Cemetery.

DEATH CERTIFICATE: NAD

1. CSR; *OR*, vol. 18:903; vol. 21:565–66; vol. 36, pt. 1:1028, 1055; vol. 40, pt. 2:661, pt. 3:775, 792; vol. 42, pt. 1:871, pt. 3:1140; vol. 51, pt. 2:893; Hamilton J. Eckenrode and Bryan Conrad, *James Longstreet: Lee's War Horse*, 8–9, 314, 320–21; William Garrett Piston, "Lee's Tarnished Lieutenant: James Longstreet and His Image in American Society" (diss.), 600–601; Sorrel, *Confederate Staff Officer*, 103, 116, 243–46, 274; Freeman, *Lee's Lieutenants* 2:239; Dawson, *Reminiscences of Confederate Service*, 115–16, 197; Eugene Alvarez, "Death of The 'Old War Horse' Longstreet," *Georgia Historical Society* 52:70–77; *Gainesville (Ga.) News*, Jan. 6, 1904.

WILLIAM WING LORING • *Born December 4, 1818*, in Wilmington, North Carolina. Served in the Florida and Mexican wars. He was commissioned directly into the regular army in 1846. On August 20, 1847, he was wounded at Churubusco, Mexico. The following month, because of a wound received at Chapultepec on September 13, 1847, his left arm was amputated at the shoulder. He was ordered home in October 1847. A colonel of the line when he resigned from the army in May 1861, he was appointed brigadier general in the Confederate service that same month and then major general in February 1862. Loring was wounded during the Atlanta campaign on July 28, 1864, near Lickskillet Road, and left his command the next day. Although expected back by late August, he did not return until September 10. He was sent to the rear on March 20, 1865, because of illness.[1] Following the war he joined the service of the Khedive of Egypt in 1869 and returned to the United States in 1879. He died December 30, 1886, in New York City and was buried in Loring Park, St. Augustine, Florida.

DEATH CERTIFICATE: Cause of death, pneumonia.

1. *OR*, vol. 38, pt. 3:688, 872, 904; General Order no. 324, Hdq., The Army of Mexico, Oct. 26, 1847, in Benjamin Huger Papers, UV; Walter A. Roher, "Confederate Generals—The View from Below," *CWTI* 18:10–13; Heitman, *Historical Register and Dictionary* 2:28; French, *Two Wars*, 219, 222; *CV* 3:20; *CMH* 11:203, Fla.

MANSFIELD LOVELL • *Born October 20, 1822,* at Washington, D.C. He graduated from USMA in 1842. During the Mexican War, he was wounded twice: at Monterey in 1846 and at Chapultepec on September 13, 1847.[1] Lovell resigned from the U.S. Army in 1854 and entered business. Later he was deputy street commissioner of New York City. When he left this position, he was commissioned major general in the Confederate Army in October 1861. After the war he returned to New York and worked as an engineer. He died June 1, 1884, in New York City and was buried there in Woodlawn Cemetery.

DEATH CERTIFICATE: (autopsy) Exhaustion from chronic spasm of diaphragm (hiccoughs) due to the irritation from the passage and impaction of renal calculi in the left ureter. Hiccoughs for seven days.

    1. Heitman, *Historical Register and Dictionary* 2:28; *CMH* 2:162, Md.

MARK PERRIN LOWREY • *Born December 30, 1828,* in McNairy County, Tennessee. In January 1848, Lowrey left New Orleans for Mexico. During the march from the mouth of the Rio Grande to join Taylor's command, Lowrey contracted measles and was disabled for some weeks. By the time he had recovered and his regiment was combat-ready, the Mexican War was over. He was mustered out of the service in July. Lacking a good education, he was taught at night by his boarder, a local teacher. He entered the Baptist ministry in 1853 and continued this profession until 1861. His first enlistment during the Civil War was terminated by loneliness, lack of conviction in the cause, and an undefined sickness. He raised a new regiment and was elected colonel of the 32nd Mississippi Infantry in April 1862. At Perryville on October 8, 1862, Lowrey was wounded in the left arm but remained on the field. On the retreat the following day, he had difficulty keeping up with the army. He obtained leave, but as it was not safe to go home because of Federal troops, he slipped through the lines and went to his brother's home, located south of Ripley, Mississippi. His family was sent for to help with his care. He moved his family south of Blue Mountain, where he recuperated for six weeks. At Wartrace, Tennessee, he took command of his regiment and fought at Murfreesborough on January 1, 1863. He was promoted to brigadier general from October 1863. Outside of Nashville in December 1864, his life was saved when an officer saw the flash of a sharpshooter's rifle and yelled to him. Lowrey stooped in time, but the minié ball killed a nearby soldier. He resigned his commission on March 14, 1865, because of ill health caused by long service and exposure. He founded the Blue Mountain Female Institute at Blue Mountain, Mississippi, in 1873. Lowrey was ill in the fall of 1882; the following year his doctors told him his heart was very weak. On February 27, 1885, at Middleton, Tennessee, while buying a train ticket, he turned suddenly, gasped for breath, and fell to the floor dead.[1] He was buried at Blue Mountain, Mississippi, at North First Street.

DEATH CERTIFICATE: NAD

    1. Larry Wells Kennedy, "Fighting Preacher of the Army of Tennessee: General Mark Perrin Lowrey" (diss.), 5, 24, 35–39, 111, 193; *SHSP* 16:356–66.

ROBERT LOWRY • *Born March 10, 1830,* in Chesterfield District, South Carolina. He was practicing law in 1861 and enlisted as a private in the Rankin Grays. Soon afterward he was elected major of the 6th Mississippi Infantry. He was wounded twice at Shiloh on April 6, 1862, and was on leave in May. That month he was elected colonel. In November he was a witness in the court of inquiry against Earl Van Dorn. He was appointed brigadier general from February 1865. Following hostilities he took part in politics and Confederate veteran affairs. Before his death he was in poor health for eighteen months.[1] He died January 19, 1910, at Jackson, Mississippi, and was buried at Brandon, Mississippi, in the City Cemetery on College Street.

DEATH CERTIFICATE: NAD

1. CSR; *OR,* vol. 10, pt. 1:581; vol. 17, pt. 1:439; Robert Lowry subject file, MDAH; *CV* 18:182.

HYLAN BENTON LYON • *Born February 22, 1836,* in what was Caldwell County, Kentucky. He graduated from USMA in 1856. Served in the Florida wars. Lyon resigned from the U.S. Army in April 1861 and entered the Confederate service as an artillery captain. He was elected lieutenant colonel of the 8th Kentucky Infantry in February 1862 and was promoted to brigadier general from June 1864. During the spring of 1864, a problem he had with his breast healed rapidly, and he was almost well by June. Not enough information is available to make a diagnosis. After the war he farmed and was involved in the Kentucky prison system. His death occurred quite suddenly on April 25, 1907, near Eddyville, Kentucky, where he was buried.[1]

DEATH CERTIFICATE: NAD

1. H. B. Lyon to wife, June 6, 16, 1864, in Hyland B. Lyon letters, Microfilm, 2 rolls, MSU; *CV* 15:560.

M

JOHN MCCAUSLAND • *Born September 15, 1836,* at St. Louis, Missouri. Teaching at the start of the war, he was commissioned colonel of the 36th Virginia in 1861. His promotion to brigadier general was from May 1864. He traveled for two years after the war and then settled on a large acreage in West Virginia. McCausland died January 25, 1927, in Mason County, West Virginia, and was buried at Henderson, West Virginia.[1]

DEATH CERTIFICATE: Cause of death, mitral insufficiency.

1. Death certificate.

WILLIAM MCCOMB • *Born November 21, 1828,* in Mercer County, Pennsylvania.[1] He left his business and enlisted as a private in the 14th Tennessee Infantry at the start of the war. A slight wound received at Cold Harbor on June 27, 1862, did not prevent him from participating in the Battle of Frayser's Farm a few days later. He was severely wounded at Sharpsburg on September 17, 1862, yet by December 10 he was listed as in command. At the Battle of Chancellorsville, on May 3, 1863, McComb was wounded again. Listed as in command of Cadmus M. Wilcox's brigade on August 31, 1863, he took part in the Overland campaign of 1864 and the siege of Petersburg. McComb passed through grades and his promotion as brigadier general ranked from January 1865. He spent the last years of his life farming in Virginia and died on July 21, 1918, near Gordonsville.[2] He was buried in Mechanicsville Cemetery at Boswells, Virginia.

DEATH CERTIFICATE: Cause of death, atherosclerosis.

1. Death certificate.

2. *OR*, vol. 19, pt. 1:1001; vol. 21:1074; vol. 25, pt. 1:926, 933; vol. 29, pt. 2:685; Head, *Sixteenth Regiment, Tennessee Volunteers*, 358; *CMH* 8:302, Tenn.

JOHN PORTER MCCOWN • *Born August 19, 1815*, in Rutherford County, Tennessee. He graduated from USMA in 1840. Served in the Florida and Mexican wars. McCown left the United States Army in May 1861 and joined Confederate service as colonel of the Tennessee Artillery Corps. His promotion to brigadier general followed in October 1861 and to major general from March 1862. Returning home after the war, he taught school in Tennessee and then moved to a farm in Arkansas. He died January 22, 1879, at Little Rock and was buried in the City Cemetery at Magnolia, Arkansas.

DEATH CERTIFICATE: NAD

BEN MCCULLOCH • *Born November 11, 1811*, in Rutherford County, Tennessee. Served in the Mexican War. As a boy, his right wrist was bitten by a young bear, which McCulloch killed with a butcher knife. There is no evidence that there was any permanent damage to his arm. In 1835 he learned of David Crockett's expedition and wanted to join up. However, he arrived too late. He continued alone as far as the Brazos River, where, in January 1836, he became ill with the measles and did not recover for several weeks. In 1839 he had a duel using rifles at forty paces with Col. Reuben Ross and was wounded in the upper portion of the right arm. Ross, an experienced duelist, shot first; McCulloch did not fire. McCulloch carried his arm in a sling for many months and never fully regained its use. As colonel of state troops in February 1861, he received the surrender of Gen. David E. Twiggs at San Antonio. He obtained his commission as brigadier general in the Confederate Army in May 1861. At Elkhorn Tavern on March 7, 1862, while reconnoitering the Federal lines, McCulloch was killed. Riding alone, he had passed out of sight in the woods. Later he was found lying on his back with a bullet hole in the right breast of his coat. A single ball had passed through his chest and lodged on the left side. A bit of powder-stained white cotton patching with a hole in the center, such as was used in the making of the cartridges of the Mississippi rifle, was sticking in the bullet hole. Reportedly he had been killed by a sharpshooter of the 36th Illinois Volunteers, who was posted behind the fence not forty yards away.[1] His remains were ultimately buried in the State Cemetery in Austin, Texas.

1. CSR; OR, vol. 8:218, 226, 281; Victor M. Rose, *Life and Services of Gen. Ben McCulloch*, 33–34, 41, 53–54, 204–5; *CMH* 11:241, Tex.; *CV* 13:551; *Houston Weekly Telegraph*, Aug. 13, 1862, in Ben McCulloch and Henry Eustace Papers, UTA.

HENRY EUSTACE MCCULLOCH • *Born December 6, 1816,* in Rutherford County, Tennessee. Served in the Mexican War. At the outbreak of the Civil War he was a U.S. marshal in Texas. He was commissioned colonel of the 1st Texas Mounted Riflemen in April 1861 and was promoted to brigadier general from March 1862. He became sick on the night of May 25, 1862, in Monroe, Louisiana, and on the twenty-sixth was scarcely able to sit up, but by June he was on duty in Tyler, Texas. Following the war he returned to his farm in Texas.[1] He died March 12, 1895, at Rockport, Texas, and was buried in San Geronimo Cemetery at Sequin, Texas.
DEATH CERTIFICATE: NAD

1. CSR; OR, vol. 3:718.

SAMUEL MCGOWAN • *Born October 9, 1819,* in Laurens District, South Carolina. Served in the Mexican War. He was a major general in the South Carolina militia when the state seceded in December 1860. During the spring of 1862, he was elected colonel of the 14th South Carolina Infantry in the Confederate service. On June 27, 1862, at Cold Harbor, McGowan was bruised on the right side by a grapeshot and was disabled for a short time. He continued on duty despite the injury until after Malvern Hill. McGowan was wounded in the thigh on August 29, 1862, at the battle of Second Manassas, but he was with the brigade in the campaign into Maryland in September. His promotion as brigadier general ranked from January 1863. While standing on the works at Chancellorsville on May 3, 1863, he was severely injured by a minié ball. Hospital records are confusing as to whether this wound was in the foot or hip, but most records and on-field observations say it was in the leg just below the knee. McGowan was hospitalized in Richmond and then transferred to Wilmington on May 11. On the twentieth, he was furloughed. In December 1863, a medical board at the general hospital in Columbia, South Carolina, found that the wound was partially healed, but McGowan was still unfit for duty. He came back in February 1864, although he had not sufficiently recovered to walk well without a cane. At Spotsylvania Court-House on May 12, 1864, he was wounded in the right forearm by a minié ball. McGowan was initially admitted to a nearby field hospital and was then transferred to a hospital in Richmond. He was furloughed in June 1864 and reported for duty on August 15. Afterward he returned home and entered politics.[1] McGowan died on August 9, 1897, in Abbeville, South Carolina, and was buried in Long Cane Cemetery two miles outside of that town.
DEATH CERTIFICATE: NAD

1. CSR; *OR*, vol. 11, pt. 2:839, 856, 869; vol. 12, pt. 2:672, 682; vol. 19, pt. 1:987; vol. 25, pt. 1:803, 807, 889, 901, 904; vol. 36, pt. 1:1092, 1094; vol. 42, pt. 2:1185; CR, 178:8, 136, 181:50, 54; C.S.A. Hospital Department. Surgical notes presented by Dr. H. McGuire to J. W. Powell and List of sick and wounded allowed to remain in private quarters and furloughed, E. S. Carrington book, 1863, Eleanor S. Brockenbrough Library, MC; Spencer Glasgow Welch, *A Confederate Surgeon's Letters to his Wife*, 26, 51, 97; Caldwell, *Brigade of South Carolinians*, 80, 122, 142; Hassler, *A. P. Hill*, 201; *CMH* 5:412.

JAMES McQUEEN McINTOSH • *Born in 1828* at Fort Brooke, Florida, which is now Tampa. He graduated from USMA in 1849. Having served on the frontier, he resigned from the army in May 1861. Initially a captain of cavalry in the Confederate Army, he was made colonel of the 2nd Arkansas Mounted Rifles in the fall of 1861 and brigadier general in January 1862. McIntosh was slightly wounded by canister shot at the battle of Wilson's Creek, Missouri, on August 10, 1861. He rode to where the surgeons were located and took off his coat. The projectile had glanced off his shoulder and, although the skin was not broken, there was a large blue lump. He was back on the field the next day. Commanding the cavalry of Gen. Ben McCulloch's wing at Elkhorn on March 7, 1862, McIntosh was shot through the heart and died soon after Ben McCulloch died.[1] He is now buried in the National Cemetery, Fort Smith, Arkansas.

1. CSR; *OR*, vol. 3:106, 118; vol. 8:281, 285; Watson, *Life in the Confederate Army*, 228.

WILLIAM WHANN MACKALL • *Born January 18, 1817,* in Cecil County, Maryland. He graduated from USMA in 1837. Served in the Florida and Mexican wars. Mackall was in poor health while at West Point; during his last winter there, he had a violent chest cold that was almost fatal. After graduation, he was stationed in Florida because duty in the North caused a return of his chest pain. On February 11, 1839, during an ambush by Indians at River Inlet, Florida, he was hit by three balls, two in the shoulder and one in the back. To escape he had to swim a nearby stream. He was in bed for a month; the ball in his back was buried so deep that it was never found. At Chapultepec, Mexico, on September 13, 1847, a spent ball hit his arm but did not inflict a wound. It just stiffened the arm for a few days. During the winter of 1851, he again had a severe chest cold. Mackall resigned from the U.S. Army in July 1861 and was appointed lieutenant colonel in the Confederate Adjutant General's Department. He went to Nashville in November 1861 and was very ill on arrival. He stayed there for nursing care and was given quinine and some type of yellow pill. His promotion to brigadier general ranked from February 1862. In the early summer of 1863 he was ill and bothered by a siege of boils. Rheumatism in the right shoulder recurred in October 1863; to obtain relief, Mackall planned on having cupping performed. During December he suffered from indigestion. He returned to his farms in Virginia following the war.[1] He died August 12, 1891, in Fairfax County, Virginia, and was buried in the Lewinsville Cemetery near McLean, Virginia.

DEATH CERTIFICATE: RNA

1. Sketch of life by wife, W. W. Mackall to Lon, Nov. 30, 1861, W. W. Mackall to wife, Oct. 3, Dec. 12, 1863, all in W. W. Mackall Papers, SHC; W. W. Mackall to Jos. E. Johnston, June 22, 1863, in Joseph E. Johnston Papers, Box 1, folder 4, CWM; Heitman, *Historical Register and Dictionary* 2:29; *CMH* 2:172, Md.

LAFAYETTE McLAWS • *Born January 15, 1821,* in Augusta, Georgia. He graduated from USMA in 1842. Served in the Mexican War. In 1845, while in Texas, he was struck by a bullet from a pepper-box pistol that glanced off of a tree. After being removed from his horse, he was spitting blood, and a hole was found where the bullet had entered his breast. Further examination revealed that his index finger had also been hit. McLaws had put it in his mouth, and this accounted for the blood he was spitting up. Because no surgeon was present, he was placed in a wagon and taken back to San Antonio. There a surgeon probed the wound and revealed that the glancing shot had taken the line of least resistance under the skin until arrested by the spine. Before long McLaws recovered and returned to Corpus Christi. After the Battle of Veracruz during the Mexican War, he was sent back to the United States on recruiting duty because of failing health. He resigned from the United States Army in March 1861 and joined the Confederacy as colonel of the 10th Georgia Infantry. In September 1861 he was promoted to brigadier general and then to major general in May 1862. McLaws was not in good health in May 1863 but participated in the battle at Gettysburg. Financially McLaws did poorly after the war.[1] He died July 24, 1897, at Savannah, Georgia, where he was buried in Laurel Grove Cemetery.

DEATH CERTIFICATE: Cause of death, heart disease.

1. *OR*, vol. 27, pt. 2:336; vol. 29, pt. 2:682; vol. 30, pt. 2:288, 505; *CMH* 6:431; French, *Two Wars,* 39; *Battles and Leaders* 3:245.

EVANDER McNAIR • *Born April 15, 1820,* near Laurel Hill, North Carolina. Served in the Mexican War. He gave up his mercantile business and raised a battalion of troops in 1861. This group was designated the 4th Arkansas Infantry when it reached full regimental strength, and he was elected colonel. His promotion as brigadier general ranked from November 1862. McNair left a sick bed and fought at the Battle of Murfreesborough. However, he became exhausted and had to leave the field on December 31, 1862. At Chickamauga, on September 20, 1863, he was disabled by a wound. He was on the field at Meridian, Mississippi, on December 9, but because of an exacerbation of the Chickamauga wound, he was not in command in May 1864. In September 1864 he was assigned to brigade command.[1] Following the war he made a number of moves and finally settled in Hattiesburg, Mississippi, where he died November 13, 1902. He was buried in the City Cemetery at Magnolia, Mississippi.

DEATH CERTIFICATE: NAD

1. *OR*, vol. 20, pt. 1:775, 913, 928, 945; vol. 30, pt. 2:24, 35, 290, 458, 500; vol. 31, pt. 3:799; vol. 41, pt. 3:952; Clark, *Histories of Several Regiments* 2:739.

DANDRIDGE MCRAE • *Born October 10, 1829,* in Baldwin County, Alabama. Prior to the Civil War he was admitted to the bar in Arkansas and was clerk of the county and circuit courts. In 1861 he entered Confederate service as a major of the Third Battalion of Arkansas Infantry. He was made colonel of the 21st Arkansas and was promoted to brigadier general in November 1862. In 1864 he resigned his commission and returned to his law practice in Arkansas. He entered into politics and was prominent in promoting his state. Following a stroke two years before his death, he was in very bad physical condition. However, his mind was strong, and he was able to carry on his work until shortly before his death, on April 23, 1899, at Searcy, Arkansas.[1] He was buried at that city in Oak Grove Cemetery.

DEATH CERTIFICATE: NAD

1. *Little Rock Arkansas Gazette,* Apr. 26, 1899.

WILLIAM MACRAE • *Born September 9, 1834,* in Wilmington, North Carolina. MacRae was a civil engineer when he enlisted in 1861 as a private in the Monroe Light Infantry. When this unit was made part of the 15th North Carolina, he was elected captain of a company. He was promoted to lieutenant colonel and colonel of the regiment, and finally was appointed brigadier general as of November 1864. Having nothing left when the war was over, he became, through hard work, general superintendent of a number of southern railroads. He died February 11, 1882, at Augusta, Georgia, and was buried in the Oakdale Cemetery at Wilmington, North Carolina.

DEATH CERTIFICATE: NAD

JOHN BANKHEAD MAGRUDER • *Born May 1, 1807,* at Port Royal, Virginia. He graduated from USMA in 1830. Served in Florida and Mexican wars. Because a bout of bronchitis made him unfit for duty in the field, Magruder did not go to Florida in 1836 and was unable to join his company there until November 1837. The climate at Hancock Barracks, Maine, severely affected his health in 1842–43. He was diagnosed as having a bronchial infection, and a warmer climate was advised. After being stationed in Baltimore on recruiting duty in October 1844, his health improved. During the Mexican War at Chapultepec on September 13, 1847, Magruder was wounded twice by grapeshot and knocked from his horse. These were apparently minor injuries. When he left the U.S. Army, he was exercising command at the brevet rank of lieutenant colonel. He was appointed brigadier general in the Confederate service in June 1861 and major general in October. Magruder was ill early in April 1862. One month later, on May 5, because there was no fighting, he turned himself over to the care of his doctor in order to reestablish his health, expecting to rejoin the army within a few days. On June 18, although quite sick, he said he would be on the field if anything of importance took place. On the morning of June 28 he had a bad attack of indigestion. At 3:30 A.M. on the twenty-ninth, the indigestion was still present, so a surgeon gave him morphine, which had an exciting effect. Magruder had approximately two hours of sleep during the seventy-two hours of this illness. Because of exhaustion, lack of sleep, indigestion, and medication, he was in a state of mental confusion. In early November 1864, unable to travel, he was confined to his bed with inflammatory rheumatism. After the end of war he went to Mexico and joined Imperial forces, but when the regime ended he returned to Texas. In February 1869 he had to discontinue a lecture tour because of arthritis. After relocating in Texas, he had poor health in 1871. For several weeks before his death he suffered from a disease of his heart. He died in Houston, Texas, on February 18, 1871, following a period of disorientation and inability to talk. His body was interred in the burial ground of his friends the Hadley family in Houston.[1] His remains were later moved to the Episcopal Cemetery at Galveston, Texas.

DEATH CERTIFICATE: RNA

1. OR, vol. 11, pt. 2:662, 665, 667, pt. 3:494, 608; vol. 41, pt. 4:1029, 1031, 1033, 1034, 1043; vol. 51, pt. 2:532; Thomas Michael Settles, "The Military Career of John Bankhead Magruder" (diss.), 30, 40–41, 137–38, 209–12, 311–13; SHSP 12:552; Galveston Daily News, Feb. 21, 24, 1871.

WILLIAM MAHONE • Born December 1, 1826, in Southampton County, Virginia. Mahone was an efficient railroad engineer and president of a railroad company before the war. Appointed colonel of the 6th Virginia Infantry in May 1861, he was promoted to brigadier general in November 1861. His health was considered delicate, so he had to nourish himself carefully, and he could not eat anything but tea, crackers, eggs, and fresh milk. A cow was always by his quarters, and laying hens were nearby. At the battle of Second Manassas on August 30, 1862, he was severely wounded in the chest by a bullet. He was absent from the army throughout September and October. He was in brigade command in November and took part in the Battle of Fredericksburg in December. He was promoted to major general to rank from July 1864. Mahone was absent due to illness during the action at Hatcher's Run in February 1865. Although back in March and April, he was still sick, and Gen. Nathaniel H. Harris had to surrender Mahone's division at Appomattox.[1] He returned to his railroad business after the war and became prominent in politics in Virginia. Mahone died October 8, 1895, at Washington, D.C., and was buried in Blandford Cemetery, Petersburg, Virginia.

DEATH CERTIFICATE: Cause of death, apoplexy, eight days' duration.

1. CSR; OR, vol. 12, pt. 2:567; vol. 19, pt. 1:842, pt. 2:683–84; vol. 21:614, 1036; vol. 46, pt. 3:1366, 1384–85, 1389; William Thomas Poague, Gunner with Stonewall: Reminiscences of William Thomas Poague, 118; Charles L. Dufour, Nine Men in Gray, 231, 242; Capt. W. N. Harris, comp., Diary of General Nat. H. Harris; "Movements of the Confederate Army in Virginia," Nathaniel H. Harris subject file, MDAH; CMH 3:634; CV 7:363; Sorrel, Confederate Staff Officer, 277, 284.

JAMES PATRICK MAJOR • Born May 14, 1836, at Fayette, Missouri. He graduated from USMA in 1856, after which he served on the frontier. He resigned in March 1861. When he entered Confederate service, he initially held staff positions but later served well as a lieutenant colonel and colonel. He was wounded while taking his men into a ditch during the attack on the Federal fort at Donaldsonville,

Louisiana, on June 28, 1863; apparently he did not leave the field. His appointment as brigadier general ranked from July 1863. He became sick while on home leave in August 1864, but was listed as in command the next month.[1] Following the war and a period in France, he returned to the United States and became a farmer in Louisiana and Texas. He died May 7, 1877, at Austin, Texas, and was buried at Donaldsonville, Louisiana, in the Ascension Catholic Cemetery.

DEATH CERTIFICATE: NAD

1. CSR; *OR*, vol. 26, pt. 1:229; vol. 41, pt. 2:1050, pt. 3:969.

GEORGE EARL MANEY • *Born August 24, 1826*, at Franklin, Tennessee. After service in Mexico, Maney practiced law in Nashville until the start of the Civil War. He was elected colonel of the 1st Tennessee in May 1861 and was promoted to brigadier general from April 1862. On November 26, 1863, near Ringgold, he was wounded in the arm. He was in command in July 1864. During September and October, Maney had a medical leave, and in the middle of January 1865, he was given another leave on surgeon's certificate for sixty days because of his arm wound.[1] He returned to Tennessee after the war and became president of a railroad. The last years of his life he held a number of diplomatic posts. He died February 9, 1901, in Washington, D.C., and was buried in Mount Olivet Cemetery, Nashville.

DEATH CERTIFICATE: Cause of death, cerebral hemorrhage; immediate, syncope.

1. CSR; *OR*, vol. 31, pt. 2:681; vol. 38, pt. 3:698, 708; vol. 45, pt. 1:667, 724.

ARTHUR MIDDLETON MANIGAULT • *Born October 26, 1824*, at Charleston, South Carolina. Manigault was injured on two occasions during the Mexican War. The first time, at Churubusco, he was struck twice. One was a spent ball that hit his left forearm, causing much pain and paralysis for a couple of days. The next ball grazed the inner part of his left thigh and passed between his legs, producing a large welt but no wound. On the second occasion, pieces of masonry splintered by a cannonball hit him on the back above the ribs and knocked him down. It was some time before he could get up, but he had only residual soreness. As a captain of a local militia company, he superintended the construction of the batteries in Charleston harbor before the Civil War. Manigault participated in the attack on Fort Sumter as a lieutenant colonel and in May 1861 was appointed colonel of the 10th South Carolina Infantry. His promotion as brigadier general dated from April 1863. On May 14, 1864, at the Battle of Resaca, he was slightly wounded in the hand by a rifle ball while standing on the brow of a ridge. He went to the rear long enough to have the wound dressed and then returned to his command. At the Battle of Franklin, on November 30, 1864, Manigault was wounded in the head. The ball entered the back part of his ear, passed under the skin, and came out about two inches behind the ear. The ball had been turned in its course by the boney projection behind the ear and made a slight groove along the bone. He could move his legs but for several hours was unable to stand without assistance. After lying on the field for an hour, he walked a mile and a half back to the hospital with the aid of two soldiers. The doctor thought the wound was not serious; however, it prevented Manigault's return to duty for the rest of the war and was postulated to have contributed to his death.[1] After his return to South Carolina, he became a rice planter. In 1880 he was elected adjutant and inspector general of South Carolina, a position he still held when he died August 17, 1886. He died at South Island, South Carolina, and was buried in Magnolia Cemetery, Charleston. Cause of death: Congestion of the brain.[2]

1. CSR; *OR*, vol. 45, pt. 1:654, 684, 688, pt. 2:643–44; Manigault, *Carolinian Goes to War*, 181, 318; A. M. Manigault to wife, Dec. 1, 1864 (typed copy supplied by R. Lockwood Tower).

2. Internment records, Magnolia Cemetery Trust, Charleston, S.C.

JOHN SAPPINGTON MARMADUKE • *Born March 14, 1833,* near Arrow Rock, Missouri. He graduated from USMA in 1857. He resigned from the U.S. Army in 1861 and was made a colonel in the Missouri militia, then a lieutenant colonel of the 1st Arkansas Battalion, and finally colonel of the Third Confederate Infantry. The second day at Shiloh, April 7, 1862, Marmaduke was disabled by a wound and was absent for a month. His promotion to brigadier general ranked from November. On June 13, 1863, he was sick and confined to his bed at Crowley's Ridge, Arkansas. He played an active role in the July 4, 1863, attack on Helena. Marmaduke mortally wounded Gen. Lucius M. Walker in a duel on September 6, 1863. He was captured at Mine Creek, Kansas, on October 25, 1864. Federal reports do not mention that he was wounded but do say he was on horseback when captured and was in a poor physical state. Others have reported he was wounded and had been thrown from his horse. He appeared to be in poor condition when he and William L. Cabell arrived at Johnson's Island, Ohio, in November, but no wound was mentioned. While a prisoner, he was seen at the U.S.A. post hospital in January 1865 with a cold. Although still a Federal prisoner, his promotion to major general ranked from March. After the war he went to Europe for his health. He later made his home in St. Louis and engaged in a number of businesses. In 1885 he was elected governor of Missouri; he died from pneumonia on December 28, 1887, in Jefferson City before the expiration of his term.[1] He was buried at that city in Woodland Cemetery.

DEATH CERTIFICATE: NAD

1. CSR; *OR*, vol. 10, pt. 2:426, 550; vol. 22, pt. 1:436, pt. 2:867; vol. 41, pt. 1:313, 357, 498, 603–4; George B. Clarke to Loudie Dorsey, Nov. 10, 1864, in Dorsey Family Papers, MHS; Jay Monaghan, *Civil War on the Western Border, 1854–1865,* 338–39; Shelby Foote, *The Civil War: A Narrative* 3:583; John F. Lee, "John Sappington Marmaduke," *Missouri Historical Society Collections* 6:31, 39–40; *CMH* 9:215, Mo.

HUMPHREY MARSHALL • *Born January 13, 1812,* at Frankfort, Kentucky. He graduated from USMA in 1832. Served in the Mexican War. At the close of the Mexican War, he weighed 194 pounds. He was a member of the United States Congress twice and was given a commission as brigadier general in the Confederate Army in October 1861. In February he was sleeping out in the open and working with the men, and he had little to eat. He had knots on his wrists and pains in his elbow, shoulder, and knee joints. He was indisposed and unable to make his report the first week in January 1863 after spending a period in the saddle. Weighing nearly three hundred pounds at the time of the Civil War, he was unfit for duty in the field. He ate frequent large meals but was temperate in the use of alcohol. Marshall would fall asleep while in the midst of a conversation, and sometimes while on his feet. On these latter occasions his eyes would be closed and he would audibly snore and appear to be asleep for a few minutes. Because of his obesity and symptom complex, which included snoring, he most likely had a form of obstructive sleep apnea. Marshall's final resignation from the Confederate Army was submitted in June 1863, and he later served in the Confederate government in a civil capacity. He was ill in December 1863. Following a period in Texas at the close of the war, he returned to Kentucky and practiced law at Louisville. His health was poor during the winter prior to his death. On March 23, 1872, he awoke with a burning and smothering sensation in his chest. Later it became so severe he returned to his home. The smothering sensation continued, and he had to sit up in bed most of the time until his death a few days later on March 28, 1872.[1] He was buried in the State Cemetery at Frankfort, Kentucky.

DEATH CERTIFICATE: Cause of death, bronchitis.

1. OR, vol. 20, pt. 1:95; "Autobiographical sketch," n.d., Charles Lanman Collection, FC; CMH 9:248, Ky.; Duke, Reminiscences, 143–45; William C. Orr, Richard J. Martin, and C. Dowell Patterson, "When to Suspect Sleep Apnea—the 'Pickwickian Syndrome,'" Resident and Staff Physician 25:101–4; Humphrey Marshall to Alexander H. Stephens, Feb. 22, 1862, and Louisville Courier Journal, n.d., both in Humphrey Marshall Papers, FC.

JAMES GREEN MARTIN • Born February 14, 1819, at Elizabeth City, North Carolina. He graduated from USMA in 1840. At Churubusco, Mexico, on August 20, 1847, he was wounded and lost his right arm. He resigned from the U.S. Army at the start of the Civil War and was made adjutant general of ten regiments of North Carolina state troops. In September 1861 he was made major general of militia, and his appointment as brigadier general in Confederate service was confirmed the following September. In June 1863, Martin reported that he could manage the Bureau of Conscription but was willing to go into the field even though it would be very difficult for him. He asked to be relieved from the field in June 1864, because each time he moved his brigade from the trenches, the exertion caused pain in his stump similar to when it had been amputated. Removed from field duty, he was transferred to the command of the District of Western North Carolina.[1] When he returned home, he became a lawyer and practiced in North Carolina until he died on October 4, 1878, at Asheville. He was buried in that city in the Riverside Cemetery.

DEATH CERTIFICATE: NAD

1. CSR; OR, vol. 18: 1089; vol. 40, pt. 2:699, pt. 3:772, 787, 788; R. E. Lee to John Mackay, Oct. 2, 1847, in R. E. and G. W. C. Lee Papers, USAMHI; Sketch of life (W. W. Mackall) by wife, in W. W. Mackall Papers, SHC; Heitman, Historical Register and Dictionary 2:30; Clark, Histories of Several Regiments 4:535; CMH 4:332.

WILLIAM THOMPSON MARTIN • *Born March 25, 1823,* in Glasgow, Kentucky. In 1844 he was admitted to the Mississippi bar and served as a district attorney for several terms before the war. He recruited a company of cavalry in 1861 and rose through the ranks of major, lieutenant colonel, and colonel of the Jeff Davis Legion. In December 1862 he was commissioned brigadier general and was promoted to major general to rank from November 1863. Following the war he was active in politics, education, and building railroads. He died March 16, 1910, near Natchez, Mississippi, and was buried in that city in the City Cemetery.
DEATH CERTIFICATE: NAD

DABNEY HERNDON MAURY • *Born May 21, 1822,* in Fredericksburg, Virginia. He graduated from USMA in 1846. That same year he was badly wounded while hunting near Camargo, Mexico, and was disabled from duty. At Cerro Gordo on April 17, 1847, Maury's left arm was shattered by a ball. Taken to the rear, he was examined by a surgeon, who stated his arm would have to be amputated. Maury found a horse and, with assistance and frequent sips of brandy, rode back five miles, apparently unwilling to undergo the amputation. Initially he was in a spacious reed house with Joe Johnston but after ten days was carried by litter to Jalapa. By the middle of May he was improving, although the wound disabled him for the rest of his life. While his arm was in splints, Maury was unable to manage his horse, and she ran away with him whenever he rode her. After the Mexican War, Maury returned to West Point, where one winter he was disabled for many weeks by a riding injury to his leg. In 1853 he became ill while at the Rio Frio, thirty miles from Fort Ewell, Texas. He lay alone all night at the ford waiting for a doctor while his condition worsened. He left the next morning in a wagon, then proceeded by buggy since there was no ambulance at the fort and he could not ride his horse. He had sick leave in San Antonio and then went home on leave. Maury arrived back in Corpus Christi in time to join Gen. Persifor Smith in the expedition into New Mexico. In June 1861 he was dismissed from the U.S. Army and in July was made a lieutenant colonel in the Confederate Provisional Army. He received his brigadier stars in March 1862 and was promoted to major general the following November. In April 1863, while at Vicksburg, Maury was confined with rheumatism. After returning home from the war, he was the founder of the Southern Historical Society and was for four years United States minister to Colombia. His last year of life was spent in Peoria, Illinois, in poor health, and he died there on January 11, 1900.[1] He was buried at Fredericksburg, Virginia, in the City Cemetery.
DEATH CERTIFICATE: RNA

1. *OR,* vol. 52, pt. 2:457; Maury, *Recollections of a Virginian,* 29, 36–40, 54, 60, 82–84; B. Huger to wife, May 13, 1847, Benjamin Huger Papers (no. 9942), UV; *CV* 8:85; *SHSP* 27:335–38.

SAMUEL BELL MAXEY • *Born March 30, 1825,* at Tompkinsville, Kentucky. He graduated from USMA in 1846. Served in Mexican War. He resigned from the U.S. Army in 1849 and became an attorney first in Kentucky and then in Texas. At the start of the Civil War, Maxey organized the Lamar Rifles. Later when this organization became part of the 9th Texas Infantry, he was made a colonel. On his way from Paris, Texas, to Richmond in August 1861, he had chills and fever. Maxey believed he had a delicate frame and that he was unable physically to stand up to much labor. His promotion to brigadier general ranked from March 1862. By May 1864, he had been on sick leave only twice, fifteen days when he was a colonel and fifteen days given to him by Braxton Bragg. However, by the last of the month, Maxey was quite feeble and scarcely able to write. After the war he returned to his law practice in Texas and served two terms in the United States Senate. In the spring of 1894, he had gastrointestinal problems, which recurred the following year. A trip to use the water at Eureka Springs, Arkansas, did not help, and he continued to feel poorly until the time of his death there on August 16, 1895.[1] He was buried in the Evergreen Cemetery at Paris, Texas.

DEATH CERTIFICATE: NAD

1. S. B. Maxey to E. Kirby Smith, Mar. 29, 1864 (p. 161), S. B. Maxey to S. S. Anderson, May 20, 1864 (p. 199), and S. B. Maxey to W. R. Boggs, May 27, 1864 (p. 214), Letter book "A," Maxey (Samuel Bell) Papers, TXSL; Louis Horton, *Samuel Bell Maxey: A Biography,* 20, 193.

HUGH WEEDON MERCER • *Born November 27, 1808,* in Fredericksburg, Virginia. He graduated from USMA in 1828. He resigned his U.S. Army commission in April 1835 and from 1841 until the start of the war was cashier of a bank in Savannah, Georgia. He entered the Confederate Army as a colonel of the 1st Georgia Volunteers and was promoted to brigadier general in October 1861. On July 24, 1864, Gen. Braxton Bragg stated that Mercer's age and physical condition made him unfit for active duty; the following day Mercer was ordered to Savannah. He was given a leave in August and, when it expired, was to report for duty with the reserves of Georgia. After the war he returned to banking in Savannah, where he remained for four years before moving to Baltimore. His health continued to deteriorate, and he spent the last five years of his life in Baden-Baden, Germany, where he died on June 9, 1877.[1] His remains were finally moved to the Bonaventure Cemetery at Savannah.

DEATH CERTIFICATE: RNA (Passport Service, U.S. Department of State).

1. CSR; *OR,* vol. 38, pt. 5:907, 911; vol. 39, pt. 2:768; vol. 49, pt. 1:1023.

WILLIAM MILLER • *Born August 3, 1820,* in Ithaca, New York. Soon after the Mexican War he moved to Florida, where he practiced law and later operated a sawmill. He joined the Confederate service in 1861 as a major in command of the 1st Florida Battalion. When this unit was merged with the 1st Florida Regiment, he was made a colonel. At Murfreesborough on January 2, 1863, he was wounded in the finger but retained command. While his wound was healing, he was placed in charge of the Confederate Conscript Bureau in southern Florida. In August 1864 he was commissioned as brigadier general.[1] After the war he returned to Florida and engaged in the lumber business and farming. Miller served in both the state legislature and senate. He died August 8, 1909, at Point Washington, Florida, and was initially buried in the yard of his home. His remains were later moved to St. John's Cemetery, Pensacola, Florida.

DEATH CERTIFICATE: RNA

1. CSR; *OR*, vol. 20, pt. 1:813; *CMH* 11:168, 206. Fla.

YOUNG MARSHALL MOODY · *Born June 23, 1822*, in Chesterfield County, Virginia. He was a clerk of the circuit court in 1861, after having been a school teacher and merchant. He entered the Confederate Army as a captain in the 11th Alabama Infantry and was then elected lieutenant colonel of the 43rd Alabama. He was promoted to colonel in November 1862. On May 16, 1864, during the battle of Drewry's Bluff, Moody received a gunshot wound through the right ankle joint. He entered a hospital in Richmond, and the lower end of the fibula was excised. The exact date of surgery was not recorded. He was furloughed August 11 and was still absent through November. He was promoted to brigadier general in March 1865. One day before the surrender at Appomattox, Moody was sick in a wagon train when he was captured. Following the war he engaged in business in Mobile. He died of yellow fever on September 18, 1886, while on a business trip to New Orleans. He was buried in that city in the Greenwood Cemetery.[1]

DEATH CERTIFICATE: NAD

1. CSR; *MSHW*, vol. 2, pt. 3:595, Case 865; *CMH* 12:426, Ala.; *New Orleans Daily Crescent*, Sept. 20, 1866; Burial Records, Greenwood Cemetery, New Orleans, La.

JOHN CREED MOORE · *Born February 28, 1824*, in Hawkins County, Tennessee. He graduated from USMA in 1849. Served in Florida wars. After resigning from the United States Army in 1855, he became a civil engineer. He left a college professorship and entered the Confederate service as a captain in the 1st Louisiana Heavy Artillery in March 1861. In April he resigned his position and accepted an appointment as captain in the Regular Confederate Army. The following September he organized and became colonel of the 2nd Texas Infantry. He was admitted to the general hospital in Galveston, Texas, on October 24, 1861, with pleurisy but returned to duty the following day. He was promoted to brigadier general in May 1862.[1] After the war he returned to Texas, where he taught and was the author of a number of magazine articles. Moore died December 31, 1910, at Osage, Texas, and was buried there in the City Cemetery.

DEATH CERTIFICATE: RNA

1. CSR.

PATRICK THEODORE MOORE · *Born September 22, 1821*, in Galway, Ireland. Moore was a merchant in Richmond when he joined Confederate service in 1861, and was commissioned colonel of the 1st Virginia Infantry. At Blackburn's Ford, Virginia, on July 18, 1861, he was wounded in the head. The injury, and his name being absent from the unit's list for reelection of officers, prevented further service with his regiment. He acted as a volunteer aide to Joseph E. Johnston and then served on James Longstreet's staff. In May 1864, Moore was temporarily assigned to duty organizing and helping place in the field the reserve forces in Virginia. His promotion to brigadier general ranked from September 1864.[1] Having lost his prior business, he returned to Richmond and opened an insurance agency. Moore died February 20, 1883, at Richmond, Virginia, and was buried there in Shockoe Cemetery.[2] DEATH CERTIFICATE: Cause of death, pleurisy.

1. CSR; *OR*, vol. 2:445, 462; vol. 36, pt. 2:1020; *CMH* 3:638; Moore, *Life for the Confederacy*, 43.
2. Death certificate.

JOHN HUNT MORGAN • *Born June 1, 1825*, in Huntsville, Alabama. Served in the Mexican War. When he was young, he was severely wounded at Lexington in a personal altercation. He was engaged in hemp manufacturing and business in Lexington and organized the Lexington Rifles in 1857. When the Civil War started, he took his unit to Bowling Green and joined the Confederate forces there. He was appointed colonel of the 2nd Kentucky Cavalry in April 1862 and brigadier general the following December. Morgan was captured during a raid into Ohio in 1863, and his health was impaired by imprisonment in the Ohio State Penitentiary. After his escape from prison, he made his last Kentucky raid in late May 1864 and came back June 20. In July Morgan was sick and unable to follow Robert E. Lee's orders. On September 4, 1864, at Greeneville, Tennessee, he was surrounded by Federal troops and was instantly killed by a shot in the chest.[1] He is buried in the City Cemetery in Lexington, Kentucky.

1. CSR; *OR*, vol. 37, pt. 2:602; vol. 39, pt. 1:489–92, pt. 2:733; Duke, *History of Morgan's Cavalry*, 19, 474, 528, 537–39; *SHSP* 31:126–27; *CMH* 9:250, Ky.

JOHN TYLER MORGAN • *Born June 20, 1824*, in Athens, Tennessee. He was an attorney and a member of the Alabama secession convention. Morgan entered Confederate service as a private in the Cahaba Rifles in 1861 and became major and lieutenant colonel of the 5th Alabama Infantry. He was made colonel of the 51st Alabama Partisan Rangers in 1862 and brigadier from November 1863. Following the war he returned to his law practice and was elected to the senate from Alabama, a position he held until his death on June 11, 1907, in Washington, D.C. He was buried at Selma, Alabama, in the Live Oak Cemetery. DEATH CERTIFICATE: Cause of death, primary, angina pectoris, one year's duration; immediate, syncope.

JEAN JACQUES ALFRED ALEXANDER MOUTON • *Born February 18, 1829*, at Opelousas, Louisiana. He graduated from USMA in 1850. Soon afterward he resigned from the army and became a railroad engineer and brigadier general of the Louisiana militia. He recruited a company at the outbreak of the war and in October 1861 was elected colonel of the 18th Louisiana Infantry. Mouton was wounded in the face at the Battle of Shiloh on April 7, 1862, and had to leave the field. A portion of his left eye was damaged. He was taken to the St. Charles Hotel in New Orleans, which had been converted into a Confederate military hospital. His promotion to brigadier general ranked from April 1862. In October he returned to duty and was assigned command of the Lafourche District in Louisiana. On April 8, 1864, while leading a charge at the Battle of Mansfield in the Red River campaign, he was killed by a sharpshooter. In another version, he was shot five times after the battle was over as he was riding up to receive the Federal troops' surrender.[1] He was first buried at Mansfield, and his remains were later moved to St. John's Cathedral Cemetery, Lafayette, Louisiana.

1. CSR; *OR*, vol. 10, pt. 1:519, 522, pt. 2:426; vol. 34, pt. 1:476, 553, 564; William Arceneaux, *Acadian General: Alfred Mouton and the Civil War*, 51–54, 132, 142; W. E. Lawrence to unknown, May 24, 1864, from the Collections of the Louisiana State Museum Historical Center, RG 56, Accession no. 11871.32, New Orleans, La.; Oates, *War between the Union and the Confederacy*, 449.

N

ALLISON NELSON • *Born March 11, 1822*, in Fulton County, Georgia. Although an attorney and politician, he took an active role in the Mexican War, the struggle for Cuban independence, the prewar troubles in Kansas, and the Indian campaigns in Texas. He entered the Confederacy as colonel of the 10th Texas Infantry. Nelson's promotion to brigadier ranked from September 1862. He developed typhoid fever on September 29, 1862, and died at Camp Hope near Austin, Arkansas, on October 7.[1] He was buried at Little Rock in Mount Holly Cemetery.

1. CSR; Warner, *Generals in Gray*, 223–24; Brown, *One of Cleburne's Command*, "Prologue," 36; McCaffrey, *Granbury's Texas Brigade*, 25.

FRANCIS REDDING TILLOU NICHOLLS • *Born August 20, 1834*, at Donaldsonville, Louisiana. He graduated from USMA in 1855. Served in the Florida wars. Although he had varicose veins, he was not prevented from entering West Point. His health, while in Florida in 1855 and in California in 1856, was poor. Nicholls resigned from the U.S. Army effective October 1, 1856, having served his obligation and because he had been having chronic gastric problems. An attorney in Louisiana at the start of the Civil War, he joined the Confederate service as captain of the Phoenix Guards. In June 1861 he was elected lieutenant colonel of the 8th Louisiana Volunteers. Although he suffered with headaches and slight indisposition in the spring of 1862, his general health was good. Near Winchester, on May 25, 1862, Nicholls received a wound to his left elbow from a minié ball. After his horse ran to the rear, Nicholls lay on the ground for a period of time before being taken into Winchester for treatment. Surgery was delayed in an attempt to save the arm, but amputation was finally performed on May 31. He was given only whiskey for anesthesia, and the surgery was a simple circular amputation. Unable to be moved, he was captured in Winchester and was paroled in June. Although unfit for field duty, he was promoted to brigadier general in October 1862. Nicholls was ordered to duty in January 1863 and arrived back in March. In the Battle of Chancellorsville on May 2, 1863, Nicholls was seriously wounded in the left foot, about six inches above the ankle, by a shell fragment. After remaining on the ground in the darkness for a while, he reached for his foot and discovered that it was gone. He expected to bleed to death, but to his surprise the wound did not bleed at all. Finally, some of his men found him and carried him on a blanket under heavy fire to a tent, where he underwent amputation of his leg. First by litter and then by ambulance, he was taken about five miles to a hospital. Later he went to Richmond and then to Lynchburg, where he was taken care of in a private home. When Nicholls had sufficiently recovered, he reported for duty in Richmond and was ordered to return to Lynchburg as commandant of the post in August 1863. Ambulation was slow with a crutch and a wooden leg. As post commander, and with only one arm and one leg, he rode out on June 17, 1864, to tell his troops that reinforcements were coming. In July he was ordered to take charge of the Bureau of Conscription in the Trans-Mississippi Department. In 1876 his party "nominated all that is left of General Nicholls" for governor of Louisiana. After serving twice as governor, he was a justice of the Louisiana Supreme Court. Capt. Joseph Demoruella, who had fought under Nicholls, was crier of the state supreme court and helped the crippled judge mount the bench. In March 1911 he resigned from the court because of his poor health. He caught a cold that he could not shake off, one that "threatened pneumonia." Although he seemed to improve for a while, he relapsed and died January 4, 1912, near Thibodeaux, Louisiana, when his heart failed.[1] He was buried there in St. John's Episcopal Church Cemetery.

DEATH CERTIFICATE: NAD

1. CSR; *OR*, vol. 21:1094; vol. 25, pt. 1:803, 1005, 1010, 1037; vol. 27, pt. 1:439, pt. 3:922; vol. 29, pt. 2:642; vol. 41, pt. 2:1026; vol. 48, pt. 1:1446; Evans J. Casso, *Francis T. Nicholls: A Biographical Tribute*, 50, 60, 62, 77–79, 86–89, 96, 107; Francis T. Nicholls, "Autobiography of Francis T. Nicholls, 1834–1881," *Louisiana Historical Quarterly* 17:51–52; Isaac Ridgeway Trimble, "The Civil War Diary of General Isaac Ridgeway Trimble," *Maryland Historical Magazine* 17:1–20; Taylor, *Destruction and Reconstruction*, 58–59, 61; *SHSP* 22:296; *New Orleans Daily Picayune*, June 5, 7, 1912.

LUCIUS BELLINGER NORTHROP • *Born September 8, 1811,* at Charleston, South Carolina. He graduated from USMA in 1831. On October 6, 1839, during the Seminole War, he accidently shot himself with his pistol, and the ball lodged in his knee. Unable to perform any duty, he was on the inactive list for almost three years. He was made an assistant commissary in the Subsistence Department in October 1842, and remained in that position for six and a half months. He applied for medical leave and began medical school in December 1843. In 1848 he continued to draw disability pay. Northrop's general health was affected by the unhealed wound and the ball that still lodged in his knee. Northrop continued on sick leave until 1861. President Jefferson Davis appointed him colonel and commissary general of the Confederacy in 1861 and brigadier general from November 1864. After the war he was bothered by dyspepsia and other illness while held in a Federal prison. After his release he returned to Virginia, where he farmed. Frequently bedridden in later years, he was paralyzed in 1890.[1] He died at Pikesville, Maryland, on February 9, 1894, and was buried in New Cathedral Cemetery, Baltimore, Maryland. Cause of death: Paralysis.[2]

1. Dufour, *Nine Men in Gray*, 200–202, 227, 229; Steiner, *Physician-Generals in the Civil War*, 87; *CV* 2:84–85; Warner, *Generals in Gray*, 225.

2. Internment Register, New Cathedral Cemetery, Baltimore, Md.

EDWARD ASBURY O'NEAL · *Born September 20, 1818,* in Madison County, Alabama. In 1861 he was a practicing attorney in Florida when he enlisted in the 9th Alabama Infantry. He was elected major and lieutenant colonel of this unit and then colonel of the 26th Alabama in 1862. At Seven Pines, on May 31, 1862, he was severely injured by a shell fragment that killed his adjutant. In the middle of July he arrived in Aberdeen, Mississippi, where he had gone to recover, and asked his wife to join him. Although his wound was still bothering him, his general health was good, and he returned to duty by late summer. O'Neal was wounded in the thigh at the Battle of South Mountain, Maryland, on September 14, 1862. Furloughed to Florence, Alabama, he reported back that winter. During the Battle of Chancellorsville on May 3, 1863, he was hit by a shell fragment. He had started on a run to the center of the brigade when he was struck, and for the balance of the day was disabled. He was back on the field in early June and took part at Gettysburg. His promotion as brigadier general from June 1863 was later canceled.[1] After the war, O'Neal returned to his law practice in Alabama and was twice elected governor. He died November 7, 1890, at Florence, Alabama, where he was buried in the City Cemetery.

DEATH CERTIFICATE: NAD

1. CSR; *OR*, vol. 11, pt. 1:970; vol. 19, pt. 1:1021, 1027, 1035; vol. 25, pt. 1:943, 948, 952; vol. 27, pt. 2:593; E. A. O'Neal to wife, July 17, 1862, and E. A. O'Neal to son (Alfred M. O'Neal), July 24, 31, 1862, both in Edward Asbury O'Neal Papers, SHC; *CMH* 12:433, Ala.

P

RICHARD LUCIAN PAGE · *Born December 20, 1807,* in Clarke County, Virginia. He became a midshipman in the United States Navy in 1824, and after extensive sea duty he rose to the rank of commander in 1855. When Virginia left the Union he resigned his commission, and in June 1861 he was appointed commander, C.S.N.

He was promoted to captain and established an ordnance and naval construction bureau. In March 1864 he was made a brigadier general in the Confederate Army and was given command of the outer defenses of Mobile Bay. Following the war he went to Norfolk, Virginia, where he was the city's superintendent of schools for a number of years. He died August 9, 1901, at Blue Ridge Summit, Pennsylvania, and was buried in Cedar Hill Cemetery, Norfolk, Virginia.

DEATH CERTIFICATE: RNA

JOSEPH BENJAMIN PALMER • *Born November 1, 1825,* in Rutherford County, Tennessee. Before the war he was an attorney, was twice elected to the Tennessee legislature, and was mayor of Murfreesborough. In 1861 he was elected colonel of the 18th Tennessee. At Murfreesborough on January 2, 1863, a minié ball passed through his right shoulder, another tore through the calf of his right leg, and a shell fragment inflicted a wound to his right knee. Despite his injuries, Palmer did not leave the field until the battle was over. Travel was uncomfortable for him, and he was left in the neighborhood of Allisonia. For more than four months erysipelas complicated his wounds. In February he was in Winchester, Tennessee, probably in a hospital, and did not return to duty until May. Erysipelas of his unhealed wounds forced him to leave the army again in July. He spent part of the time in a hospital in Chattanooga until his return in August. During the Battle of Chickamauga on September 19, 1863, he received a shoulder wound and barely escaped bleeding to death on the field, as a large artery had been severed. He had to apply local pressure to stop the bleeding. For the remainder of the day, and during the succeeding night, he lay on the battlefield, cold and neglected. Finally he was taken to an old stable, where he remained until he was moved again to other quarters. At the time of his wound he was already sick, complicating his problem. This wound caused him great suffering, and his right arm remained partially paralyzed. Although he returned in February 1864, he was not fit for duty until July. He was slightly wounded at Jonesborough on August 31, 1864. His promotion as brigadier general ranked from November. He received his final flesh wound at Bentonville on March 19, 1865. When the war ended, he returned to his law practice in Tennessee. His death on November 4, 1890, at Murfreesborough, was unexpected and occurred suddenly from a heart attack.[1] He was buried at that city in Evergreen Cemetery.

DEATH CERTIFICATE: NAD

1. OR, vol. 20, pt. 1:805, 808–9; vol. 30, pt. 2:371, 374–75; Robert O. Neff, *Tennessee's Battered Brigadier.* (*The Life of General Joseph B. Palmer*), 67, 69, 71–72, 75–76, 85–86, 88–90, 93, 104, 149, 184.

MOSBY MONROE PARSONS • *Born May 21, 1822,* in Charlottesville, Virginia. Served in the Mexican War. He was attorney general of Missouri from 1853 to 1857 and was then elected to the state senate. In 1861 he commanded the 6th Division of the Missouri State Guard, and he was appointed brigadier in the Confederate Army in November 1862. He was absent from his post in both December 1863 and January 1864 due to illness. On January 31 he was listed as present but not in command because he was sick. In February he asked for an additional leave on surgeon's certificate for restoration of his health. Parsons participated in the battles of Mansfield and Pleasant Hill in April 1864. For a few days in early May, he was sick while near McNutt's Hill, Louisiana. At the close of the Civil War, he went to Mexico and was killed on August 15, 1865, in an engagement at Camargo on the San Juan River.[1] He was supposedly buried near to where he was killed.

DEATH CERTIFICATE: RNA (Passport Service, U. S. Department of State).

1. CSR; *OR*, vol. 34, pt. 1:601, 626–28, pt. 2:933; *CMH* 9:217, Mo.

ELISHA FRANKLIN PAXTON • *Born March 4, 1828*, in Rockbridge County, Virginia. As a boy, he was blinded in one eye by an injury. Before the Civil War, he abandoned his law practice because of failing eyesight. He joined the Confederacy as a lieutenant of the Rockbridge Rifles. In April 1861, Paxton stated that increased strain from writing would injure his vision. A ball went through his shirt and bruised his arm at First Manassas on July 21, 1861. During the rest of the year, he complained of pain in his eye brought on by increased use, but he did not mention any difficulty seeing. The following October he was commissioned major of the 27th Virginia Infantry. In January 1862 he was absent sick for a few days in Winchester. He was appointed brigadier general in November. Paxton was ill for most of the winter of 1862–63 and often had to spend a day or two in bed. When he ate rice and bread he did well, but he became sick when he ate a hearty meal. His condition improved in March, after he started living on a half-bushel of dried peaches obtained from Richmond. At Chancellorsville on May 3, 1863, marching in front of his brigade, he was killed almost instantly by a minié ball through his chest. The night before, he had said that he would be killed the next day.[1] He was initially buried near the battlefield, but his remains were later moved to Jackson Memorial Cemetery, Lexington, Virginia.

1. CSR; *OR*, vol. 25, pt. 2:768, 775; James I. Robertson, Jr., *The Stonewall Brigade*, 165–66; John Gallatin Paxton, *The Civil War Letters of Gen. Frank "Bull" Paxton—a Lieutenant of Lee and Jackson*, 4, 11, 16–17, 39, 58, 72–78, 84–87.

WILLIAM HENRY FITZHUGH PAYNE • *Born January 27, 1830*, in Fauquier County, Virginia. Payne was elected Virginia commonwealth attorney in 1856 and in April 1861 enlisted as a private in Confederate service. During October he was absent on sick leave. In the battle of May 5, 1862, at Williamsburg, he was severely wounded in the mouth and was taken prisoner. Payne was bleeding profusely, and Dr. E. S. Pendleton saved his life. Payne later reported that from the time he fell until he was put in the ambulance, the chances of death to both of them from enemy fire was a "thousand to one." After Payne was exchanged, he returned to duty early in September 1862 and, although not fully recovered, was assigned to the temporary command of the 2nd North Carolina Cavalry Regiment. In November he was ordered to go into the hospital at Lynchburg, but on his application he was given command of the troops at that post. In February 1863 he was able to rejoin the army in the field. At the engagement at Kelly's Ford, Virginia, on March 17, Payne fought unmindful of his former wound. At Hanover, Pennsylvania, on June 30, 1863, Payne's horse was killed under him. He received a severe saber cut in the side and was captured again. While at Johnson's Island in May 1864, he was admitted to the hospital because of chronic diarrhea. Following his exchange, and still in a feeble condition, he was appointed on August 30 as a recorder for a court of inquiry. After passing through grades he was appointed brigadier general from November 1864. On Christmas Day, Payne participated in an attack on Custer's camp near Harrisonburg. He received his last wound on March 30, 1865, near Five Forks and Dinwiddie Court-House, Virginia, and his arm was badly fractured. Lying helpless in his home in Warrenton, he was captured and again imprisoned.[1] He returned to his law practice in Virginia following the war and later moved to Washington, D.C., where he was general counsel for the Southern Railway. He died March 29, 1904, in that city and was buried in the City Cemetery in Warrenton, Virginia.

DEATH CERTIFICATE: Cause of death, primary, arteriosclerosis, duration ten years; immediate, cerebral hemorrhage, two days' duration.

1. CSR; *OR*, vol. 11, pt. 1:572; vol. 25, pt. 1:62; vol. 39, pt. 1:80–81; vol. 46, pt. 1:1275, 1299; *CMH* 3:645; *SHSP* 36:290; *CV* 18:177; Dawson, *Reminiscences of Confederate Service*, 137, 142.

WILLIAM RAINE PECK · *Born January 31, 1818*, in Jefferson County, Tennessee. Peck was a landowner in Louisiana; in July 1861 he enlisted as a private in the 9th Louisiana Infantry. He was absent sick during the last of August 1862 but returned to duty by the last of September. In late July and August 1863 he was hospitalized at Charlottesville with a contusion. After passing through grades, he was promoted to colonel in October. Peck arrived with his command at the Rappahannock River on November 6, 1863. At Winchester on September 19, 1864, he was wounded in the right thigh by a shell. After being hospitalized at Charlottesville, he was transferred to a hospital in Richmond in early October. He returned in December and participated at Hatcher's Run on February 6, 1865. Peck's promotion to brigadier general ranked from that month.[1] Following the war he returned to his plantation in Jefferson County, Tennessee, where he died January 22, 1871. He was buried in a family plot in the Old Methodist section of Westview Cemetery, which is now on Andrew Johnson Highway.

DEATH CERTIFICATE: NAD

1. CSR; *OR*, vol. 29, pt. 1:627.

JOHN PEGRAM · *Born January 24, 1832*, at Petersburg, Virginia. He graduated from USMA in 1854. After resigning from the U.S. Army in May 1861, he entered Confederate service as lieutenant colonel of the 10th Virginia Infantry. On July 11, 1861, at Rich Mountain, Virginia, Pegram was thrown from his horse and injured. He returned to the field later in the day, but the accident confined him to his bed in Beverly, Virginia, for a few days. He surrendered his forces on the thirteenth and was released from the Federal prison in January 1862. Soon after his exchange was completed in April, he was promoted to colonel; in November he was commissioned brigadier general. Pegram was severely wounded in the leg at the Wilderness on May 5, 1864, and did not report back for duty until August. In the fight on the west side of Hatcher's Run on February 6, 1865, he was struck by a musket ball. The ball hit him near the heart, and he died almost as soon as he touched the ground. He was killed just a few days after his wedding.[1] Pegram was buried in Hollywood Cemetery, Richmond, Virginia.

1. CSR; *OR*, vol. 2:245, 257–58, 261, 264–68; vol. 36, pt. 1:1028, 1071, 1074, pt. 2:960; vol. 43, pt. 1:568; vol. 46, pt. 1:381, 390; Douglas, *I Rode with Stonewall*, 312; Clark, *Histories of Several Regiments* 3:282.

JOHN CLIFFORD PEMBERTON · *Born August 10, 1814,* in Philadelphia, Pennsylvania. He graduated from USMA in 1837. Served in the Florida and Mexican wars. He was wounded twice in the assaults before the capture of Mexico City. In April 1861 he resigned from the U.S. Army and rose rapidly in the Confederate service— to brigadier general in June 1861, to major general ranking from January 1862, and to lieutenant general from October 1862. He resigned his lieutenant general commission in 1864 and was appointed a lieutenant colonel of artillery. He served in this position until the end of the war, when he settled in Virginia and farmed. He later returned to Pennsylvania, and in the spring before his death his health began to fail.[1] He died July 13, 1881, at Penllyn and was buried in Laurel Hill Cemetery at Philadelphia.

DEATH CERTIFICATE: RNA

1. John C. Pemberton, *Pemberton: Defender of Vicksburg*, 10, 13, 277.

WILLIAM DORSEY PENDER · *Born February 6, 1834,* in Edgecomb County, North Carolina. He graduated from USMA in 1854. Following graduation, Pender served in New Mexico and on the Pacific coast. He left the U.S. Army in March 1861 and joined the Confederate service as colonel of the 3rd North Carolina. On December 7, 1861, he was ill and felt as though he would have a recurrence of dysentery. However, in such situations he would follow a diet, which would make the feeling pass and enable him to continue on duty. On March 13, 1862, he was exceedingly hoarse and had a sore throat brought on by drilling in cold weather. By the eighteenth, he could not drill because he was suffering from a cold and sore throat. He developed a cough that lasted for the next week. He was promoted brigadier general to rank from June. Probably on June 27, 1862, during the Seven Days' battles, Pender received a flesh wound of his arm. Although this wound, according to others, occurred on July 1, Pender mentioned that it happened before the twenty-ninth, and that they were not engaged on the twenty-eighth. Unfortunately, he did not provide a date in his official report. By the first of July his arm was much better. Later that month, while visiting his wife, he had an unspecified illness. However, he had improved by the twenty-ninth while he was in Richmond and thought that after he proceeded to where the water was better he would be cured. He was knocked down by the explosion of a shell at Second Manassas on August 29, 1862, but refused to leave the field. Because his heavy felt hat provided some protection, he received only a small cut on the top of his head; however, some of his hair had to be removed. Pender had diarrhea in October, which was followed by some ailment resembling rheumatism. At Fredericksburg on December 13, 1862, a bullet passed through his left arm, but no bones were broken. He continued to ride along the line with the injured limb hanging down and blood dripping from his fingers. Although he had to go to the rear to have his wound dressed, he soon returned to the field. On May 4, 1863, following the battle at Chancellorsville, Pender was hit by a spent ball while standing behind an entrenchment. The ball, which had killed an officer in front of him, produced only a slight bruise to his right arm near the shoulder. However, in a few days the arm was stiff and he was ill. He improved when medication was administered and on May 13 was able to resume command of the brigade. The arm was still very painful two weeks after the injury, and he admitted that the wound had been a little deeper than he had first thought. In May 1863 he was promoted to major general. At Gettysburg on July 2, while riding down his line, he was struck in the thigh by a two-inch-square shell fragment. The next day he tried to get back on his horse but found it was impossible. On July 5 he was in an ambulance along with Gen. Alfred M. Scales, who was also wounded. Gen. John D. Imboden shared a little bread and meat with them at noon. When the column finally started, they were placed behind the advanced guard during the retreat. Pender appeared to have improved and was taken by ambulance to Staunton. The first night he was there the wound began to hemorrhage; using a towel and a hairbrush as a tourniquet, he managed to stop the bleeding. A surgeon attempted to mend the artery, but it bled again, and he amputated the leg on July 18. Pender survived only a few hours.[1] He was buried in the yard of the Calvary Church at Tarboro, North Carolina.

1. CSR; OR, vol. 11, pt. 2:839, 898–902; vol. 12, pt. 2:671; vol. 21:634, 647, 648; vol. 25, pt. 1:803, 926; vol. 27, pt. 2:298, 320, 447, 608, 658; A. L. Diket, Wha Hae Wi' (Pender) . . . Bled, 53, 67, 99, 157–58; Hassler, General to His Lady, 107, 123, 125, 126, 160–61, 169, 171, 260; S. T. Pender, "Life of General Pender," W. D. Pender Papers, SHC; W. D. Pender to Fanny Pender, Oct. 29, 1862, May 7, 9, 23, 1863, in W. D. Pender letters, SHC; Clark, Histories of Several Regiments 2:690; CV 33:96; CMH 4:334.

WILLIAM NELSON PENDLETON • Born December 26, 1809, in Richmond, Virginia. He graduated from USMA in 1830. While at Fort Moultrie in November 1830, Pendleton was confined to his bed with a violent ague followed by a high fever. He had been through the swamps in Carolina, and the doctor stated that he "almost" had yellow fever. Treatment consisted of a physic every two hours. Traveling across New Jersey in the summer of 1832, he developed fever and nausea and began vomiting. His limbs were paralyzed, and his hands and feet contracted in an unusual manner. Camphor and sugar made him feel better, but the fever continued and he required hospitalization. In October 1833 he resigned from the U.S. Army. He engaged in teaching and was ordained an Episcopal minister in 1837. He was very ill at Newark in 1838 with derangement of his liver and digestive tract. Despite vigorous internal and external treatment, Pendleton suffered considerably and was depressed. He was subjected to cupping and leeches for months. During 1839 he had a less serious bout of fever. For the next few years he taught and had a parish until 1853, when he became rector of a church in Lexington, Virginia. In May 1861 he was elected captain of the Rockbridge Artillery and in July was promoted to colonel on the staff of Gen. J. E. Johnston as chief of artillery. At the battle of First Manassas on July 21, 1861, Pendleton had his horse shot from under him. A bullet nipped his ear and another grazed his back. The first part of November he had deep jaundice, which had the characteristics of viral hepatitis. Although feeling weak and good-for-nothing, he was not as sick as he had been with previous illness. He remained in his room most of the time but walked a few yards every day, and his diet consisted of tea and dry toast. He used a number of remedies in an attempt to find a cure. Internally, he took calomel powders with a little carbonate soda after meals and tried a few tablespoonsful of bitter wine of iron. Externally, he put mustard plaster over the region of the stomach, duodenum, and liver and rubbed diluted nitromuriatic acid over the same area. None of these remedies helped, and he remained as yellow as "any white human being ever was." He intended to try a more effective purgative and warm sponge baths if he didn't improve. The vigorous doses of calomel and oil made him sicker for a few days, but by the middle of the month he was on horseback and able to be in camp. His appetite had obviously improved, as he had a breakfast of toast, broiled chicken, and tea, and his dinner consisted of cold mutton, roast turkey, roast beef, ham, sweet potatoes, pickles, and jellies. Surprisingly, he reported no discomfort. By November 21, 1862, the yellow tint of his eyes and skin had lessened and, except for an occasional bout of indigestion, he was strong enough to be about. After four days in the saddle in March 1862, he developed piles and had to rest and apply cold water to the area. That same month he was promoted to brigadier general. He had a fever on June 29 and took a blue pill, apparently a purge. He returned to the field the next day. On July 3, he had an injury to his right ankle from a horse kicking him and was incapacitated for a few days. The last of August, Pendleton had an episode of diarrhea, but with medical aid he was able to continue. Gen. Robert E. Lee urged him to find some place to rest and get well. Pendleton went with some of his staff to Mr. Foote's plantation, two miles north of Hay Market, where Gen. Isaac R. Trimble was recovering from a leg wound. On August 31, he was confined to his bed. His right side was blistered, supposedly to act on the liver. The side was very sore when he rode, but a quiet day relieved it greatly. He was physically exhausted on September 3 but gradually returned to his regular form by the seventh. Following the war he returned to his rectorship in Lexington, Virginia. In February 1873 his doctor reported that Pendleton's health required special care and that he would benefit by prudent travel.[1] He died January 15, 1883, at Lexington and was buried there in Jackson Memorial Cemetery.

DEATH CERTIFICATE: Cause of death, old age.

1. OR, vol. 11, pt. 2:536; vol. 12, pt. 3:926; vol. 19, pt. 1:829; vol. 51, pt. 1:36; Susan (Pendleton) Lee, *Memoirs of William Nelson Pendleton, D.D.*, 37–38, 50–51, 71, 73, 161–62; Edwin G. Lee to mother, July 22, 1861, W. N. Pendleton to wife, Nov. 5, 7, 21, 1861, Mar. 13, June 29, July 4, Aug. 31, 1862, and W. N. Pendleton to daughter, Nov. 16, 1861, all in W. N. Pendleton Papers, SHC; W. N. Pendleton to Joseph E. Johnston, Feb. 15, 1873, in Joseph E. Johnston Papers, CWM; Freeman, *Lee's Lieutenants* 2:226.

ABNER MONROE PERRIN · *Born February 2, 1827*, in Edgefield District, South Carolina. After the Mexican War he became a lawyer in South Carolina. Perrin entered Confederate service as a captain of the 14th South Carolina Brigade. While a captain, he was left sick at Leesburg on September 5, 1862. He was made a colonel in February 1863 and was commissioned brigadier general from September 1863. In the early morning hours of May 12, 1864, at Spotsylvania, Perrin was killed. He had come up leading his brigade through heavy fire and, pierced by seven balls, fell from his horse.[1] He was buried in the City Cemetery in Fredericksburg, Virginia.

1. CSR; OR, vol. 36, pt. 1:1030, pt. 2:993; CV 17:438.

EDWARD AYLESWORTH PERRY · *Born March 15, 1831*, in Richmond, Massachusetts. Perry was practicing law in Florida in 1861 when he raised a Florida company that became part of the 2nd Florida Infantry. Initially a company captain, he was elected colonel of the regiment in May 1862. He was severely wounded at Frayser's Farm on June 30, 1862, during the Seven Days' battles. His promotion to brigadier general ranked from August 1862. That autumn, when he had recovered, he was put in command of the newly organized Florida Brigade, which he led at Chancellorsville in May 1863. Soon afterward he contracted typhoid and was not at Gettysburg. He returned to his brigade in late September. In the Battle of the Wilderness on May 6, 1864, Perry was wounded again. He rode up to his men quite slowly and, bleeding freely, had to be helped from his horse. He was transferred from Howard's Grove Hospital to a general hospital in Alabama on June 5 and given a forty-day furlough. On September 3, 1864, he returned but was not able to go on duty in the trenches as his wound made him unfit to serve on foot. Finally, on September 28, he was ordered to report for duty with the reserves of Alabama. After the war he returned to his law practice and was elected governor of Florida in 1884. Perry died suddenly from a stroke on October 15, 1889, while visiting Kerrville, Texas.[1] He was buried at Pensacola, Florida, in St. John's Cemetery.

DEATH CERTIFICATE: NAD

1. CSR; OR, vol. 11, pt. 2:760; vol. 14:629; vol. 39, pt. 2:883; vol. 42, pt. 2:1232–33; Oates, *War between the Union and the Confederacy*, 350; CMH 11:105, 156–57, 207, Fla.; *Dictionary of American Biography*, s.v. "Perry, Edward Aylesworth."

WILLIAM FLANK PERRY · *Born March 12, 1823*, in Jackson County, Georgia. Self-educated, he was elected Alabama's first superintendent of public instruction and became president of the East Alabama Female College in 1858. In May 1862 he left this position and enlisted as a private in the 44th Alabama. By the middle of May he had become major of the regiment; as of September of that year he was lieutenant colonel. His appointment to colonel, which was made in 1864, was back dated to September 1862. In the Devil's Den at Gettysburg on July 2, 1863, a spherical case shot exploded near his head. Later when he tried to get to his feet, he was unable to stand without support. This disability continued until after nightfall and prevented him from seeing much of the fighting. In August 1864 at New Market Heights, some two miles below Drewry's Bluff, he tumbled into a hole made by a Federal gunboat shell and sprained his ankle. He received a medical furlough through September. His promotion to brigadier general ranked from February 1865. After the war, he spent two years as a farmer and then went to Kentucky, where he again became a teacher. In October 1900, because of poor health, he resigned his professorship at Ogden College, Bowling Green, Kentucky.[1] He died at Bowling Green on December 17, 1901, and was buried there in Fairview Cemetery. Cause of death: Pneumonia.[2]

1. CSR; *OR*, vol. 46, pt. 1:1277; Oates, *War between the Union and the Confederacy*, 228–29, 373; Jesse B. Johnson and Lowell H. Harrison, "Ogden College: A Brief History," *Register of the Kentucky Historical Society* 68:189–220.

2. Burial permits, Warren County, Ky., 1877–1913, 2.

JAMES JOHNSTON PETTIGREW • *Born July 4, 1828*, in Tyrrell County, North Carolina. Sickly as an infant and during early childhood, Pettigrew, due to an "unfortunate exposure," was weak and could not tolerate temperature extremes. Precocious in spite of continued episodes of poor health, he passed the examination for the University of North Carolina a month before his fifteenth birthday. In May 1848, while he was studying law in Baltimore, he had an attack of chills and fever, which was followed the next summer by measles. He undertook a prolonged trip to Europe; following an episode of ague while in Berlin in 1850, he spent a month in a spa near Frankfurt. He was in Paris in April 1852 when the ague returned, and he was under a doctor's care for six weeks. He returned to the United States that same year and again was ill with the ague. In addition to his usual medical problems he had an eye infection in the summer of 1854, yellow fever in 1858, and "break-bone fever" in 1860. In November 1860, Pettigrew became a colonel of the First Regiment of Rifles of South Carolina and in January was with his troops at Fort Morris, not far from Fort Sumter. He resigned from the militia, was elected colonel of the 22nd North Carolina in July 1861, and was promoted to brigadier in February 1862. At Seven Pines on May 31, 1862, Pettigrew was wounded. The first ball entered the lower part of his throat, struck the windpipe, passed under the collarbone, and tore the bones of the shoulder. It cut an artery, and he would have bled to death had it not been for Colonel Bull. By this time Pettigrew was unconscious. Subsequently, he received another shot in the left arm and a bayonet wound in the right leg. When he regained consciousness, he thought he had been mortally wounded and refused to be taken to the rear. Insensible, he lay on the field all night and woke up a prisoner. He was taken to a farmhouse that had been converted to a hospital and was locked in the smoke-house. A physician who examined him sent him, limping and under guard, to the rear. Finally, he arrived at a house where he remained for over a week. He was transported to Fortress Monroe and then to Baltimore by steamer. Here he was allowed to remain at Guy's Monument House Hotel under medical treatment until his quarters became a public issue. He was ordered to Fort Delaware in spite of some question of his being able to withstand the trip because of his condition. He requested to be sent back to Baltimore on parole in July to have a galvanic battery applied to his paralyzed arm. The application was not granted. He was exchanged at Aiken Landing, Virginia, on August 5. After arrival back to duty, he was assigned to the command of Petersburg on August 11 and given a brigade. At Gettysburg on July 3, 1863, his horse was killed. The bones of Pettigrew's right hand were crushed by a grapeshot, but he remained on the field with his hand in splints. With assistance, he was one of the last to leave the field. In the retreat to the Potomac, Pettigrew was in command of a portion of the rear guard. He was fatally wounded on July 14, 1863, at Falling Waters, Maryland, during an attack by Federal cavalry. At the beginning of the fight, Pettigrew's horse was frightened by the gunfire and plunged. Pettigrew, who because of his injured right hand and prior shoulder wound had trouble managing the horse, fell with him. Rising in pain, Pettigrew saw a Federal soldier in the act of firing on his men. Drawing his pistol, he approached the soldier when a pistol ball hit him in the left side of the abdomen just above the hip, passed downward, and came out in the back. Medical officers reported that his chance of recovery depended on quiet care. They suggested placing him in a nearby barn and entrusting him to the Federal surgeons, but he would not consent to being a prisoner again. Placed on a litter, he was carried across the river and, over a two-day period, was taken to the Boyd home near Bunker Hill, a distance of twenty-two miles. He expired there on July 17, 1863, probably from peritonitis.[1] He was buried at the family home, "Bonarva," which is now in the Pettigrew State Park in Tyrrell County, North Carolina.

1. CSR; *OR*, vol. 9:480; vol. 11, pt. 1:749, 810, 991, 992, pt. 3:672; vol. 27, pt. 2:310, 323, 640–41, 644, 651; ser. 2, vol. 4:18, 25–26, 40, 313–14; Paul E. Steiner, "Medical-Military Studies in the Civil War. 6. Brigadier General James Johnston Pettigrew, C.S.A.," *Military Medicine* 130:930–37; Walter Clark, "General James Pettigrew, C.S.A.," *North Carolina Booklet* 20:171–80; Clyde N. Wilson, *Carolina Cavalier: The Life and Mind of James Johnston Pettigrew*, 6, 27–28, 33, 44, 59–60, 67, 79, 82–85, 164–69; *CMH* 4:196–97; *SHSP* 26:144; Clark, *Histories of Several Regiments* 2:334, 358, 366, 375–77, 4:559–61.

EDMUND WINSTON PETTUS · *Born July 6, 1821, in Limestone County, Alabama.* A practicing attorney, he was elected major of the 20th Alabama following secession. In October 1861 he was elected lieutenant colonel of the regiment. During the summer of 1863 he was promoted to colonel, and his obvious courage earned his brigadier's stars in September 1863. Near Bentonville, North Carolina, on March 19, 1865, he received a flesh wound in the right leg. However, he remained with his brigade until it was withdrawn to its original line. He was hospitalized on March 20 in Raleigh and sent to Greensboro in April. After the war he returned to his law practice in Alabama and entered politics. During the summer of 1874 he was ill. In 1896 he was elected to the United States Senate and served in this capacity until his death on July 27, 1907, at Hot Springs, North Carolina.[1] He was buried at Selma, Alabama, in Live Oak Cemetery.

DEATH CERTIFICATE: NAD

1. CSR; *OR*, vol. 47, pt. 1:1091, 1096; *CMH* 12:436, Ala.; E. W. Pettus to Jos. E. Johnston, June 25, 1874, in Joseph E. Johnston Papers, CWM.

GEORGE EDWARD PICKETT · *Born January 28, 1825,* at Richmond, Virginia. He graduated from USMA in 1846. Served in the Mexican War. Pickett resigned from the U.S. Army in June 1861 and was appointed major of artillery in the Confederate Regular Army. In July he was made a colonel and was promoted to brigadier general to rank from January 1862. In an assault at Cold Harbor on June 27, 1862, Pickett was wounded in the shoulder. John Haskell, who saw Pickett standing in a deep hollow after he was wounded, thought he was capable of taking care of himself and did not send for a litter. However, recovery took three months, part of which he spent in Richmond with his sister. Pickett resumed brigade command in late September. On his return, his shoulder and arm were still stiff and he could not wear a coat sleeve on his injured arm. Because he could not lift his hand very high, he had to bend his neck way over to reach his mouth while eating, and someone had to assist in buttoning his collar. In October 1862 he was promoted to major general. At Petersburg, on May 5, 1864, Pickett collapsed and took to his bed with nervous exhaustion, which was vaguely diagnosed as fever. Although back in the field by the middle of June, he was sick again for a few days in August.[1] Pickett returned to Virginia after the war and became an insurance agent. He died July 30, 1875, at Norfolk, Virginia, and was buried in Hollywood Cemetery at Richmond.

DEATH CERTIFICATE: Cause of death, abscess of liver.

1. CSR; *OR*, vol. 11, pt. 2:564, 758–59, 767, 980; vol. 40, pt. 1:760, pt. 2:659; Haskell, *Memoirs*, 32; George Edward Pickett, *Soldier of the South: General Pickett's War Letters to his Wife*, 18, 23–25, 96, 114; *SHSP* 25:206; William Glenn Robertson, *Back Door to Richmond: The Bermuda Hundred Campaign, April–June 1864*, 128, 140.

ALBERT PIKE · *Born December 29, 1809,* in Boston, Massachusetts. Served in the Mexican War. Traveling with a wagon train along the east slope of the Sangre de Cristo mountains on the way to Santa Fe in November 1831, Pike suffered frost-bitten feet during a blizzard. He arrived at Fort Smith in December 1832 suffering from malaria and with his legs lacerated and infected. He stayed there to improve his health, but after a brief remission, his recovery was delayed when his chills and fever recurred in January. Prior to his marriage in the fall of 1834, he had another bout of malaria. As a practicing lawyer in Little Rock, Pike, a compulsive eater who weighed between 275 and 300 pounds, would starve himself when plagued with a troublesome case. When the problem was resolved, he would fill a wagon with food and along with a cook go into the woods. There he would gorge himself around the clock for days. On July 29, 1847, on a sandbar in the Arkansas River near Fort Smith, Pike met future Confederate general John Selden Roane for a duel. The argument was prompted by Roane belittling Pike's participation in the Battle of Buena Vista in Mexico. Each combatant had fired two shots without anyone being hit before an armistice was called. Pike was commissioned a Confederate brigadier general in August 1861 and was to negotiate with the Indians so they would join the South. While conducting treaty negotiations with the Plains Indians in the summer of 1861, he was stricken with such severe cramps from drinking gyp water that he had to be taken back to the Wichita Agency. In July 1862, Pike complained that he was too corpulent to ride a horse very much, and that he had sudden attacks of neuralgia in his back that disabled him for days at a time. Because of his health and trouble with other Confederate officers, he resigned his commission that month. He lived in Memphis a few years after the war but then moved to Washington, D.C., where he wrote and was active in Masonic affairs. His health began to fail in the fall of 1889, and he was afflicted by a number of medical problems all at once. He had headaches, fevers, gout, boils, rheumatism, neuralgia, and dyspepsia. Even picking up a pen caused pain in his fingers. The attacks continued during the spring and summer of 1890. He took to his bed in October and never left it again. By the first of the year, his voice had become hoarse, and he could take only liquids. A diagnosis of esophageal stricture was made, but he refused any dilatations. In March there were further bouts of gout, fever, and rheumatism, and he continued to weaken. Finally, when nothing would go through his esophagus, five attempts at dilatation were made, but all failed. Starvation contributed to his death on April 2, 1891, in Washington, D.C.[1] He was buried there in Oak Hill Cemetery.

DEATH CERTIFICATE: Cause of death, primary, esophageal stricture, about one year's duration; immediate, pyaemia, about ten days' duration. Total illness about five months.

1. OR, vol. 13:957; Robert Lipscomb Duncan, *Reluctant General: The Life and Times of Albert Pike*, 29, 53–54, 56, 78, 129–30, 147, 179–81, 272–73; Donovan, *Governors of Arkansas*, 17–22.

GIDEON JOHNSON PILLOW · *Born June 8, 1806*, in Williamson County, Tennessee. He was appointed brigadier general of volunteers in 1846 and was later advanced to the grade of major general. At Churubusco, Mexico, on August 20, 1847, he was wounded in the arm and never recovered from its effects. During the attack at Chapultepec on September 13, 1847, Pillow was wounded in the ankle by grapeshot. He convalesced in Mexico City in the winter of 1847–48 and was discharged in July 1848. Pillow was made the senior major general of Tennessee's provisional army when that state seceded from the Union; the following July he was commissioned brigadier general in the Confederate Army. Following the Civil War he was an attorney in Memphis, Tennessee. Pillow died of yellow fever on his plantation near Helena, Arkansas, on October 8, 1878.[1] He was buried in Elmwood Cemetery at Memphis.

DEATH CERTIFICATE: NAD

1. *CV* 1:329–30; Cummings, "Seven Ohio Confederate Generals," 414–16; French, *Two Wars*, 87; *Memphis Press-Scimitar*, Mar. 11, 1878.

CAMILLE ARMAND JULES MARIE PRINCE DE POLIGNAC • *Born February 16, 1832*, at Millemont, Seine-et-Oise, France. Polignac served in the French army from 1853 to 1859. Through his acquaintance with P. G. T. Beauregard, he offered his service to the Confederacy and was appointed a lieutenant colonel of infantry in July 1861. He had a headache on June 15, 1862, and was unfit for duty. The following January he was promoted to brigadier general. On May 30–31, 1863, he had inflammation of his mouth, tongue, palate, and lips. The suggested therapy was three drams of borax and two ounces of pure rose water with an equal weight of honey. His promotion as major general ranked from April 1864. Early in August 1864, de Polignac had his second attack of fever in two years. The following month the fever recurred along with chills, which came every couple of days for a week.[1] He returned to France after the war and studied mathematics for the rest of his life, except for a period in which he fought in the Franco-Prussian War. He died November 15, 1913, at Frankfort-on-Main, Germany.

DEATH CERTIFICATE: NAD

1. Camille Polignac Diary of the War Between the States, *CWTI* Coll., USAMHI.

LEONIDAS POLK • *Born April 10, 1806*, in Raleigh, North Carolina. He graduated from USMA in 1827, after which he resigned and entered the Episcopal ministry. He was in poor health during the late 1820s and 1830s, having inherited a tendency to pulmonary problems, and traveled frequently for his health. In March 1836 he woke up partially paralyzed and with his speech impaired. He had a similar attack the following month. Treatment consisted of bleeding, cupping, and nux vomica, and his recovery was slow. In the spring of 1849 he had cholera, and in the fall of 1854 he had yellow fever. He was appointed major general in the Confederate Provisional Army in June 1861. At Columbus, Kentucky, in November 1861, an eight-ton rifled Dahlgren gun called the "Lady Polk" had a shot left in it after the battle ended. As it cooled, the gun contracted on the retained shot. Later, on November 11, when Polk was watching the gunfire, the "Lady Polk" burst, killing some of the nearby troops. Polk was knocked down and his eardrums were injured. Stunned, he was carried to his headquarters. On the thirteenth, Polk's physician said that rest was an absolute necessity. By the twenty-sixth Polk's system was shocked, and there were indications of a more serious injury than was first supposed. At last, he was able to assume command again in December 1861. By the end of the month, although his health was good, it was thought he needed more exercise. He was promoted to lieutenant general to rank from October 1862. Polk was not well and suffered from rheumatism in September 1863, and again was in poor health in December. He was killed instantly at an outpost on Pine Mountain near Marietta, Georgia, on June 14, 1864. A Parrott shell passed through his left arm, body, and right arm before emerging to explode against a tree. The trunk of the chestnut tree struck by the shell was still standing in 1902.[1] Polk was first buried in Augusta, Georgia. Later, his remains were moved to the Christ Church Cathedral in New Orleans, Louisiana.

1. CSR; *OR*, vol. 3:313, 330, 739; vol. 4:550; vol. 7:692, 694–95, 705, 758; vol. 30, pt. 1:72, 77; vol. 38, pt. 1:223, 243; vol. 52, pt. 2:206, 242; Joseph Howard Parks, *General Leonidas Polk, C.S.A.: The Fighting Bishop*, 74, 109, 112; *CV* 3:88, 10:204, 12:118–19, 277–78, 439; *CMH* 1:663; *SHSP* 18:381; Buck, *Cleburne and his Command*, 223–24.

LUCIUS EUGENE POLK • *Born July 10, 1833*, in Salisbury, North Carolina. Leaving his farm in Arkansas in 1861, he enlisted as a private in the Yell Rifles. He was wounded in the face at Shiloh in April 1862. Polk was promoted from second lieutenant to colonel of his regiment that same month and was back on the field in command in May. He was wounded in the head at Richmond, Kentucky, on August 30, 1862, and was as "wild as a March hare." While he was being taken to the rear, Patrick Ronayne Cleburne stopped to talk to him and was wounded himself. Polk reported back the day before the Battle of Perryville, where on October 8, 1862, he was wounded in the foot. In December he was promoted to brigadier general and was ordered to report for assignment. He was able to take part in the battle at Murfreesborough. He was ill for a short time in March 1864. On June 16, 1864, east of Mud Creek, Georgia, his horse was shot from under him, and he was wounded. (Other reported dates for this wound include May 17, June 14, June 17, and June 27.) A cannonball had passed over the outer portion of Polk's left leg and fractured the bone. The head of the fibula was surgically removed, along with the fractured portions, and the wound was dressed on the field. Litter bearers carried him to Cleburne's headquarters. On June 20, the bandages were removed and the wound was redressed. By July 1, the wound was doing well; all the dead portions had sloughed off, and there was healthy granulation tissue. His general health was good. The wound permanently incapacitated him for further field duty, however, and he returned to his home on crutches. He entered politics in Tennessee after the war and was elected state senator in 1887. Four weeks after returning to Columbia, Tennessee, following his son's marriage in Pennsylvania, he became ill and died December 1, 1892, from typhoid-dysentery.[1] He was buried in St. John's Churchyard at Ashwood near Columbia.

DEATH CERTIFICATE: NAD

1. *OR*, vol. 10, pt. 2:520; vol. 16, pt. 1:936, 946, 950; vol. 20, pt. 1:852, pt. 2:449; *CR*, 764:102; James Cooper Nisbet, *Four Years on the Firing Line*, 199; *CMH* 10:410, Ark.; Liddell, *Liddell's Record*, 96; Brown, *One of Cleburne's Command*, 95–96; Buck, *Cleburne and his Command*, 203, 224; *CV* 1:295; *Columbia (Tenn.) Maury Democrat*, Dec. 8, 1892.

CARNOT POSEY • *Born August 5, 1818*, in Wilkinson County, Mississippi. He was slightly wounded on February 23, 1847, in the fighting at Buena Vista during the Mexican War. After returning home from the war he was appointed United States district attorney in Mississippi and held this position until 1861. He recruited the Wilkinson Rifles and was elected its captain. The following June he was elected colonel of the 16th Mississippi Infantry. At the Battle of Cross Keys, Virginia, on

June 8, 1862, he was wounded and carried by litter bearers to the rear. Incapacitated from active duty for two months, he reported back before he was fully recovered. A surgeon later told William L. Brandon that he had expected Posey to die from this wound because he was so despondent, nervous, and easily depressed. He stated that he had told Posey that half of his regiment would be glad to have a similar wound if they could get a thirty-day furlough. His promotion to brigadier general ranked from November 1862. At Bristoe Station, Virginia, on October 14, 1863, Posey was wounded in the left thigh by a shell fragment. He was admitted to the receiving hospital at Gordonsville, Virginia, on October 23 and transferred the same day to the hospital at Charlottesville. Infection set in, and he died in the home of a friend on November 13, 1863. He was buried in the University Cemetery on the grounds of the University of Virginia.[1]

1. CSR; OR, vol. 12, pt. 1:784; vol. 29, pt. 1:427, 429; Wm. L. Brandon in J. F. H. Claiborne Papers, SHC; Register Book, Receiving Hospital, Gordonsville, Va., June 1, 1863–May 5, 1864, 305, Eleanor S. Brockenbrough Library, MC; CMH 12:265, Miss.; Nisbet, Four Years, 53.

JOHN SMITH PRESTON • Born April 20, 1809, at Salt Works near Abingdon, Virginia. A prewar attorney and member of the South Carolina state senate, he lived in Europe from 1856 to 1860. When the war started he was appointed lieutenant colonel and served on P. G. T. Beauregard's staff. He was made colonel in April 1863 and brigadier general in June 1864. During the war he mainly served in conscription. Preston moved to England after the war and returned to the United States in 1868. He died May 1, 1881, at Columbia, South Carolina, and was buried in the cemetery at the Trinity Episcopal Church.

DEATH CERTIFICATE: NAD

WILLIAM PRESTON • Born October 16, 1816, near Louisville, Kentucky. After serving in the Mexican War, Preston was engaged in politics. He served in Congress from Kentucky and was appointed minister to Spain in 1858. He joined the Confederacy as a colonel on the staff of Albert S. Johnston, and in April 1862 he was appointed brigadier general. During July and August 1862, Preston remained in Vicksburg because he was prostrated with fever. He left Chattanooga on September 20 for Kentucky and in December was given brigade command. In early June 1863 he had a bout of fever. By the middle of the month, although his strength had improved, he had pain in his left eye, and his doctor reported he had iritis. At the close of the war he traveled to Mexico, England, and Canada before returning to Kentucky in 1866 and reentering politics. He died on September 21, 1887, in Lexington, Kentucky, and was buried in the Cave Hill Cemetery in Louisville, Kentucky.[1] Cause of death: Rheumatic gout.[2]

1. OR, vol. 16, pt. 2:862; vol. 20, pt. 2:417, 448; William Preston Johnston to wife, Aug. 11, 1862, and William Preston to William Preston Johnston, June 18, 1863, both in Johnston Family Papers (1798–1943), FC; CMH 9:76, Ky.; Thompson, History of the Orphan Brigade, 368.
2. Burial records, Cave Hill Cemetery Company, Inc., Louisville, Ky.

STERLING PRICE • *Born September 20, 1809,* in Prince Edward County, Virginia. During the Mexican War, before arriving with his men at Santa Fe on September 28, 1846, he became seriously ill with cholera. In late October, Price had recovered sufficiently to assume command of the territory. However, he had a relapse and was very ill in November and December. During the mid-1850s his chronic diarrhea improved for a while. He was governor of Missouri from 1853 to 1857 and was in command of the Missouri militia in May 1861. In June, Price had dysentery and had to be carried to Lexington. By late July he was able to be taken in an ambulance to Cowskin Prairie near Cassville. On August 10, 1861, at Wilson's Creek, Price was slightly wounded in the side but did not leave the field. The next day he moved his troops to Springfield. He received a flesh wound in the arm at the Battle of Elkhorn on March 7, 1862, but put on a sling and would not leave the field. During the retreat, he rode in an ambulance because of weakness from loss of blood. His commission as major general in the Confederate Army ranked from March. On April 29, he was in the Tishomingo Hotel in Corinth, Mississippi, which was being used as a hospital. When introduced to nurse Kate Cumming, he had to offer her his left hand because his right arm was disabled by the wound. Although in bad health, he could not be induced to stay there longer and left the next day to be with his troops. The last of July 1864, Price wanted his two physicians to go with him to Shreveport because he had been sick and might need them. In January 1865 there were many rumors about Price's death. Following the war he went to Mexico. While at Veracruz in May 1866, his old intestinal problem recurred, along with weight loss. That August, while he and his family were in Córdoba, he had typhoid fever and his condition deteriorated. His family feared for his life, and in December they all left Mexico for Missouri. In January 1867, he was described as a bald, bent, shrunken old man. A short recovery period occurred in March; however, the disease relapsed and he went to a spa at Baden Springs, Indiana. Severe diarrhea forced him to return to St. Louis. Cholera-like symptoms continued until his death on September 29, 1867, in St. Louis. He was buried in Bellefontaine Cemetery in that city.[1]

DEATH CERTIFICATE: Cause of death, chronic diarrhea.

1. *OR,* vol. 3:106; vol. 8:281, 285; vol. 48, pt. 1:1320, 1342; Shalhope, *Sterling Price,* 59–62, 130, 167, 177–79, 205–7, 286–90; Horn, *Army of Tennessee,* 22–23; *CMH* 9:58, Mo.; Cumming, *Kate,* 27–28; Bevier, *History of First and Second Missouri,* 113–14; William H. McPheeters Civil War Diary—June 1, 1863, to June 20, 1865, July 30, August 1, 1864, William M. McPheeters Papers, MHS.

ROGER ATKINSON PRYOR • *Born July 19, 1828,* near Petersburg, Virginia. After establishing his law practice, he developed a serious problem with his throat in 1850. Ordered to a warmer climate and not to speak in or out of court, he became a journalist. During the surrender of Fort Sumter in April 1861, Pryor, a volunteer aide to P. G. T. Beauregard, was sent as an emissary to the fort. He saw a bottle on the table in the unused hospital that he thought contained brandy. After drinking some of it, he read the label and discovered it was potassium iodine. The Federal surgeon treated him with purging, pumping, and puking. Pryor entered

Confederate service as colonel of the 3rd Virginia Infantry and was promoted to brigadier general in April 1862. Following the Battle of Seven Pines in June 1862, Pryor had malaria and was confined to his tent a few miles outside of Richmond. Mrs. Pryor went out, brought him back into Richmond, and put him in the Spotswood Hotel. His doctor reported that all Pryor wanted was buttermilk. Although still weak and not yet discharged by his doctor, he returned on July 26, when orders came requesting he rejoin his troops. He resigned from the Confederate Army on August 18, 1863, and served without rank as a cavalry courier. Following the war in late 1895, while serving on the New York Supreme Court, he had much pain, and surgery was recommended. Some nights the pain was so severe that he could not sleep and walked about the room all night. However, he wanted to finish the January court docket before he had any surgery. On February 7, 1896, under an anesthetic, he had what was called, without any further details, a dangerous operation. The procedure was performed in his home with a number of surgeons in attendance. He slept soundly the next two nights without the need for narcotics. His diet was restricted to chicken broth until February 9, when he was allowed a small bird and a cold bottle. Early in 1919, he developed an illness that lasted for several weeks before his death. He died in New York City on March 14, 1919, and was buried in Princeton, New Jersey, in the Princeton cemetery.[1]

DEATH CERTIFICATE: Cause of death, pneumonia with pulmonary embolism; contributory, old age.

1. Robert S. Holtzman, *Adapt or Perish: The Life of General Roger A. Pryor, C.S.A.*, 14, 19–20, 60, 132, 156; Mrs. Roger Pryor, *Reminiscences of Peace and War*, 172–74; *New-York Daily Tribune*, Feb. 10, 1896.

WILLIAM ANDREW QUARLES • *Born July 4, 1825*, near Jamestown, Virginia. Quarles practiced law, was a circuit court judge, state bank supervisor, and president of a railroad before the war. In 1861 he was elected colonel of the 42nd Tennessee Infantry. He suffered with chronic diarrhea, which relapsed in March 1863. His promotion as brigadier general ranked from August 1863. Quarles was severely wounded on July 28, 1864, in the battle around Atlanta on the Lickskillet Road. Bishop Quintard nursed him back to health. At Franklin, on November 30, 1864, the middle third of his left humerus was fractured by a cannonball. Unable to get away, he was captured on December 18 in a house by the roadside at which he was recovering and was taken to a hospital in Nashville. Continuing to suffer from his wound, he was paroled in May 1865.[1] Quarles returned to his law practice and politics in Tennessee after the war. He died December 28, 1893, in Logan County, Kentucky, and was buried in the Cumberland Presbyterian graveyard in Christian County, Kentucky.

DEATH CERTIFICATE: NAD

1. CSR; *OR*, vol. 45, pt. 1:654, 685, 708, 721, 722, pt. 2:250, 252; vol. 49, pt. 2:581; Head, *Sixteenth Regiment, Tennessee Volunteers*, 326–27.

R

GABRIEL JAMES RAINS • *Born June 4, 1803*, in Craven County, North Carolina. Graduated from USMA in 1827. Near Fort King during the Florida War on April 28, 1840, he was severely wounded.[1] He resigned from the United States Army and was appointed a Confederate brigadier in September 1861. His greatest contribution was the development of the antipersonnel mine and of various torpedoes. Following the war he was a chemist in Augusta and continued his interest in explosives. Rains died August 6, 1881, in Aiken, South Carolina, and was buried there in the St. Thaddeus Cemetery.

DEATH CERTIFICATE: NAD

1. Heitman, *Historical Register and Dictionary* 2:34; *CMH* 4:339; *SHSP* 10:39.

JAMES EDWARDS RAINS • *Born April 10, 1833*, in Nashville, Tennessee. He had been a district attorney general when, at the outbreak of the war in 1861, he enlisted as a private in the 11th Tennessee Infantry. His election as colonel of the regiment occurred in May 1861 and his promotion to brigadier in November 1862. During the Battle of Murfreesborough, on December 31, 1862, he was killed almost instantly by a minié ball, which cut the gauntlet on his right hand and passed into his chest. He fell from his horse, and his body was captured by the Federal troops. Rains was first buried on the battlefield; later his remains were removed to Mt. Olivet Cemetery, Nashville.[1]

1. *OR*, vol. 20, pt. 1:670, 775, 913, 927, 938–39; Clark, *Histories of Several Regiments* 2:489.

STEPHEN DODSON RAMSEUR • *Born May 31, 1837*, at Lincolnton, North Carolina. Graduated from USMA in 1860. While at West Point he was on the sick list thirty-seven times. During his third year there, he had chronic headaches that made him unfit for duty. He resigned his commission in April 1861, and by May he was a major of artillery in the Confederate service. On July 25, 1861, at Raleigh, Ramseur broke his collarbone when he was thrown from his horse during a severe storm. He was able to return to duty on the twenty-ninth. In September he had a severe bout of typhoid fever and was cared for by a couple in Smithfield. He was elected colonel of the 49th North Carolina in April 1862. During the charge at Malvern Hill on July 1, 1862, a ball broke his right arm above the elbow, rendering it useless. He did not want to leave the field, but because of the serious nature of the wound, he was transported that night to a private home in Richmond. The median nerve was either damaged or severed. He was given a sixty-day leave on July 10. After a month he was able to withstand the journey home, but severe pain in his arm continued. Still bothered by paralysis of the arm and severe enough pain to require frequent morphine, he returned to Richmond for treatment on October 25. The surgeon thought that the ball had carried clothing into the wound, and that surgery would be required for complete healing. In November he was promoted to brigadier general, and in the middle of the month he returned to North Carolina. Early in January 1863 he was in Richmond with his arm in a sling. His arm looked as though it would be useless for a long time, but he returned to his command that month. Although he had to write with his left hand, he had fewer episodes of severe pain that winter. At Chancellorsville on May 3, 1863, Ramseur was hit on the leg by a shell fragment but remained on the field for the whole action. He was admitted to a general hospital in Richmond and treated for a severe and painful contusion of the shin. After recuperating in North Carolina, he rejoined his command in late May. In June, with his arm still in a sling, he was of so little use that a woman with whom he dined had to cut his food. However, he fought at Gettysburg the following month. At the Bloody Angle of Spotsylvania Court-House on May 12, 1864, a ball passed through his right arm below the elbow. Although painfully wounded, Ramseur refused to leave the field, but he could not participate in the charge. On the fourteenth he had difficulty keeping up with the troops, but by the nineteenth he was able to lead an attack against the Federal flank. His nomination to the command of Jubal A. Early's division in late May depended on his health being equal to the duty. By May 31, the arm was almost healed. He was assigned to temporary command and promoted to major general in June 1864 but was ill from lack of sleep, poor food, and bad water. During the summer he lost some of his hair. At the Battle of Cedar Creek, on October 19, 1864, Ramseur received a minor wound, and two of his horses were killed. Later, Ramseur was mounting his third horse when it too was shot. Immediately afterward, Ramseur was wounded by a minié ball. As this occurred behind Federal lines, he was taken to the rear first by horseback, with an officer running alongside to prevent him from falling, and then by ambulance. Travel was slow because the road was clogged with other vehicles. He was taken prisoner south of Strasburg and surrendered to a Federal surgeon. Taken to Belle Grove, Philip H. Sheridan's headquarters, he was visited by many of his old West Point friends. The ball had entered the right side of his chest, traversed the right and left lung, and had lodged near the left chest wall. A Confederate surgeon, assisted by a Federal surgeon, attended him, but apparently because of the nature of his wound, no active treatment was undertaken. The surgeon gave him wineglass after wineglass full of laudanum or opiate until he was unconscious, and he remained in this state until he died the following day. The night before the battle, Ramseur had told John B. Gordon that he thought he would die the next day. He was buried in St. Luke's Church Cemetery at Lincolnton, North Carolina.[1]

1. CSR; *OR*, vol. 11, pt. 2:793, 795; vol. 25, pt. 1:889, 947, 994; vol. 36, pt. 1:1073, 1082, pt. 3:873–74; vol. 43, pt. 1:553, 560, 562, 564; Gallagher, *Stephen Dodson Ramseur*, 21, 25, 32–33, 44–50, 64–65, 110, 117, 120, 138, 162, 179; Special Order no. 159, Richmond, July 10, 1862, R. R. Hutchinson to Mrs. S. D. Ramseur,

Oct. 20, 1864, and Address by Col. Henry A. DuPont given Sept. 16, 1920, Stephen D. Ramseur Papers, NCSA; J. A. Young to Bryan Grimes, Jan. 25, 1863, in Bryan Grimes Papers, NCSA; Paul E. Steiner, "Medical-Military Studies on the Civil War. 7. Major General Stephen D. Ramseur, C.S.A.," *Military Medicine* 130:1016–22; *SHSP* 18:185–88, 229, 256–57; *CMH* 4:341; Gordon, *Reminiscences*, 63–64.

GEORGE WYTHE RANDOLPH • *Born March 10, 1818,* at "Monticello" near Charlottesville, Virginia. While a young midshipman aboard the United States *Constitution* in early 1836, Randolph had influenza and required hospitalization at Smyrna, Turkey. It has been postulated that this actually was acute tuberculosis and the onset of the condition that was later to contribute to his death. Randolph resigned from the navy in 1839 and studied the law. A case of mumps in the summer of 1841 caused him to be quarantined. In late July 1851, terrible pain just below the chest, accompanied by severe prostration, was self-diagnosed by Randolph as dyspepsia. That year he moved to Richmond where he soon started participating in local militia affairs and organized the Richmond Howitzers. Similar episodes of dyspepsia bothered him periodically during the prewar years. His health was poor in the summer of 1858, and the following fall he had attacks of laryngitis and spat up a blood clot. In April 1861, Randolph and his militia unit were officially taken into state service. By 1861 he already had the appearance of a man with poor health. Ill from bronchitis in the autumn of 1861, Randolph was forced to take sick leave to recuperate at his family's estate. He was promoted to brigadier general to rank from February 1862 and the following month accepted a position in the Confederate cabinet. In 1862, his Virginia medical consultants advised that by limiting his activities and avoiding cold and damp conditions, his tuberculosis could be stabilized. In November 1862 he reported that he was too ill for a field command and desired a staff position. His bronchial troubles continued to bother him during the war years, and in 1864 he consulted two professors of the University of Virginia Medical School. They diagnosed his case as chronic tuberculosis and noted that his right lung had partly solidified. He was advised to move to a different climate and to consult pulmonary specialists in London. Although only in his late forties, his face was very wrinkled. He and his wife first took a blockade runner and then a British steamer, arriving in Liverpool in November 1864. He caught a cold, which caused his voice and cough to worsen. The specialists, however, reported that his bronchitis was more of a threat than the tuberculosis, which they thought was arrested. The disease had supposedly cleared from the right lung, and the left lung was much improved. They advised he winter in southern France and return the next spring for an examination. In February 1865, while in France, he experienced a series of hemorrhages, apparently from his lungs, and was completely debilitated. Since he was feeble, his wife fed him beef essence and wine whey. When reexamined in London in June, his condition was considered to have worsened; rather than go back home to Virginia, he was advised to return to France for the climate. Finally, in September 1866 he and his wife traveled to New York. The following month his condition became worse, and he never spoke again above a whisper. Because he was weak, his wife had to wash and almost dress him. On April 3, 1867, the day of his death, while at the family estate near Charlottesville, he supposedly regained his voice long enough to repent his former agnosticism. He was buried at Monticello, Virginia, near his grandfather, President Thomas Jefferson.[1]

DEATH CERTIFICATE: NAD

1. George Green Shackelford, *George Wythe Randolph and the Confederate Elite*, 14, 23, 27–28, 34, 49, 62, 78, 148–49, 151, 153, 160–61.

MATT WHITAKER RANSOM • *Born October 8, 1826*, in Warren County, North Carolina. He served in the lower house of North Carolina from 1858 to 1861. After enlisting as a private, he was commissioned lieutenant colonel of the 1st North Carolina ranking from May 1861. Ransom was absent from Camp Bee, Virginia, in September 1861 because of illness but returned in October. His promotion to colonel ranked from April 1862. At Malvern Hill on July 1, 1862, a wound in his right arm rendered it useless. He also was hit on the right side by a shell fragment. Unable to continue on the field, he had to be carried to the rear. During the Maryland campaign in September, he was present with his arm in a sling. Not fully recovered from his wound, he left on a thirty-day sick furlough on October 14 and returned in December. On April 12, 1863, Ransom was in Wilmington, North Carolina, on court-martial duty. His promotion to brigadier general ranked from June. While rallying his sharpshooters at Wooldridge's Hill on May 14, 1864, he was struck by a ball, which shattered both bones of his left forearm. Although the surgeons initially stated that an amputation would be required, Ransom wanted his arm saved even at the expense of his life. A surgeon removed the shattered ends of the bones and left the remaining ones for nature to heal. Although shorter than before, the arm was later serviceable, and use of the hand was retained. He recuperated in Richmond and returned to duty on October 13. At Five Forks on April 1, 1865, with his left arm in a sling, he had two horses killed under him. The last horse pinned him to the ground. With only one strong arm, Ransom was in danger of being injured from the struggles of the dying horse until he was freed.[1] He resumed his law practice after the war and served in the United States Senate from 1872 until 1895 and as ambassador to Mexico from 1895 to 1897. Ransom died October 8, 1904, near Garysburg, North Carolina, and was buried on his plantation near Jackson, North Carolina.

DEATH CERTIFICATE: NAD

1. CSR; *OR*, vol. 11, pt. 2:794; vol. 18:982; vol. 19, pt. 1:916, 919; Clark, *Histories of Several Regiments* 2:600, 603, 609, 619–20, 626.

ROBERT RANSOM, JR. • *Born February 12, 1828*, in Warren County, North Carolina. Graduated from USMA in 1850. As a child in the summer of 1834, Ransom suffered a broken left arm between the wrist and the elbow when his horse fell. It was fractured again the following winter and for the third time the succeeding spring. These injuries left him with a weak left arm for the rest of his life. An episode of fever and inflammation of the bowels in the summer of 1856 prompted a one-month leave from the army. He went to Carlisle and then Washington, D.C., until December, when he was assigned to Fort Leavenworth. Ransom had pneumonia in February 1857, and he returned to the east on another sick leave. There was hemorrhage from his lungs in March 1858, and he was given an indefinite leave of absence. While in Virginia the following August, he had typhoid fever. His health was poor in the spring of 1859, but when it improved, he took recruits to Fort Riley, Kansas. Ransom resigned from the U.S. Army in May 1861 and was appointed colonel of the 1st North Carolina cavalry in July. He was promoted to brigadier general in March 1862. During the war, Ransom's health continued to be bad and necessitated frequent sick leaves. He was ill in Kinston, North Carolina, in April 1863, and it was not certain whether he could remain in command. However, he returned on May 22, and his promotion to major general ranked from that month. He was on duty at Richmond until July, when he was disabled by illness and given a leave. In October he took command in eastern Tennessee. In August 1864, President Jefferson Davis stated that Ransom's health rendered it necessary to remove him from duty. Accordingly, he was relieved on the tenth and given a leave to regain his health. During September he served as president of a court of inquiry. He was assigned to Charleston in November 1864, but just after Christmas was compelled by illness to abandon his post. He never returned to duty. On April 14, 1865, he was at his home on sick leave.[1] Following the war he had a number of occupations; his final profession was as a civil engineer at New Bern, North Carolina, where he died on January 14, 1892. He was buried there in Cedar Grove Cemetery.

DEATH CERTIFICATE: NAD

1. OR, vol. 18:255, 1023; vol. 27, pt. 3:1065; vol. 43, pt. 1:990, 993, 1001; David Sweet, ed., "Autobiography," Robert Ransom Papers, SHC; Clark, *Histories of Several Regiments* 3:327, 5:277; Wharton J. Green, "Confederate General Robert Ransom," an address before the Ladies Memorial Association, May 10, 1899; *CMH* 4:345.

ALEXANDER WELCH REYNOLDS • *Born April 1816* in Clarke County, Virginia. Graduated from USMA in 1838. Served in the Florida and Mexican wars. Although he did not offially leave the U.S. Army, he was appointed a captain in Confederate service in March 1861. Reynolds was appointed colonel of the 15th Virginia Infantry in July 1861 and was promoted to brigadier general ranking from September 1863. He was wounded during the Atlanta campaign near New Hope Church on May 27, 1864. In September he was assigned to the headquarters of the District of Northeast Georgia and was in the field trying to improve discipline. After the war in 1869, he entered the service of the Khedive of Egypt and died in Alexandria on May 26, 1876. He was found dead in bed, supposedly from a heart attack, but some of his comrades thought that excessive alcohol had played a role. He was probably buried in Alexandria.[1]

DEATH CERTIFICATE: RNA (Passport Service, U.S. Department of State).

1. *OR*, vol. 38, pt. 3:814; vol. 49, pt. 1:974; William B. Hesseltine and Hazel C. Wolf, *The Blue and the Gray on the Nile*, 58, 217–18.

DANIEL HARRIS REYNOLDS • *Born December 14, 1832,* at Centerburg, Ohio. Reynolds left his law practice in Arkansas and raised a company that made him captain in 1861. He was promoted to major in April 1862 and to lieutenant colonel in May. His assignment as colonel ranked from September 1863 and as brigadier from March 1864. Reynolds was slightly wounded at Franklin on November 30, 1864, but remained on the field. In December he was placed in brigade command. Near Bentonville on March 19, 1865, a Federal cannonball that passed through his horse's chest shattered Reynolds's left leg. The condition of the leg necessitated amputation above the knee. He was transported by ambulance and finally arrived in Charlottesville, Virginia, where he signed a parole on May 29, 1865.[1] After the war he returned to his law practice and served one term in the Arkansas state senate. He died March 14, 1902, at Lake Village, Arkansas, and was buried there in Lake Village Cemetery.

DEATH CERTIFICATE: NAD

1. *OR*, vol. 45, pt. 2:696, 715; vol. 47, pt. 1:1101, 1103–4; Cummings, "Seven Ohio Confederate Generals," 670; *History of Southern Arkansas*, 1083–85; *CV* 19:211.

ROBERT VINKLER RICHARDSON • *Born November 4, 1820,* in Granville County, North Carolina. Richardson was both an attorney in Memphis and brigadier general in the militia at the start of the war. In September 1862 he organized a regiment of partisan rangers and in February 1863 was elected colonel of the 1st Tennessee Partisan Rangers. He was ill November 2 and 3, and unable to command. He was promoted to brigadier general in December 1863. After the war he was involved in levee and railroad building. On a trip concerning railroad business, he stopped at a tavern in the village of Clarkton, Missouri. About ten o'clock at night on January 6, 1870, he stepped outside of the door to get a drink from a pail of water on the porch. He was instantly shot and killed by someone who fired a shotgun loaded with buckshot. The cause of the killing and the identity of the murderer were never determined. Richardson was buried in Elmwood Cemetery, at Memphis, Tennessee.[1] Cause of death: Gunshot wound.[2]

1. *OR*, vol. 31, pt. 1:249, 253; *Memphis Public Ledger*, Jan. 11, 1870.
2. Burial record, Elmwood Cemetery, Memphis, Tenn.

ROSWELL SABINE RIPLEY • *Born March 14, 1823,* at Worthington, Ohio. Graduated from USMA in 1843. Served in the Florida and Mexican wars. Because of illness he was not fit for duty while at Fort Henry in Baltimore Harbor in December 1843. He resigned from the U.S. Army in 1853 and established a business in Charleston, South Carolina. A lieutenant colonel of state troops, he occupied first Fort Moultrie and then Fort Sumter after their evacuation by Federal forces. He was appointed brigadier general in the Confederate Army in April 1861. At Sharpsburg on September 17, 1862, he was wounded in the throat by a minié ball. It would have been fatal had it not passed first through his cravat. He returned to the field an hour and a half after the wound was dressed; however by afternoon he had to leave because of exhaustion and weakness. About one month later he assumed command of the first military district of South Carolina. After the war he went to England and entered into a manufacturing venture, which failed. He returned to the United States and engaged in business and writing. In later years, Ripley had severe asthma and had to walk at night when difficult breathing prevented him from sleeping. He suffered a fatal stroke after breakfast in the dining room of the New York Hotel on March 29, 1887. Ripley was buried in Magnolia Cemetery at Charleston, South Carolina.[1]

DEATH CERTIFICATE: Cause of death, cerebral apoplexy.

1. CSR; *OR*, vol. 14:635; vol. 19, pt. 1:1027, 1033; *CMH* 5:418; Cummings, "Seven Ohio Confederate Generals," 404, 563–64, 594, 736.

JOHN SELDON ROANE • *Born January 8, 1817*, in Wilson County, Tennessee. Served in the Mexican War. In 1847, he publicly insulted Albert Pike about his Mexican War experiences, and Pike challenged him to a duel. They exchanged pistol shots on a sandbar in the Arkansas River on July 29 without either hitting the other. The attending surgeon brought about a reconciliation before they fired their third shots. He served as governor of Arkansas from 1849 until 1852. In March 1862 he was commissioned a brigadier general in the Confederate Army and served most of his time in garrison duty.[1] He returned to Arkansas after the war and died April 8, 1867, at Pine Bluff. He was buried in Oakland Cemetery at Little Rock.

DEATH CERTIFICATE: NAD

1. Donovan, *Governors of Arkansas*, 17–22.

WILLIAM PAUL ROBERTS • *Born July 11, 1841*, in Gates County, North Carolina. He left his position as a teacher and enlisted in a cavalry company in June 1861. Roberts was promoted from orderly sergeant through ranks to major in the 2nd North Carolina. At Haw's Shop, Virginia, on June 3, 1864, he received a slight gunshot wound to the head. The next day he was admitted to a Richmond hospital. He returned to duty in less than a week following his promotion to colonel. His appointment as brigadier general ranked from February 1865. Roberts returned to North Carolina after the war and served as state legislator and state auditor. He died in a hospital at Norfolk, North Carolina, on March 28, 1910, as the result of a fall in his home. Roberts was buried in the Old City Cemetery at Gatesville, North Carolina.[1]

DEATH CERTIFICATE: RNA

1. CSR; Clark, *Histories of Several Regiments* 2:101; *CV* 18:342.

BEVERLY HOLCOMBE ROBERTSON • *Born June 5, 1827*, in Amelia County, Virginia. Graduated from USMA in 1849. He was dismissed from the U.S. Army after having been appointed a captain in Confederate service to rank from March 1861.

In September he was elected colonel of the 4th Virginia Cavalry. During early May 1862, Robertson was sick in Richmond but was back on the field by May 27. He obtained his brigadier stars in June 1862. At his request, he was relieved as being unfit for active duty in August 1863. He reported for temporary duty October 15 and was authorized to go to Richmond to arrange his staff.[1] After the war he moved to Washington, D.C., and opened an insurance business. He died November 12, 1910, in that city and was buried in Amelia County, Virginia.

DEATH CERTIFICATE: Cause of death, immediate, syncope, duration a few days; primary, arteriosclerosis with myocardial degeneration, duration, some years.

    1. *OR*, vol. 11, pt. 1:445, 572, 742; vol. 27, pt. 3:1007, 1075; vol. 28, pt. 2:421.

FELIX HUSTON ROBERTSON • *Born March 9, 1839,* at Washington, Texas. He resigned from West Point in January 1861 to join the Confederacy and was appointed second lieutenant of artillery in March 1861. Passing through the ranks of captain and major, he was promoted to lieutenant colonel in January 1864. His promotion to brigadier general was from July 1864. While acting as Joseph Wheeler's chief of staff, Robertson was severely wounded at Buck Head, Georgia, on November 28, 1864. (Although some sources give the twenty-ninth as the date of his wound, the twenty-eighth is probably correct.) Fighting on horseback, he had emptied his gun and was using his saber when a bullet broke his left elbow and carried away pieces of two of the bones. He raised himself up in his stirrups and with all of his strength delivered a blow with his saber on the head of the man who had shot him. The force broke the stirrup leather, and only by catching his right heel in his saddle was he able to stay on his horse, which was in full gallop. His left hand was useless and he had his saber in his right hand, but by taking the reins in his teeth he was able to take control of the horse and bring it to a stop. Robertson rode his horse back to a house about a half mile from the battlefield. He lay on the gallery floor while a surgeon gave him morphine and surgically removed the bullet. Robertson awoke the next morning and was taken by buggy to the hospital in Augusta. He was transferred to private quarters for three weeks, where his care was continued by his landlady's brother-in-law, who was a physician. When Robertson was able to travel, he went to Columbia, Georgia, to visit friends and then on to Macon. In January 1865 he was reported to be recovering rapidly. However, Gen. Joseph Wheeler reported in March that Robertson was still disabled from his wound, and he saw no more action. In 1896, many years after the war, Robertson was shot at with a shotgun when he tried to evict a tenant, and some of the shot grazed his arm. Taking his Winchester rifle, Robertson killed the man. Later his action was ruled as self-defense. Robertson was the last general officer of the Confederacy to die. He died April 20, 1928, at Waco, Texas, and was buried there in Oakwood Cemetery.[1]

DEATH CERTIFICATE: Cause of death, natural causes and senility.

    1. *OR*, vol. 44:375, 411, 910–11 (incorrectly indexed in part as B. H. Robertson); vol. 47, pt. 1:1132, pt. 2:1028; from the interview conducted by Helen Pool Baldwin, "The Life Story of Brig. General Felix

Robertson," *Texana* 8:154; William Carey Dodson, *Campaigns of Wheeler and his Cavalry*, 291; Lawson, *Wheeler's Last Raid*, 404–6.

JEROME BONAPARTE ROBERTSON • *Born March 14, 1815*, in Woodford County, Kentucky. Robertson studied medicine and graduated from Transylvania University in 1835. After service in the Army of the Republic of Texas, he practiced medicine in Texas until 1840, when his health failed and he took up farming. Robertson joined the Confederate Army as a captain in the 5th Texas Infantry and was promoted to lieutenant colonel in November 1861, colonel in June 1862, and brigadier in November 1862. He was slightly wounded in the shoulder at the Battle of Cold Harbor on June 27, 1862, and he was wounded in the groin at the battle of Second Manassas on August 30. Robertson was able to be at Boonsboro Gap on September 14, after which his physical exhaustion was so great that he had to be carried from the field. Subsequently he was unable to take part in the Battle of Sharpsburg. Following his return he participated in the December battle of Fredericksburg. On July 2, 1863, at Gettysburg, Robertson was wounded above the right knee while leading the Texas Brigade. This injury prevented him from getting about the field and he went back about two hundred yards. He was in brigade command at Chickamauga in September. On June 24, 1864, he was ordered to take command of the reserve forces of the state of Texas, but he required an ambulance for transportation. Returning to Texas after the war, he practiced medicine and was superintendent of the state bureau of immigration; after moving to Waco, he was involved in building railroads in West Texas. He died January 7, 1891, at Waco from a progression of his cancer of the face, which had developed about ten years before his death. Robertson was buried in Waco at Oakwood Cemetery.[1]

DEATH CERTIFICATE: NAD

1. CSR; *OR*, vol. 11, pt. 2:564, 596; vol. 12, pt. 2:606, 618–19, 622; vol. 21, 621; vol. 27, pt. 2:406; vol. 30, pt. 2:290, 358, 510; vol. 34, pt. 4:692; *CMH* 11:253; Harold B. Simpson, *Touched with Valor*, 7, 12, 21.

PHILIP DALE RODDEY • *Born April 2, 1826*, at Moulton, Alabama. At the start of the war, Roddey was engaged in steamboating and became captain of a cavalry company he organized in 1861. He was ill and barely able to sit up in April 1862. He was commissioned colonel in December 1862 and was promoted to brigadier general in August 1863. Although lame in one ankle, he dismounted from his horse and marched with his men as they left Newnan on July 30, 1864. Roddey was sick September 20, 1864, but was assigned to the command of the District of North Alabama on the twenty-fourth. After the war he established a business in New York. While on a business trip to England, he died of uremina on July 20, 1897, in Westminster Hospital in London. He was later buried in Greenwood Cemetery, Tuscaloosa, Alabama.[1]

DEATH CERTIFICATE: RNA (Passport Service, U.S. Department of State).

1. *OR*, vol. 39, pt. 2:859, 869; Jordan, *N. B. Forrest*, 561, 582; Henry, *"First with the Most" Forrest*, 352; Lawson, *Wheeler's Last Raid*, 33; Warner, *Generals in Gray*, 262.

ROBERT EMMETT RODES • *Born March 29, 1829,* at Lynchburg, Virginia. Rodes taught at the Virginia Military Institute, his alma mater, until 1851, when he engaged in civil engineering. He joined the Confederacy as colonel of the 5th Alabama Infantry and was promoted to brigadier general in October 1861. At Seven Pines on May 31, 1862, Rodes received a gunshot wound in the arm and a contusion but did not leave the field until sunset. After hospitalization at Lynchburg and treatment in private quarters, he returned to duty on the twentieth of June. At Cold Harbor on June 27, Rodes was present but still too weak from his unhealed wound and a fever to remain on the field. He was carried to Richmond on the night of June 29 and did not rejoin his unit until September 6. At Sharpsburg on September 17, 1862, he helped a wounded aide to a barn and had just turned to go back when he was struck on the thigh by a shell fragment. However, it was only a slight wound, and he returned to the battle. In May 1863 he was commissioned major general. Rodes was killed at Winchester on September 19, 1864, while directing a counterattack. He had been trying to control his horse when a shell burst over him. A fragment struck him behind the ear and he died within a few hours. Some reported that he had been killed by a bullet rather than a shell fragment. He had just finished talking to John B. Gordon when he was mortally wounded, and fell near the feet of Gordon's horse. He was buried in the Presbyterian Cemetery at Lynchburg.[1]

1. CSR; *OR*, vol. 11, pt. 1:940–41, 974, 977, pt. 2:626, 628, 632; vol. 19, pt. 1:1023–24, 1027, 1038; vol. 43, pt. 1:574; Charles D. Walker, *Memorial, Virginia Military Institute Biographical Sketches,* 443; *CMH* 12:441, Ala.; *SHSP* 2:25–29; Gordon, *Reminiscences,* 321.

LAWRENCE SULLIVAN ROSS • *Born September 27, 1838,* at Bentonsport, Iowa. A student, he spent his vacations from the university in service against the Indians. At the Battle of Wichita, on October 1, 1858, Ross was wounded while fighting the Comanches. First an arrow went through his shoulder and then a 0.58 caliber ball hit him in the body. The bullet entered the chest and came out the back between his shoulder blades. He fell off his horse partially paralyzed. An Indian friend pulled a silk handkerchief through the arrow tract so there was free bleeding and put something into the wounds. Because Ross was too badly injured to be moved, he lay on the battlefield for five days. The wounds became infected and so painful that he asked to be killed. Finally, he was moved ninety miles to the nearest post, first on a litter with mules, then on the men's shoulders, and lastly by an ambulance. During the rest of 1858, Ross experienced great difficulty from these wounds. Also in 1858, he joined the Texas Rangers. In May 1860, he had an acute attack of bronchitis and, too ill for duty, went to private quarters. After Texas separated from the Union, Ross left the Texas Rangers and entered the Confederate service as a private. He was promoted to colonel of the 6th Texas Cavalry in May 1862. While at Corinth that month he had a bad cold with a fever. Unwell and in spite of the exertion and heat, he participated in the fighting. The illness continued into June and, although his weight was down to 125 pounds, he was able to attend to his duties. In January 1863 Ross felt ill, a condition made worse by his homesickness. Starting September 26, 1863, and continuing at least into April 1864, he had fever and chills almost every three days. In spite of what was apparently malaria, he was not off duty for even an hour. He was appointed brigadier general ranking from December 1863. In January 1865, Ross was so sick for two or three days that he was unable to leave his room and was taken care of by friends. This illness led to chronic attacks of bronchitis for the rest of his life. After the war he returned to Texas and started farming. He was elected county sheriff in 1873 and state senator in 1881 and 1883. In 1878 and 1881, he again had respiratory problems and fever. A popular individual in the state, he was elected governor in 1887. During the Christmas season of 1897, Ross had indigestion and a chill. The gastrointestinal symptoms continued, and he died with "acute congestion of the stomach and bowels" on January 3, 1898, at College Station, Texas. Ross was buried in Oakwood Cemetery at Waco.[1]

DEATH CERTIFICATE: NAD

1. Bessie Ross Clarke, "Literary Productions: Biographical Sketch of S. P. Ross and L. S. Ross," 50–51, 56, Ross Family Papers, BU; Judith Ann Benner, *Sul Ross: Soldier, Statesman, Educator,* 29–31, 37, 39–40, 231–32; Sul Ross to Lizzie Ross, May 16, June 2, 14, 1862, Sul Ross to wife, Jan. 24, 1863, Apr. 26, 1864, Jan. 29, 1881, Ross to Victor M. Rose, June 1, 1878, July 9, 1881, all in Ross Family Papers, BU.

THOMAS LAFAYETTE ROSSER • *Born October 15, 1836,* in Campbell County, Virginia. Rosser was on the sick list forty-eight times in four years at West Point and resigned in April 1861, prior to graduation. He joined the Confederacy the next month and was appointed first lieutenant; he was made a captain in September. Rosser received a severe flesh wound in the arm during a skirmish at Mechanicsville on May 23, 1862. In early June 1862 he was made a lieutenant colonel and within a few weeks was elected colonel of the 5th Virginia Cavalry. He was listed as in command on July 23 and took part in the operations in August. At the start of the Battle at Kelly's Ford, Virginia, on March 17, 1863, Rosser was on court-martial duty. However, he rode immediately to the front, where he was severely wounded in the foot and disabled. He rejoined the army at Orange Court-House in May. His promotion to brigadier general ranked from September. He had a severe cold the first part of October 1863. On the twelfth of that month near Fleetwood, Rosser received a slight wound and started to the rear to have it dressed. Seeing his men waver, he went back into action. When he wrote his wife on the twenty-first, he was not sure he could write, apparently because of the wound. While leading a charge on June 11, 1864, at Trevilian Station, he was wounded in the leg. Although he had not recovered from his injury after recuperating in private quarters for more than a month, Rosser participated in the fight at Reams' Station on August 25. In November 1864 he was promoted to major general. During the first part of 1865, Rosser was still riding each day with his leg wound draining. On March 31, 1865, the Confederates attacked the Federal troops at Five Forks; while driving them almost to Dinwiddie Court-House, Rosser was slightly wounded in the arm. In the battle of the High Bridge on April 6, he was wounded in the arm once more but ignored his injury. He was not paroled at Appomattox Court-House as has been recorded, but escaped the morning of April 9 and reported at Staunton early in May for parole. Following the close of the war he became a chief engineer for a railroad. In June 1889 he was appointed a brigadier general of the United States Volunteers and was mustered out four months later. He died March 29, 1910, at Charlottesville, Virginia, and was buried there in Riverview Cemetery.[1]

DEATH CERTIFICATE: RNA

1. CSR; OR, vol. 11, pt. 1:664; vol. 12, pt. 2:730, pt. 3:652; vol. 25, pt. 1:59; vol. 36, pt. 1:1096; vol. 42, pt. 1:944–46; vol. 46, pt. 1:512, 1279, 1299; Paul E. Steiner, "Medical-Military Studies on the Civil War. 10. Major General Thomas L. Rosser, C.S.A," Military Medicine 131:72–80; T. L. Rosser to Betty, May 12, 1863, T. L. Rosser to wife, Oct. 8, 21, 1863, and Disability Leave on Surgeon's Certificate, July 5, 1864, all in Rosser Family Papers (no. 1171), UV; CR, 145:117, 127; CMH 3:658; Battles and Leaders 4:233, 238; Dawson, Reminiscences of Confederate Service, 139; Freeman, Lee's Lieutenants 3:252, 709.

DANIEL RUGGLES · *Born January 31, 1810*, in Barre, Massachusetts. Graduated from USMA in 1833. Served in the Florida and Mexican wars. At the time of the outbreak of the Civil War, he was on sick leave in Virginia, and he resigned from Federal services in May 1861. He was commissioned brigadier general in August. On November 19, 1861, he was reported to have been sick since his October arrival in New Orleans and was thus unable to perform his duties. However, by late December he was serving with his troops. He assumed command of the District of North Alabama on February 23, 1862. Although present at the time of the Battle of Shiloh in April 1862, he was sick afterward. In May he was assigned to command. He was made commissary general of prisoners in March 1865. After the war, except for a four-year period in Texas, Ruggles spent the rest of his life in Virginia. He died June 1, 1897, at Fredericksburg, Virginia, after a lingering illness of several months, and was buried there in the City Cemetery.[1]

DEATH CERTIFICATE: RNA

1. CSR; OR, vol. 6:751, 770, 790; vol. 7:905; vol. 10, pt. 1:470, 475, pt. 2:529; CMH 3:660; Freeman, Lee's Lieutenants 1:718; CV 5:415.

ALBERT RUST · *Born in 1818* in Fauquier County, Virginia. He had two terms in the Arkansas state legislature and two terms in Congress. He resigned his United States congressional seat in March 1861 and was elected to the Confederate Provisional Congress. In July he was appointed colonel of the 3rd Arkansas Regiment, and his promotion as brigadier general was from March 1862. Postwar he returned to his farm in Arkansas and again entered politics. He died April 4, 1870, near Little Rock and was buried there in Oakland Cemetery.[1]

DEATH CERTIFICATE: NAD

1. Sexton Book, Oakland Cemetery.

S

ISAAC MUNROE ST. JOHN · *Born November 19, 1827,* at Augusta, Georgia. Engaged as a railroad engineer in 1861, he enlisted in a militia company. Gen. John B. Magruder recognized his talents and made him his chief engineer. He was made captain of engineers in February 1862 and was commissioned major of artillery in October. St. John was given charge of the Nitre Corps and in 1863 was promoted to both lieutenant colonel and colonel. The Confederate Congress made him brigadier general and commissary general in February 1865. After the war he continued as a civil engineer. He died April 7, 1880, at White Sulphur Springs, West Virginia, and was buried in Hollywood Cemetery at Richmond, Virginia. Cause of death: Pneumonia.[1]

1. Burial register, Hollywood Cemetery, Richmond, Va.

JOHN CALDWELL CALHOUN SANDERS · *Born April 4, 1840,* at Tuscaloosa, Alabama. He left his studies at the University of Alabama when the Civil War started and was elected captain of a company in the 11th Alabama Infantry. At Frayser's Farm on June 30, 1862, a shell fragment tore the deep tissues of his leg; however, he remained on the field until after dark. He rejoined the regiment on August 11. At the Battle of Sharpsburg on September 17, Sanders received a facial wound from pebbles thrown up by a cannonball. His promotion from major to colonel ranked from that month. He was wounded in the knee by a minié ball at Gettysburg on July 2, 1863. In August and September he was listed as in command. During the winter, Sanders served as a member of a general court-martial. He was commissioned brigadier general in May 1864. On August 21, 1864, he was advancing on foot along the Weldon Railroad when a minié ball passed through both his thighs and severed the femoral arteries. While being removed a short distance, Sanders asked to be laid down and, within a few minutes, bled to death. He was buried in Hollywood Cemetery at Richmond, Virginia.[1]

1. CSR; *OR*, vol. 27, pt. 2:619; vol. 29, pt. 1:400, pt. 2:685, 821; vol. 38, pt. 3:692; *CMH* 12:443, Ala.; Warner, *Generals in Gray*, 268.

ALFRED MOORE SCALES · *Born November 26, 1827,* at Reidsville, North Carolina. Scales served in the North Carolina legislature and was a representative in Congress before the war. He entered Confederate service as a private in April 1861 and was elected captain of a company of the 13th North Carolina in May. In October he was elected colonel of the regiment. During the late winter of 1861, he was sick in his quarters. Following the battle at Malvern Hill on July 1, 1862, he collapsed from exhaustion and was close to death. He did not return to duty until the middle of November. At Chancellorsville on May 3, 1863, he was shot through the thigh but continued on the field until loss of blood forced him to halt. Two men carried him to the rear on a litter. He went home to recover and in June was promoted to brigadier general and ordered to report to A. P. Hill. On July 1, during the first day's fighting at Gettysburg, Scales was wounded in the leg by a shell fragment. On July 5 he was in an ambulance with Gen. William D. Pender, who was also wounded. While waiting for the column to move, Gen. John D. Imboden shared a little bread and meat with them. Scales and Pender were carried back to Virginia in the ambulance, and Scales was left in Winchester to recover. He was back in October, but at the time of the surrender in 1865 he was at home on sick leave. Following the end of the war he returned to his law practice in North Carolina and took an active role in politics. After serving in the state legislature and in Congress, he was governor from 1884 to 1888. He was never in good health after he left Raleigh in 1888. In spite of visiting medical specialists in the North and going to various springs, there was no improvement in his condition. Prior to being confined to his bed he visited the Tate Springs in Tennessee but became so much worse that he had to return home. His condition was diagnosed as Bright's disease, and as time went on his brain became affected so that for several months before he died he was conscious only at intervals. He died February 8, 1892, at Greensboro, North Carolina, and was buried there in Green Hill Cemetery.[1]

DEATH CERTIFICATE: NAD

1. CSR; OR, vol. 19, pt. 1:1045; vol. 25, pt. 1:936; vol. 27, pt. 2:670, pt. 3:909; CMH 4:349; SHSP 8:518; Clark, Histories of Several Regiments 1:670, 4:184; CV 33:96; Greensboro (N.C.) Patriot, Feb. 10, 1892.

THOMAS MOORE SCOTT • *Probably born in 1829* at Athens, Georgia. Scott left his farm in 1861 and was elected colonel of the 12th Louisiana Infantry. He was promoted to brigadier general from May 1864. Disabled by the explosion of a shell at Franklin on November 30, 1864, he fell and had to be carried to a house in the rear. In January 1865 Scott was still unfit for duty because the concussion had injured his spine and kidneys, and it was believed he would not return to duty for at least six months. After the war he returned to his farm in Louisiana. Scott was found dead at seven o'clock in the morning in the Sample Coffee House at the corner of Jackson and Magazine streets in New Orleans on April 21, 1876. Scott had been at the saloon about seven o'clock the night before and left after having had several drinks. He returned at about half past eight and drank some more. He went to sleep in a chair and was found dead in the same position the next day. The coroner's jury said his death was due to "congestion of the brain brought on by alcohol." He was buried at New Orleans in the Tomb of the Soldiers Home in Greenwood Cemetery.[1]

DEATH CERTIFICATE: NAD

1. CSR; OR, vol. 45, pt. 1:654, 684, 708; CMH 10:316, La.; CV 5:600; New Orleans Daily Picayune, Apr. 22, 1876.

WILLIAM READ SCURRY • *Born February 10, 1821,* at Gallatin, Tennessee. Served in the Mexican War. Scurry was appointed a commissioner from Texas in 1860 to work on the Texas–New Mexico boundary line and was a member of the Texas secession convention the following year. He entered the Confederate service in the 4th Texas Cavalry as a lieutenant colonel in 1861. During the engagement at Glorieta, New Mexico Territory, on March 28, 1862, his cheek was grazed twice by minié balls. He was promoted to brigadier general in September. The last of October 1862, he reported to Theophilus H. Holmes that he was sick. He was ill again in March 1863. While in command of the Subdistrict of Texas in June 1863, Scurry had to take sick leave because of inflammation of his eyes. Confined to the house, he had difficulty seeing. On the evening of April 9, 1864, near Pleasant Hill, Louisiana, he was grazed again by a minié ball but continued on the field. He was killed on April 30, 1864, in the battle at Jenkins' Ferry. Refusing to be taken to the rear, he bled to death on the field. He was buried in the Texas State Cemetery at Austin.[1]

1. CSR; OR, vol. 9:541; vol. 13:899; vol. 26, pt. 2:73; vol. 34, pt. 1:537, 549, 568, 817; Joseph P. Blessington, *The Campaigns of Walker's Texas Division*, 196; CMH 11:256, Tex.; Warner, *Generals in Gray*, 270–71.

CLAUDIUS WISTAR SEARS • *Born on November 8, 1817,* in Peru, Massachusetts. Graduated from USMA in 1841, resigned one year later, and was engaged in teaching until 1861, when he entered Confederate service. He was first elected a captain of a company in the 17th Mississippi Infantry and was later appointed colonel of the 46th Mississippi Infantry. When his regiment was ordered to Port Gibson, Mississippi, on April 28, 1863, he had to remain in bed because of chills. The next day he was able to ride and followed the troops. Sears was on the field on the thirtieth but, because of continuing illness, had to use an ambulance. His promotion as brigadier general ranked from March 1864. Although he had chills again in April, he was able to drill his troops. He awoke June 19, 1864, with bad sciatica from sleeping on a rock on the ground. Lame and sick, he had difficulty performing his duty. In the middle of July the surgeon sent him to private quarters in Eufaula, where he remained for a month. He returned to the field hospital south of Atlanta in August and remained there a few days before going back to duty. In the middle of November, Sears was sick again and had to go to private quarters in town for a couple of days. He sprained his back on December 7 and was off duty until the tenth. When Samuel G. French was injured, Sears assumed command of the division on the thirteenth. The troops were falling back on December 15, 1864, during the Battle of Nashville, when Sears mounted his horse and marched his command in the near darkness. When he felt something strike his foot, he looked down and saw his leg swinging helplessly. A cannonball had passed through his horse and crushed his left leg. As he was taken off the horse, it fell over dead. Years later one of his soldiers said that Sears ignored his own condition and, standing on his one foot on the frozen ground, cried over his horse, which had been with him during the whole war. There was no surgeon present to help him, so his comrades put him in an ambulance. He was taken to Ewing's place on the Franklin Pike, and his leg was amputated just below the knee. Immediately after surgery he was put in an ambulance and taken farther to the rear. He traveled south from the sixteenth of December through the nineteenth and finally stopped eight miles below Pulaski. The wound was dressed by a surgeon on the twentieth and twenty-first. Sears had trouble sleeping because of the discomfort, but on the twenty-ninth was able to sleep after taking morphine. He was captured a few days later and was not paroled until June 23, 1865.[1] Sears returned home and taught mathematics at the University of Mississippi. He died February 15, 1891, at Oxford, Mississippi, and was buried there in Saint Peter's Cemetery.

DEATH CERTIFICATE: NAD

1. CSR; *OR*, vol. 38, pt. 3:904; vol. 45, pt. 2:389, 774; vol. 49, pt. 2:581; Claudius W. Sears Diaries, MDAH; *CV* 11:327.

PAUL JONES SEMMES • *Born on June 4, 1815*, at Montford's Plantation, Wilkes County, Georgia. Besides his banking and farming interests in Georgia, he was a captain in a local militia unit until 1861. Semmes entered Confederate service as colonel of the 2nd Georgia Infantry; his promotion as brigadier general ranked from March 1862. Following the battle at Malvern Hill on July 1, 1862, he was so exhausted that he could not reach the camp that night without the assistance of two of his men. He was mortally wounded in the thigh during the fighting at Gettysburg on July 2, 1863. A tourniquet was applied, and he was taken off of the field and then back to Martinsburg, West Virginia, where he died. It is of interest that there are no blood stains at the thigh level of the coat Semmes was wearing at the time he was mortally wounded. Many reports have his date of death as July 10. However, other records, including a letter from his wife, give the date as the ninth. He was temporarily buried at Martinsburg, and his remains were later moved to Linnwood Cemetery at Columbus, Georgia.[1]

1. CSR; *OR*, vol. 11, pt. 2:723–24; vol. 27, pt. 2:299, 310–11, 320, 359, 362; Warner, *Generals in Gray*, 272–73; *CMH* 6:435; Freeman, *Lee's Lieutenants* 3:191–94; CSR of Benjamin Grubb Humphrey; Harry W. Pfanz, *Gettysburg—The Second Day*, 286, 523–24; Letter to author from Howard O. Hendricks, Jan. 31, 1991.

JACOB HUNTER SHARP • *Born on February 6, 1833*, at Pickensville, Alabama. Sharp was an attorney in Mississippi when he enlisted as a private in the 1st Battalion Mississippi Infantry; he was soon elected captain. His unit became part of the 44th Mississippi, and he was elected colonel. Sharp's promotion to brigadier general was from July 1864. He did not confine himself to his law practice when he returned home but also purchased a newspaper and entered politics. He was in poor health the last years of his life. He died September 15, 1907, at Columbus, Mississippi, and was buried there in Friendship Cemetery.[1]

DEATH CERTIFICATE: NAD

1. Mrs. Mary Sharp Owens, "Biographical Memorandum," Jan. 9, 1935, in Nathaniel H. Harris subject file, MDAH; *CV* 15:516.

JOSEPH ORVILLE SHELBY • *Born on December 12, 1830*, in Lexington, Kentucky. As the result of his rope manufacturing business and an inheritance, he was wealthy and prominent in Missouri before the war. He raised a cavalry company in 1861 and was elected its captain. During the summer of 1862 he was made a colonel. At Hartville, Missouri, on January 11, 1863, Shelby's life was saved when a bullet hit the gold badge he wore on his hat. The incident was not mentioned in his report. A minié ball hit his elbow and then passed through his forearm and came out at the wrist at Helena, Arkansas, on July 4, 1863. Faint from shock and loss of blood, Shelby returned to the fight after the wound had been dressed. He did not make a report on the battle and was under a surgeon's care in Batesville for several weeks. In September he left his bed and, in spite of the fact his arm was still suppurating, led his troops on the road to Little Rock. Reduced to almost a skeleton and with his shattered arm in a sling, Shelby was given troops for the purpose of proceeding into Missouri. In the middle of October his arm gave him a lot of pain and continued to suppurate. During the expedition, he traveled more than one thousand miles through enemy country. His promotion to brigadier general was from December 1863. While in Mexico after the war, his stiff arm continued to bother him. However, his health was generally good following his return to the United States in 1867 except for brief illness in late 1879 and in August 1885. On February 1, 1897, he continued with his duties as a U.S. marshal at Adrian, Missouri, in spite of a bad cold. He developed a fever and was ordered to bed by his physician. Within a short time he contracted pneumonia and was not able to recognize any of his family. Although a specialist was called in from Kansas City, it was concluded that nothing more could be done for Shelby. He became comatose and died ten days after the onset of his illness on February 13, 1897. He was buried at Kansas City, Missouri, in the Forest Hill Cemetery.[1] Cause of death: Inflammation of brain.[2]

1. CSR; *OR*, vol. 22, pt. 1:199–205, 412, 437; Daniel O'Flaherty, *General Jo Shelby: Undefeated Rebel*, 184–89, 200, 275, 321, 352, 394–95; *SHSP* 24:199–200; *CMH* 9:114, 135, 139–40, 149, Mo.

2. Internment Record, Int. no. 1488, no. 15 of 1897, Forest Hill Cemetery, Kansas City, Mo.

CHARLES MILLER SHELLEY • *Born December 28, 1833*, in Sullivan County, Tennessee. A professional builder, Shelley was made a lieutenant of the Talladega Artillery when Alabama left the Union. In the reorganization of the unit into an infantry unit and its incorporation into the 5th Alabama Infantry Regiment, Shelley was elected captain. He recruited the 30th Alabama in January 1862 and was appointed colonel. His promotion to brigadier general ranked from September 1864. After the war he returned to Alabama and entered politics. He died on January 20, 1907, at Birmingham, Alabama, and was buried in Oak Hill Cemetery at Talladega, Alabama.

DEATH CERTIFICATE: NAD

FRANCIS ASBURY SHOUP • *Born March 22, 1834*, at Laurel, Indiana. Graduated from USMA in 1855. Served in the Florida wars. He resigned from the U.S. army in 1860; after studying the law he became an attorney in Florida. In March 1861 he was commissioned a lieutenant of artillery in the Confederate service and was promoted to major in November. His promotion to brigadier general ranked from

September 1862. On his arrival at Mobile on September 25, 1863, he was assigned to command of a brigade. However, he was unable to perform his duties and had to leave because of illness. In February 1864 he was back on duty. Following the war he became an Episcopal priest in 1868, and he served as rector of a number of churches and taught primarily at Sewanee, Tennessee. He was sick the entire summer before his death on September 4, 1896, at Columbia, Tennessee, from heart failure. He was buried on the grounds at the University of the South at Sewanee.[1]

DEATH CERTIFICATE: NAD

1. *OR*, vol. 31, pt. 3:851–52; vol. 32, pt. 2:692; Garrett, *Obituaries from Tennessee Newspapers*, 350.

HENRY HOPKINS SIBLEY · *Born on May 25, 1816*, at Natchitoches, Louisiana. Graduated from USMA in 1838. Served in the Florida and Mexican wars. During the summer of 1840, he was granted a week's leave from Carlisle Barracks because of illness and went to Governor's Island. His illness continued and he received additional leave. Medications prescribed by two New York physicians seemed only to make his condition worse. Recovery was slow, and he did not return to duty until August. While in Mexico in 1847–48 he had short periods of illness and, with other officers, suffered from snow blindness while climbing Mt. Popocatepetl in 1848. He burned his hand in April 1855 and had to return to Fort Belknap, Texas, from a scout up the Clear Fork of the Brazos River. Sibley's application on medical certificate for sick leave from Fort Bridger in August 1858 was rejected until his physician provided an assurance that a change of climate would benefit his health. He was finally able to leave in September and went to New York, where he remained on sick leave and detached service. It was not until August of the next year that he returned to Fort Bridger. By 1861 his general health was poor and he was drinking in excess. He resigned from the United States Army in April 1861 and in June was appointed a brigadier general in Confederate service. Because of illness, he was unable to go up the Rio Grande Valley from Fort Bliss on January 13, 1862. He did depart the next day, but he had to rest for a day at Mesilla (Territory of Arizona) because of continued sickness. According to his doctor, Sibley had to retire to his tent the night of February 16 because of acute colicky abdominal pain, nausea, and vomiting. The following day he gave up command of his troops, and for the next five days remained in either his tent or ambulance, drinking heavily throughout the period. On the twenty-first, against the advice of his doctor, he took to his saddle to participate in the Battle of Valverde. Exhausted, suffering with the colic, and still drinking, he could hardly stay on his horse and had to give up the command again that afternoon. During the operations in western Louisiana in April 1863, Sibley was sick and asked permission to go on the line of retreat in advance of the column. After the war, from December 1869 until November 1873, he was out of the country and was a general of artillery in the Egyptian Army. His colic became more severe and his drinking was even more of a problem during this period. Following his return to the United States, his health continued to deteriorate, and by 1883 he was practically an invalid. Incapacitating dizziness made it impossible for him to stand for long periods, while loss of control of his bowels and kidneys forced him to wear a diaper. His last years were full of excruciating pain, which he tried to alleviate by heavy drinking and by chewing various local herbs. It has been suggested that his colic was due to renal stones, but there is no more evidence to support this diagnosis than an intestinal origin for his pain. He died on August 23, 1886, at Fredericksburg, Virginia, and was buried there in the City Cemetery.[1]

DEATH CERTIFICATE: Cause of death, fistula.

1. *OR*, vol. 9:505–12, 522; vol. 15:393, 1093; vol. 53:793; Jerry Thompson, *Henry Hopkins Sibley: Confederate General of the West*, 39, 60, 69, 73, 75, 102, 168–70, 228, 246–47, 251–52, 257, 260–61, 338, 340, 367–68; W. C. Nunn, ed., *Ten More Texans in Gray*, 141; Martin Hardwick Hall, "The Army of New Mexico: Silbey's Campaign of 1862" (diss.), 157–58, 166; *Southern History of the War*, 178.

JAMES PHILLIP SIMMS • *Born January 16, 1837*, at Covington, Georgia. Simms left his law practice in Georgia and was a major in the 53rd Georgia Infantry in September 1862. In October he was promoted to colonel. In July 1863, Simms was debilitated with febris communicus. He was admitted to the general hospital in Richmond and obtained a thirty-day furlough on the twentieth. He was wounded during the assault on Fort Lowdon at Knoxville on November 29, 1863, and obtained leave. On December 31 he was listed as in command. His promotion to brigadier general ranked from December 1864. After the war he returned to his law practice in Covington. Having been afflicted for some time with some unspecified disease, he was unconscious for a number of days prior to his death on May 30, 1887. However, he regained consciousness on the twenty-ninth and was able to recognize his family and friends. That night he again had a violent attack with great suffering but was peaceful at the time of his death. He was buried in the City Cemetery at Covington.[1]

DEATH CERTIFICATE: NAD

1. CSR; *OR*, vol. 31, pt. 1:495, pt. 3:890; CR, 178:36, 181:73; *Covington (Ga.) Star*, May 31, 1887.

WILLIAM YARNEL SLACK • *Born August 1, 1816*, in Mason County, Kentucky. Served in the Mexican War. He studied law and was an attorney in 1861 when the governor appointed him a brigadier general of the Missouri State Guard. He was severely wounded in the left hip at Wilson's Creek on August 10, 1861, but rejoined his command in October. On March 7, 1862, at the Battle of Elkhorn, Slack was struck by a ball in almost the same place as he had been wounded at Wilson's Creek. He was taken to a house a mile east of the battlefield and seemed to improve for the first few days. Later he was moved about seven miles farther east to Moore's Mill, Arkansas, because of fear of capture. His condition worsened, and he died early in the morning of March 21. Slack's promotion as brigadier general in the Confederate service was granted posthumously by the senate and ranked from April 1862. He was initially buried in the yard at Moore's Hill. Later his remains were moved to the Confederate Cemetery at Fayetteville, Arkansas.[1]

1. CSR; *OR*, vol. 3:101, 106, 186; vol. 8:285, 305, 312; Bevier, *History of First and Second Missouri*, 48; *CMH* 9:82, Mo.; Warner, *Generals in Gray*, 278.

JAMES EDWIN SLAUGHTER • *Born in June 1827* in the middle of what was later the battlefield of Cedar Mountain. Slaughter remained in the U.S. Army following the Mexican War until he was dismissed in May 1861. He entered Confederate service as a captain of artillery and was promoted to major in November and to brigadier general in March 1862. He asked for a thirty-day leave on a surgeon's certificate on June 14. In November 1862 Slaughter was sick in Mobile with laryngitis, which lasted for twelve months. Because he had only been able to attend to duty for a little more than half the time the previous winter, he was recommended by his surgeon to go to a warm, dry climate. His health had been poor ever since his arrival at Fort Brown, Texas, and in October 1863 he was supposedly suffering from dengue. His physician again told him that a warm and dry climate was very necessary if he hoped to recover his health.[1] After the war he lived in Mexico until 1867, when he returned and settled in Mobile. Slaughter engaged in civil engineering and was postmaster. He died on January 1, 1901, while on a visit to Mexico City, and was buried there.

DEATH CERTIFICATE: RNA (Passport Service, U.S. State Department).

1. CSR; *OR*, vol. 20, pt. 2:417.

EDMUND KIRBY SMITH • *Born on May 16, 1824*, at St. Augustine, Florida. Graduated from USMA in 1845. Served in the Mexican War. At the time of his graduation, he failed his eye examination because he was nearsighted and thus was refused his commission. Smith, however, was able to obtain certificates from his instructors and others that at no time had the visual defect been obvious from the way he had performed his duties. For the rest of his life he wore spectacles. Following a visit with family and friends in 1845, he became sick after having two teeth filled with an amalgam that caused him some type of problem with the two teeth and his eye. In the summer of 1849, while at St. Louis, he was ill for some weeks with an attack of bilious fever, which was accompanied by symptoms suggesting cholera. He was again sick in the summer of 1851, but by the fall he was doing better and had regained the weight that he had lost. Being a firm believer in the beneficial effects of cold water, he planned to take the baths at Brattleboro the next year. Along with many others he had yellow fever while on the lower Rio Grande in the summer of 1853. He was totally helpless for a month but had recovered by January. During a battle with Comanches near Old Fort Atchison, Texas, on May 13, 1859, he was shot at close range. The ball passed through the upper part of his thigh, missed all large vessels, and left a wound about four or five inches all the way through. Hating litters, he had refused to ride on one and remained in the saddle during the eighteen-day trip back to camp. Smith joined the Confederate Army as a lieutenant colonel and was commissioned brigadier general in June 1861. At First Manassas on July 21, 1861, he was struck by a minié ball and fell from his horse. The ball entered behind the right collarbone, passed below the muscles, and exited near the left shoulder, leaving a twelve-inch-long wound. Smith was taken care of in private quarters about thirty miles from the battlefield. On August 5, the wound was considered not too serious; in fact, Smith thought he might be back by September. During his recovery, he met his future wife, who helped nurse him. He was promoted to major general in October 1861 and assumed command of the troops of East Tennessee in February 1862. In late June, Smith had typhoid fever and was unable to take the field. He went to Montvale, Tennessee, to convalesce, and by mid-July reported he would soon be able to return. On June 4, 1863, he was in Shreveport, Louisiana, for ten days with a bilious attack. Supposedly by taking quinine, blue mass, and rest, Smith was able to ward it off and felt quite well again. However, ill health detained him at Shreveport again in late August. In September 1863, following his return from Marshall, Texas, he was confined to his room with an inflamed eye and was prohibited from giving his full attention to business. In late August 1864, he was sick for over ten days with an attack of acute dysentery. After the war he was president of the Pacific and Atlantic Telegraph Company for two years. He then held positions as president, chancellor, and professor at different institutions of higher learning. For the last two years of his life, Smith was in poor health. He developed fever and chills on March 10, 1893, while visiting his cousin in New Orleans, and was confined to bed for five days. He recovered enough to visit his daughter in Vicksburg before going back to Sewanee, Tennessee, on March 20. Two days later, he caught a cold and had a relapse with congestion of the right lung. He died soon afterward on March 28, 1893. Smith was buried on university grounds at the University of the South at Sewanee.[1]

DEATH CERTIFICATE: NAD

1. OR, vol. 2:476, 496, 522; vol. 7:908; vol. 16, pt. 2:710, 727; vol. 22, pt. 1:26, pt. 2:855, 983, 988; vol. 34, pt. 1:482; vol. 51, pt. 2:222; Arthur Howard Noll, General Edmund Kirby Smith, 20–21, 85, 124; Joseph Howard Parks, General Edmund Kirby Smith, C.S.A., 42, 69, 76, 80, 98; newspaper clipping, n.i., n.d., n.p., in Smith-Kirby-Webster-Black-Danner Family Papers, Gen. and Mrs. Ed. Kirby Smith and daughter Nina folder, USAMHI; CMH 1:655; CV 1:99, 3:55–56, 7:63, 108, 310; Randolph H. McKim, A Soldier's Recollections, 360; Columbia (Tenn.) Maury Democrat, Apr. 6, 1893.

GUSTAVUS WOODSON SMITH • Born either November 30 or December 1, 1821, at Georgetown, Kentucky. Graduated from USMA in 1842. Served in the Mexican War. Smith left the U.S. Army in 1854 and became a civil engineer. At the start of the Civil War he was street commissioner of New York City. Not fully recovered from a stroke that caused paralysis, Smith was detained for some time on his way south to join the Confederacy, and in May 1861 was physically unfit to take command. After his arrival in Richmond, he was commissioned major general in the Confederate Army in September. Episodes of poor health recurred in December and in March 1862. In April his physician reported that his state of health made him unfit for the climate of the South Carolina coast. During the battle around Fair Oaks Station on June 2, 1862, Smith became acutely ill and had to leave the field. Later in the day he developed partial paralysis. It was stated that he was unable to endure the mental excitement incident to his presence with the army. The same day he was taken to Richmond, and his condition worsened during the next two or three weeks. His physician suggested that complete quiet, mountain air, and the free use of sulphur waters offered the only chance for his recovery. Smith improved slowly. On July 18, he said, "I do not get straight in brains and nerves as fast as I hoped." In these respects there had been little improvement, but his general health was good. In August 1862 Smith was well enough to take command again. However, his surgeons doubted that his physical condition would permit him to discharge more than post command in a healthful climate. By special orders on August 10, 1862, on reporting for duty, he was assigned to a division. In January 1863, Smith's health was not as good as he wished. He was in Richmond in February, and the secretary of war reported that Smith would be there for some time. In November 1864 he was at Savannah and almost broke down with fatigue and the need for rest. He returned to duty on December 7. Following the war he was a superintendent of an ironworks in Tennessee and insurance commissioner of Kentucky before finally moving to New York City. Years later, he still had not fully recovered from the illness he had during the war. He died on June 24, 1896, at New York City and was buried in New London, Connecticut, in Cedar Grove Cemetery.[1]

DEATH CERTIFICATE: Cause of death, myocarditis; contributing, chronic endocarditis, age and mitral insufficiency.

1. CSR; *OR*, vol. 5:1008; vol. 9:454; vol. 11, pt. 1:993, pt. 3:671, 685–86; vol. 12, pt. 3:832; vol. 14:597, 746; vol. 18:855–56, 895; vol. 51, pt. 2:594; vol. 53:36; William Preston Johnston to wife, June 2, 1862, in Johnston Family Papers, FC; Jasper S. White to R. E. Lee, June 2, 1862, in W. N. Pendleton Papers, SHC; Smith, *Battle of Seven Pines*, 17, 27, 166; *SHSP* 26:79–80; Haskell, *Memoirs*, 9; *CMH* 9:254, Ky.; Freeman, *Lee's Lieutenants* 1:262.

JAMES ARGYLE SMITH • *Born on July 1, 1831*, in Maury County, Tennessee. Graduated from USMA in 1853. Smith resigned from the U.S. Army in May 1861 and joined the Confederate Army as a lieutenant of infantry. He was promoted to major and then to lieutenant colonel in March 1862. The following July he was commissioned colonel; his promotion to brigadier ranked from September 1863. He was wounded in both thighs on November 25, 1863, at Missionary Ridge while leading a charge against the Federal artillery. In March 1864 he was listed as in command. Near Atlanta, on July 22, 1864, Smith was wounded and assisted from the field. When he returned to active duty, he took part in the operations in middle Tennessee during November and December.[1] He farmed in Mississippi following the war and in 1877 was elected state superintendent of public education. Smith died December 6, 1901, at Jackson, Mississippi, and was buried there in Greenwood Cemetery.

DEATH CERTIFICATE: NAD

1. *OR*, vol. 31, pt. 2:750; vol. 32, pt. 3:595; vol. 38, pt. 3:747, 753; vol. 45, pt. 1:739; Buck, *Cleburne and his Command*, 239; *CMH* 12:269, Miss.

MARTIN LUTHER SMITH • *Born September 9, 1819,* at Danby, New York. Graduated from USMA in 1842. Served in the Mexican War. Although Northern born, he had married a Southern woman and resigned from the United States Army in April 1861. Initially commissioned major in the Confederate corps of engineers, he was promoted to colonel from February 1862, to brigadier general in April, and finally to major general from November 1862. He settled in Savannah, Georgia, and he died there soon after the war, on July 29, 1866, following a brief illness. Smith was buried in Oconee Hill Cemetery at Athens, Georgia.[1]

DEATH CERTIFICATE: RNA

1. *CV* 6:530.

PRESTON SMITH • *Born December 25, 1823,* in Giles County, Tennessee. Smith was a successful lawyer in Memphis in May 1861 when he was elected colonel of a militia regiment, the 154th Tennessee. The unit was mustered into Confederate service under the same designation. At Shiloh, on April 7, 1862, he was wounded in the right shoulder by a minié ball that disabled his arm, and he had to leave the field. He was told to report back May 14. His promotion as brigadier general was from October 1862. At Chickamauga during a night attack on September 19, 1863, Smith rode into a Federal brigade. They recognized him as a Confederate and fired a volley that mortally wounded him. One bullet struck the gold watch in front of his heart but was just diverted to another area of his body. Transported to the rear, he died in less than an hour. Initially buried at Atlanta, his remains were later moved to the Elmwood Cemetery at Memphis, Tennessee.[1]

1. *OR,* vol. 10, pt. 1:411, 449; vol. 30, pt. 2:24, 35, 79, 108, 112–13; *CMH* 8:331; Gordon, *Reminiscences,* 204.

THOMAS BENTON SMITH • *Born on February 24, 1838,* at Mechanicsville, Tennessee. Before the war he worked in the shops of a railroad. Later he was elected a company lieutenant of the 20th Tennessee. When the unit was reorganized in May 1862, he was elected colonel. He was severely wounded at Murfreesborough on December 31, 1862, and carried off the field. By late January he was back in brigade command. In the Battle of Chickamauga, he was wounded severely in the arm early on September 19, 1863, and had to leave the field. In December he was listed as in command. He was promoted to brigadier general to rank from July 1864. On December 16, 1864, in front of Nashville, Smith was struck on the head with a sword after he had surrendered. He was taken to a Federal field hospital where it was found that his brain was exposed. Death was anticipated momentarily. However, he recovered and spent the last years of his life in a state asylum at Nashville. At a Confederate veteran reunion held there in 1897, Smith, although in a deep depression, was able to command a drill and short parade and took the men through the manual of William J. Hardee's tactics. He died May 21, 1923, at Nashville and was buried there in Mount Olivet Cemetery.[1]

DEATH CERTIFICATE: Cause of death, chronic myocarditis (Sudden); contributory, traumatic psychosis.

1. *OR*, vol. 20, pt. 1:777, 784, 813, 821–22; vol. 23, pt. 2:620; vol. 30, pt. 2:384, 387, 399; vol. 31, pt. 3:806; vol. 45, pt. 1:442, 660; Confederate States Army Casualties, Roll 1; *CV* 2:118, 18:577, 20:522; *CMH* 8:332; Johnson, *Partisan Rangers*, 197; Warner, *Generals in Gray*, 284.

WILLIAM SMITH · *Born on September 6, 1797,* in King George County, Virginia. After operating a postal service, he served as a member of the Virginia senate, as a United States congressman, and as governor of Virginia before the war. He was commissioned colonel of the 49th Virginia Infantry in 1861. Smith was elected to the First Regular Confederate Congress, attended a few sessions, but resigned in 1863. On May 31, 1862, at Seven Pines, he was wounded twice; one injury was a severe contusion of the thigh from a minié ball. He was back on the field by late June. At Sharpsburg, on September 17, 1862, Smith was wounded three times but refused to relinquish command. Early said he saw blood streaming from Smith's left shoulder and thought that he was also hit by a ball in the arm and one in the leg. Although standing up, Smith was unable to move and was subsequently carried off in a helpless condition. The last of January 1863, after a ball had been removed, he was improving rapidly. He was ordered to report for assignment to the command of a brigade on May 19, 1863. He was promoted to brigadier general from January 1863 and to major general from August. In January 1864 he was elected governor of Virginia and held that position until the end of the war.[1] Afterward he returned to his farm in Virginia but could not completely stay out of politics. Smith died May 18, 1887, near Warrenton, Virginia, and was buried in Hollywood Cemetery at Richmond. Cause of death: Natural causes.[2]

1. CSR; *OR*, vol. 11, pt. 1:959; vol. 19, pt. 1:971; vol. 25, pt. 2:809; Virginia Laura Hale and Stanley S. Phillips, *History of the Forty-Ninth Virginia Infantry, C.S.A.,* 29–31; *CV* 4:304, 8:162–63.
2. Burial Register, Hollywood Cemetery, Richmond, Va.

WILLIAM DUNCAN SMITH · *Born July 28, 1825,* in Augusta, Georgia. Graduated from USMA in 1846. During the Mexican War he was severely wounded at Molino del Rey on September 8, 1847. In January 1861, Smith returned from a leave of absence in Europe and resigned from the U.S. Army. He was commissioned colonel of the 20th Georgia Infantry in July. He was on sick leave in Georgia during the first two months of 1862. By the end of February, Smith certified, because no surgeon was present, that his health was still not good enough for him to come back to duty. He was promoted to brigadier general to rank from March 1862. In April he reported for duty and was ordered to report to the general commanding at Savannah. His final illness, which began nine weeks before his death, occurred while he was in Charleston, South Carolina. He died there on October 4, 1862, and was buried in Magnolia (City) Cemetery at Augusta.[1] Cause of death: Lung hemorrhage.[2]

1. CSR; *OR*, vol. 6:433; vol. 14:552, 632; Heitman, *Historical Register and Dictionary* 2:37; *CMH* 6:437.
2. Burial Records, Magnolia Cemetery, Augusta, Ga.

GILBERT MOXLEY SORREL · *Born on February 23, 1838,* at Savannah, Georgia. When the Civil War started, Sorrel went to Virginia and served as James

Longstreet's aide-de-camp with the rank of captain. At Sharpsburg on September 17, 1862, a shell burst over his head, and he was struck by a fragment. He was carried on a stretcher to a less-exposed place and received whiskey. After being placed in an ambulance, he was sent to a field infirmary. He had a contusion below the right shoulder, and the whole side of his body was black and blue with extravasated blood. He was moved some fifteen miles to a safer location and within two weeks returned to duty rather stiff. Sorrel, an excellent staff officer, passed through grades and was promoted to lieutenant colonel to rank from June 1863. On July 2, 1863, at Gettysburg, a shell burst directly over him again and a fragment struck him below the same shoulder. This paralyzed the arm for about ten days, and he was quite black from the shoulder down to the wrist. His appointment as brigadier general occurred in October 1864. In January 1865, near Petersburg, Sorrel was knocked out of his saddle when a bullet passed through the many folds of his clothing and struck him on the hipbone. The ball, however, glanced off and only bruised him. At Hatcher's Run, Virginia, on February 7, 1865, a bullet passed through Sorrel's right lung, smashing the ribs in front and back. Air gushed through the orifice, and the surgeon plastered the holes shut and sent him back that night. He was borne on a litter on the soldiers' shoulders for eight miles over rough and frozen roads to a small shanty. After being transferred to quarters near Petersburg, Sorrel was taken care of by his brigade surgeon. Two weeks later he was moved to Richmond, and the wound healed well. In March he was moved to Roanoke County, and in April he went to Lynchburg, where he was given an ambulance and a mule to get out of the reach of Federal forces. His wound broke down as he went through the mountains. His condition would not permit him to make the journey home on horseback, and he had to go by sea. After the war he spent most of his remaining years in Savannah, where he wrote his reminiscences. He died on August 10, 1901, near Roanoke, Virginia, and was buried in Laurel Grove Cemetery at Savannah.[1]

DEATH CERTIFICATE: RNA

1. CSR; Sorrel, *Confederate Staff Officer,* 14, 114, 117–20, 169, 283–85, 288–90.

LEROY AUGUSTUS STAFFORD • *Born April 13, 1822,* near Cheneyville, Louisiana. Served in the Mexican War. Stafford at the start of the Civil War was a prominent farmer. He was elected captain of a militia company that entered Confederate service as part of the 9th Louisiana Infantry with Stafford as lieutenant colonel. In October 1861 he was promoted to colonel of the unit. He received a contusion of his foot at the Battle of Sharpsburg on September 17, 1862, and had to give up his command. Apparently he was absent for only a short time. He was commissioned brigadier general in October 1863. In January 1864, Stafford went to Richmond to have some type of surgery performed and was furloughed until the first of March. On May 5, 1864, the first day of the Battle of the Wilderness, a bullet injured his spinal cord. He was admitted to a hospital in Richmond, Virginia, on the seventh and died the next day. He was first buried in Hollywood Cemetery at

Richmond, but his remains were later moved to the Greenwood Plantation near Cheneyville.[1]

1. CSR; *OR*, vol. 19, pt. 1:1014, 1017; vol. 33:1187–88; vol. 36, pt. 1:1028, 1071, pt. 2:951, 960; CR, 178:614; *CMH* 10:317, La.

PETER BURWELL STARKE · *Born in 1815* in Brunswick County, Virginia. Active in politics, he was a member of the Mississippi senate in 1862. Starke was commissioned colonel of the 28th Mississippi Cavalry in February of that year. He was absent on sick leave in late August 1863. After his return in mid-September, he was placed on detached service as a member of a general court-martial. His promotion as brigadier general ranked from November 1864.[1] Following the war he settled in Mississippi and was a member of the board of state levee commissioners until 1872. The following year he returned to Virginia, where he remained for the rest of his life. He died July 13, 1888, near Lawrenceville, Virginia, and was buried in the Percival Family Cemetery on what was formerly the farm of his second wife's family.
DEATH CERTIFICATE: Cause of death, debility.

1. CSR.

WILLIAM EDWIN STARKE · *Born in 1814* in Brunswick County, Virginia. Starke was a cotton broker in New Orleans, and at the outbreak of the war he returned to Virginia. He entered Confederate service and was aide to Robert S. Garnett until after Garnett's death, when he was commissioned colonel of the 60th Virginia. On June 26, 1862, during the Seven Days' battles, Starke was wounded in the hand but returned to command three days later. He was still suffering from the wound and was forced to relinquish command on the thirtieth. He was promoted to brigadier general in August 1862. At Sharpsburg on September 17, 1862, he fell, hit by three minié balls, and survived less than an hour. He was buried in Hollywood Cemetery at Richmond, Virginia.[1]

1. CSR; *OR*, vol. 11, pt. 2:836, 839, 841, 849–50; vol. 19, pt. 1:147, 956, 1008, 1015, 1017; *CMH* 3:663.

WILLIAM STEELE · *Born on May 1, 1819*, at Albany, New York. Graduated from USMA in 1840. Served in the Mexican and Florida wars. Steele left the U.S. Army in May 1861 and was appointed colonel of the 7th Texas Cavalry. His promotion to brigadier general ranked from September 1862. At the end of the war he returned to Texas where, while serving as state adjutant general, he was instrumental in the efficient organization of the Texas Rangers. He was having breakfast in San Antonio on January 10, 1885, when he suffered a stroke. He died the next day and was buried in Oakwood Cemetery, Austin, Texas.
DEATH CERTIFICATE: Cause of death, apoplexy.[1]

1. San Antonio Metropolitan Health District, San Antonio, Tex.; *Austin Daily Statesman*, Jan. 13, 1885.

GEORGE HUME STEUART · *Born on August 24, 1828*, at Baltimore, Maryland. Graduated from USMA in 1848. He resigned from the U.S. Army in April 1861 and was appointed captain of cavalry in Confederate service. Steuart was made lieutenant colonel on the formation of the 1st Maryland Infantry and was promoted to colonel in July 1861. His commission as brigadier ranked from March 1862. On June 8, 1863, at the Battle of Cross Keys, Steuart was struck by grapeshot or a canister in the muscles of the neck and back, and his collarbone was broken. An ambulance carried him off the field to safe quarters. The projectile was cut out in August, and he improved. Although still unfit for active field duty in September, he was ordered to Winchester and given command of the Maryland Line. After serving as post commander, he went on sick leave to Savannah on November 24, 1862, because the unhealed fractured collarbone gave him continued difficulty. It was not until May 1863 that he was able to report again for assignment to duty. Steuart was struck on the arm near the shoulder by a ball at Payne's Farm on November 27, 1863. When his coat was taken off, it was found that there was only a contusion, which turned very dark in a few minutes.[1] Following the war he settled on a farm in Maryland. He died November 22, 1903, at South River, Maryland, and was buried in Green Mount Cemetery at Baltimore.

DEATH CERTIFICATE: Cause of death, primary, gastric ulcer; immediate, hemorrhage.

1. CSR; *OR*, vol. 12, pt. 1:714, 782, 784, 818; vol. 18:1070; vol. 19, pt. 2:614; vol. 25, pt. 2:810, 817, 830; vol. 29, pt. 1:848; *SHSP* 10:257; Howard, *Recollections*, 178, 182–83, 242; McKim, *Soldier's Recollections*, 115, 119–25.

CLEMENT HOFFMAN STEVENS · *Born August 14, 1821,* in Norwich, Connecticut. He served at sea for a number of years as secretary to two of his relatives, both of whom were commodores in the United States Navy. From 1842 until the start of the Civil War he was cashier of a bank in Charleston, South Carolina. Stevens was serving as a volunteer aide to his cousin, Gen. Bernard E. Bee, at the battle of First Manassas on July 21, 1861, when he was severely wounded. Returning home as soon as he had recovered from his wound, he took charge of a militia regiment at Charleston. In January 1862 he was serving as a volunteer aide-de-camp. He was commissioned colonel of the 24th South Carolina Infantry in April. At the Battle of Chickamauga on September 20, 1863, Stevens was wounded and sent to the hospital at Marietta, Georgia. He was still absent recuperating through December 1863. In January 1864 he was promoted to brigadier general and was listed as in command on April 30. Stevens was mortally wounded by a bullet at the Battle of Peachtree Creek on July 20, 1864; the two officers who carried him to the rear were also wounded. He was admitted to the Ocmulgee Hospital in Macon, Georgia, on July 22. The minié ball had hit him in the head, fracturing the curvature of the right mastoid process, the minor table of the temporal bone, and the auditory process. Cerebral matter was oozing from the wound. Using chloroform anesthesia, the surgeon extracted the ball and bone spicules. Stevens died on the twenty-fifth. He was first buried in Magnolia Cemetery, Charleston, South Carolina, but his remains were later moved to the St. Paul's Episcopal Church Cemetery in Pendleton, South Carolina.[1]

1. CSR; *OR*, vol. 6:82; vol. 30, pt. 2:242, 246, 247; vol. 32, pt. 3:868; vol. 38, pt. 5:894, 911; E. Capers to Marcus J. Wright, June 17, 1889, in Ellison Capers Papers, SCL; *CMH* 5:419; M. D. Surgical Cases, Ocmulgee Hospital, Macon, Ga.; Mar.–July 1864, CR, 754.

WALTER HUSTED STEVENS • *Born August 24, 1827,* at Penn Yan, New York. Graduated from USMA in 1848. His resignation from the U.S. Army was not accepted, and he was dismissed in May 1861. He received a captaincy of engineers in the Confederate Army and was later promoted to major and to chief engineer of the Army of Virginia. In January 1862, after being in poor health and unfit for duty for some months, Stevens's recovery was still uncertain. In May he was appointed colonel. The next month he was in the field helping select gun positions near Malvern Cliff. By July 1862, there was some question as to whether he could perform his duties because of his health. In early August, Robert E. Lee sent him to Petersburg to make an examination of the country; that same month Stevens received his promotion as brigadier general.[1] He left the country after the war and went to Mexico, where he died November 12, 1867, at Veracruz. He was buried in Hollywood Cemetery, Richmond, Virginia. Cause of death: Yellow fever.[2]

1. *OR*, vol. 5:948, 1016; vol. 11, pt. 2:910, pt. 3:641, 663.
2. Burial Register, Hollywood Cemetery, Richmond, Va.

CARTER LITTLEPAGE STEVENSON • *Born September 21, 1817,* near Fredericksburg, Virginia. Graduated from USMA in 1838. Served in the Mexican and Florida wars. Dismissed from the U.S. Army in June 1861, he joined the Confederate service as colonel of the 53rd Virginia. He was promoted to brigadier general from February 1862 and to major general from October 1862. After the war he returned to Virginia and was engaged as a civil and mining engineer. He died August 15, 1888, in Caroline County, Virginia, and was buried in the City Cemetery at Fredericksburg.
DEATH CERTIFICATE: RNA

ALEXANDER PETER STEWART • *Born October 2, 1821,* in Rogersville, Tennessee. Graduated from USMA in 1842. In 1845, he resigned from the U.S. Army because of poor health and returned to Tennessee. From that time until the start of the war he held a number of prestigious university teaching positions. When he joined the Confederacy, he performed general duties until promoted to brigadier general in November 1861. His promotion as major general ranked from June 1863. He was reported to have been slightly wounded at Chickamauga, but in his report, written from near Chattanooga in October, he did not mention a wound. In June 1864 he was promoted to lieutenant general. During the Battle of Ezra Church before Atlanta on July 28, 1864, a ball made a V-shaped wound in the middle of Stewart's forehead. Blinded by the flow of blood, he had to be led from the battlefield. He was able to return to duty by the middle of August. Stewart returned to teaching after the war until 1886, when he was appointed a commissioner of the Chickamauga and Chattanooga National Military Park. He served in this capacity until his death. When he was more than seventy years of age, he learned to ride a bicycle. On one occasion, while riding about Chickamauga Park, he had a fall that confined him to bed for several days. On March 30, 1893, an empty freight train knocked him off a trestle bridge, and he fell some twenty feet. His right arm was broken at the wrist and above the elbow, and he was severely bruised. Even toward the end of July of that year he wrote with great difficulty and some pain. During the middle of 1895, he had a three-month siege of malarial fever and for a while was not expected to live. In January 1898 his doctor reported he had a heart condition but later reversed this diagnosis. While on vacation in August 1903 at Epsom Springs in Tennessee, Stewart had a stroke, which deprived him of the power of speech and paralyzed the right side of his face and the left side of his body. Although his powers of reasoning and memory were not impaired and he made a complete recovery, he relinquished personal supervision of the Chickamauga Park. Having great faith in the therapeutic value of natural spring waters, he visited the Borden-Wheeler Springs in Alabama before moving to St. Louis. His son, Dr. Alexander P. Stewart, Jr., who had given up his medical practice, devoted himself to caring for his father. Stewart died August 30, 1908, in Biloxi, Mississippi, from organic heart disease and the infirmities of his age. He was buried in Bellefontaine Cemetery at St. Louis, Missouri.[1]

DEATH CERTIFICATE: NAD

1. *OR*, vol. 30, pt. 2:360; vol. 38, pt. 3:688, 872, 904, 927, 943; Marshall Wingfield, *General A. P. Stewart*, 73–77, 112–13, 125–26, 143, 149, 170, 178–79; *Columbia (Tenn.) Maury Democrat*, Sept. 19, 1895; Alex. P. Stewart to S. G. French, Nov. 19, 1896, in Samuel G. French Papers, MDAH; *CV* 3:260–61, 12:392, 16:594–95; *CMH* 1:693; Burial Records, Bellefontaine Cemetery, St. Louis, Mo.

MARCELLUS AUGUSTUS STOVALL • *Born September 18, 1818*, in Sparta, Georgia. Served in the Florida wars. He entered the U.S. Military Academy in 1836 but was prevented from graduating because of severe attacks of rheumatism. Serving as captain of a militia artillery unit, he was made colonel of artillery in the Georgia militia in 1861. In October 1861 he was appointed lieutenant colonel of the 3rd Georgia Battalion in the Confederate Army. His promotion as brigadier general ranked from January 1863. He required a leave because of rheumatism in December 1863. During the Atlanta campaign on the night of May 15, 1864, Stovall was so ill that he had to turn over the command. He was not able to return until June 1. He was absent sick during the last of July, but on August 31 he fought at Jonesborough with his brigade.[1] With the close of the war he returned to Georgia and engaged in the chemical business. He died August 4, 1895, at Augusta, Georgia, and was buried there in the Magnolia (City) Cemetery. Cause of death: Valvular heart disease.[2]

1. CSR; *OR*, vol. 38, pt. 3:822–25; vol. 52, pt. 2:713; *CMH* 6:441.
2. Burial Records, Magnolia Cemetery, Augusta, Ga.

OTHO FRENCH STRAHL • *Born June 3, 1831*, at McConnelsville, Ohio. Strahl was practicing law in Tennessee at the start of the Civil War and in May 1861 joined the Confederate Army as a captain of the 4th Tennessee Volunteer Infantry. Elected lieutenant colonel the same month, he was promoted to colonel from April 1862.

In the middle of February 1863, he received a thirty-day sick leave on surgeon's certificate. His promotion as brigadier general ranked from July 1863. When Strahl entered the Tennessee campaign, he was recovering from a wound received at the Battle of Atlanta on July 22, 1864. At Franklin on November 30, Strahl was standing in a ditch handing guns up to troops who were posted above. He was shot in the neck but able to talk and crawl down into the ditch. A staff officer started carrying him to the rear when he was shot again. The third and last shot struck him in the back of the head, killing him instantly. He was first buried at St. John's Church, Ashwood, Tennessee, but his remains were later removed to the Old City Cemetery at Dyersburg, Tennessee.[1]

1. CSR; *OR*, vol. 45, pt. 1:654, 686, 737; *CV* 1:102, 9:149, 12:347; *CMH* 8:334.

JAMES EWELL BROWN STUART • *Born February 6, 1833,* in Patrick County, Virginia. Graduated from USMA in 1854. He was wounded by Indians at the Battle of Solomon's River, Kansas, on July 29, 1857. While charging a warrior, Stuart was hit in the center of the chest by a pistol shot fired from only two feet away. The bullet was deflected and lodged under the left nipple. Unable to continue the fight, he was taken to a small field fortification and a tent fly was stretched out. He had to stay on his back for hours because movement caused pain. Stuart was able to walk some by August 5 and was riding by the eighth. On August 17, he arrived at Fort Kearny. He had recovered by November though the bullet was not removed.[1] When Virginia left the Union, Stuart resigned his commission and entered the Confederate Army as colonel of the 1st Virginia Cavalry. He received his brigadier stars in September 1861 and was promoted to major general in July 1862. In Upperville, Virginia, on November 3, 1862, Stuart was slightly injured by a falling chimney that had been struck by a shell, sending shattered stones and bricks flying. On May 11, 1864, having intercepted Philip H. Sheridan's raid at Yellow Tavern in front of Richmond, he was mortally wounded. He had been waiting on horseback when one of the dismounted Federal troops, only ten to fifteen yards away, fired one bullet at him with a pistol. He was hit in the right side of the abdomen, but the missile velocity was not sufficient to unseat him from his horse. The .44 caliber bullet weighed about 180 grains and had a muzzle velocity of approximately seven hundred feet per second. Also, his horse became unmanageable, and Stuart was placed on the ground to rest against a tree. Another horse was obtained and he was lifted on it to facilitate moving if another charge occurred. Finally his surgeon arrived, and he was placed in an ambulance. Stuart agreed to take some whiskey, although apparently he had never drunk any before. It was possible to make an examination of the wound about a half hour after he had been hit. The doctor said Stuart was close to complete prostration, which was probably shock, and due to its rapidity, was neural in origin. To avoid the Federal troops, men constructed a detour over poor roads. Stuart died in Richmond on May 12, 1864, about twenty-seven hours after he had been shot. During the last few hours of his life, he himself applied the ice that was intended to relieve pain; he also ate a large quantity. Because his mind was clear, he was able to make final disposition of his personal effects. A combination of infection and hemorrhage probably were the factors that caused death within this period of time. The bullet had entered the right flank below the ribs, passed into the peritoneal cavity, perforating the intestine in one or more places, and severed blood vessels of the mesentery. Stuart was buried in Hollywood Cemetery at Richmond.[2]

1. J. E. B. Stuart to Flora, Aug. 19, 1857, in Personal Papers Collection, VSL; J. E. B. Stuart to Hon. Henry A. Wise, Nov. 11, 1857, in Murray J. Smith Collection, USAMHI; *SHSP* 8:437–38; Emory M. Thomas, *Bold Dragoon: The Life of J. E. B. Stuart*, 48–52.

2. Von Borcke, *Memoirs of the Confederate War* 2:29–30, 313–14; Freeman, *Lee's Lieutenants* 3:424–28, 761–63; *SHSP* 7:107–10, 140–43.

T

WILLIAM BOOTH TALIAFERRO · *Born December 28, 1822,* in Gloucester County, Virginia. He was commissioned a captain of infantry in the United States Army in February 1847 during the war with Mexico, and when mustered out had reached the rank of major. In November 1847, while at Pueblo, Mexico, he was extremely sick with an awful disease, which was known as "the scrooge" of Mexico. For many days he had to subsist entirely on calf's feet jelly, which, difficult to procure, cost him about three dollars a day. By the next month he was almost well. A practicing attorney, he commanded a Virginia militia before the Civil War and entered Confederate service as colonel of the 23rd Virginia Infantry. His promotion as brigadier general ranked from March 1862. In June he was ill and away from his troops. At Groveton on August 28, 1862, Taliaferro was shot in the foot, neck, and arm, the last being the most severe of the wounds. On the advice of his surgeons, he left the army for Richmond on the twenty-ninth. He visited his family during September and returned to Richmond in late October. In November his arm was sore; the doctor who examined him was certain that the ball was still in the arm. Taliaferro was back in December, and in March 1863 was assigned to the District of Georgia. In December 1863, Taliaferro was sick and went to the country to recover. In February 1864 he was commanding the Seventh Military District. At the close of the war, he returned to Virginia and resumed his law practice, served in the state legislature, and was a county court judge. He was feeble for a year or so before his death; because of failing vision, he gave up his position as judge. In November 1897, when his horse almost upset the buggy, Taliaferro had an attack resembling apoplexy. Prostrate in the bottom of the vehicle, he was taken to his home in Gloucester County and for days was almost insensible. Although he improved in December and January and was able to recognize friends, he could not carry on a conversation for more than a few minutes. He died February 27, 1898, and was buried in Ware Church Cemetery in Gloucester County.[1]

DEATH CERTIFICATE: RNA

1. *OR*, vol. 12, pt. 2:645, 654, 658; vol. 14:787, 814; vol. 19, pt. 2:683–84; vol. 21:675–77, 1036; vol. 35, pt. 1:112, 150; W. B. Taliaferro to wife, Nov. 13, 1862, in Mrs. Sally Lyon Taliaferro Diary, 1859–74, typescript copy; Wm. H. Manny to J. W. Taliaferro, Dec. 17, 1862 (1863), and "A Soldier Sleeps," Letters and notes pertaining to Gen. William Booth Taliaferro, all in William Booth Taliaferro Papers, CWM; Freeman, *Lee's Lieutenants* 2:109; Aztec Club Archives Historical Papers, General Information, W. M. Booth Taliaferro, Diary, typed, USAMHI.

JAMES CAMP TAPPEN • *Born on September 9, 1825,* at Franklin, Tennessee. After studying the law, he moved to Arkansas where he served in the state legislature and was elected circuit court judge. Tappen entered the Confederate Army as colonel of the 13th Arkansas in May 1861. He was absent sick on April 3, 1862, prior to the Battle of Shiloh, and rejoined his command on April 7. He was appointed brigadier in November 1862 and was transferred to the Trans-Mississippi Department.[1] After the war he returned to politics and his law practice in Arkansas. He died March 19, 1906, at Helena, Arkansas, and was buried there in Maple Hill Cemetery.

DEATH CERTIFICATE: NAD

1. *OR*, vol. 10, pt. 1:427, 429.

RICHARD TAYLOR • *Born January 27, 1826,* near Louisville, Kentucky. Despite poor health, he joined his father, Gen. Zachary Taylor, in Texas in 1846 when the Mexican War started. The climate did not suit him, however, and his father sent him back to New Orleans when he developed inflammatory rheumatism. In the spring of 1847 he had a recurrence of his symptoms, and in August he went to White Sulphur Springs, where he obtained some benefit after a month or two. During August 1850 he had what he called congestion of the brain produced by anxiety and exposure to the sun. Barely able to sit up, he went to Pass Christian, where he had to get around in a wheelchair. He was sick again in January and the first part of February 1853. Taylor was a member of the Louisiana state senate at the start of the Civil War, and he was appointed colonel of the 9th Louisiana Infantry. He became ill after the battle of First Manassas; a persistent low-grade fever was accompanied by loss of strength and the use of his limbs. To improve his health, he was ordered to go to the springs some twenty miles south, where his sister joined him. With her nursing care and the sulphur water, he slowly regained his health. The cold winter of 1861–62 was very hard on Taylor, who suffered with rheumatism and headaches. He was bedridden with arthritis during the last of September 1861, and given a leave in October, he was again nursed by his sister. He was promoted to brigadier general in October 1861. When he went to Richmond to talk to President Davis on April 30, he had to travel in an ambulance because of his pain. During the day and night of June 25, 1862, Taylor had severe pains in his loins and head. The next day he was unable to mount his horse; although the brigade marched off without him, they left behind a small ambulance in case he needed it. Lying on the floor of a vacant house, he was barely conscious enough to understand the messages sent to him. There was continuous pain in his head and neck and he had weakness of his extremities. After only a few hours of sleep on the twenty-seventh, he heard the sounds of battle and in a bouncing ambulance followed the troops to Cold Harbor. To preserve his strength, he used the ambulance throughout the Seven Days' battles. Paralysis of the lower extremities complicated his condition, and after the battles he was sent to Richmond, where he stayed for a month. Taylor's promotion as major general ranked from July 1862. In mid-July, Taylor was still an invalid and was sent to Louisiana to recruit troops. On October 19, 1862, he left Alexandria and proceeded to Jackson, Mississippi, then went with J. C. Pemberton to Vicksburg on the twenty-sixth. Illness prevented him from visiting the works on the Red River on January 19, 1864. In late April he had a low-grade fever; although quite sick, he was able to stay in the saddle. By May his poor health made it almost impossible for him to conduct the affairs of his command, and he again requested that he be relieved from duty. In June it was thought that his mind had been affected by his previous paralytic illness. He was on leave at Natchitoches, Louisiana, on July 28 when he was ordered to go to Alexandria. Because it was not possible to cross the Mississippi River, he was ordered to proceed to his departmental headquarters at Meridian. His health was such that it was uncertain if he could travel to see P. G. T. Beauregard in October.[1] An interesting detailed analysis of Taylor's wartime symptoms has been made, and it has been speculated that they were the result of a conversion reaction.[2] After the war he returned to New Orleans and worked against the detrimental effects of Reconstruction. Soon after moving to Winchester, Virginia, in the summer of 1875, he had a recurrence of his arthritis and spent several weeks in bed. Taylor died April 12, 1879, in the New York City home of a friend, where he had once again been nursed by his sister. He had dropsy and was aroused long enough to take communion before he died. Taylor was buried in Metairie Cemetery at New Orleans.[3]

DEATH CERTIFICATE: Cause of death, great engorgement and infarction of spleen, thrombosis of splenic and portal veins, ascites and hematemesis of six weeks' duration.

1. OR, vol. 9:731; vol. 11, pt. 2:620; vol. 12, pt. 3:918; vol. 15:174, 789; vol. 34, pt. 1:540, 543–45, 584, pt. 2:891; vol. 41, pt. 1:90, 118; vol. 52, pt. 2:771; Taylor, Destruction and Reconstruction, 23, 79, 83–84, 90, 93, 99, 196; SHSP 10:259; Freeman, Lee's Lieutenants 1:668; Liddell, Liddell's Record, 184; T. Michael Parrish, Richard Taylor, Soldier Prince of Dixie, 21–22, 35, 42, 45, 134–35, 153, 481.

2. Harris D. Riley, Jr., "General Richard Taylor, C.S.A.," Southern Studies: An Interdisciplinary Journal of the South (Spring 1990):67–86.

3. Maury, Recollections of a Virginian, 229–30; New Orleans Daily Picayune, Apr. 13, 1879.

THOMAS HART TAYLOR · Born July 31, 1825, at Frankfort, Kentucky. Served in the Mexican War. Before the Civil War, Taylor practiced law for a short time, was a cattle drover to California, and was a farmer and a businessman. He enlisted in the Confederacy in 1861 as a captain of cavalry. He was made lieutenant colonel of the newly organized 1st Kentucky Infantry and was elected colonel to rank from October 1861. Taylor's appointment as brigadier general in November 1862 was not sent to the Confederate Senate, and he had little field duty the rest of the war. He returned to Mobile after the war and engaged in business. In 1870 he went to Kentucky, where he served in law enforcement. He died April 12, 1901, at Louisville, and was buried in the State Cemetery at Frankfort.

DEATH CERTIFICATE: Cause of death, typhoid fever.

JAMES BARBOUR TERRILL · *Born February 20, 1838*, in Bath County, Virginia. Terrill, who was nearsighted, was practicing law in Virginia in May 1861 when he was elected major of the 13th Virginia. During 1863, Terrill was on sick leave for twenty-one days in February and for eight days in April. His promotion as colonel ranked from May 1863. He was killed in an encounter near Bethesda Church on May 30, 1864, and his body was taken by the Federal troops, who buried him at the Bethesda Church on the battlefield. Having already been nominated as brigadier to the Confederate Senate, his promotion ranked from May 31, 1864.[1]

1. CSR; *OR*, vol. 51, pt. 1:245; *CV* 13:21; *CMH* 3:672.

WILLIAM TERRY · *Born on August 14, 1824*, in Amherst County, Virginia. Terry started a law practice in Virginia in 1851 and was a member of a local militia group before the war. In April 1861 his unit was incorporated into the 4th Virginia, and he was made a lieutenant and the following April promoted to major. He was wounded in the left elbow and side at Groveton in August. By October he had returned, and he took part in the Battle of Fredericksburg in December. In September 1863 he was promoted to colonel. He sustained a contusion of the shoulder from a bullet at Payne's Farm, Virginia, on November 27, 1863, and went on sick leave in December. On May 12, 1864, at Spotsylvania, Terry received two slight wounds but was in command of Kemper's brigade on the seventeenth. His promotion as brigadier general ranked from that month. Although seriously wounded at Winchester on September 19, 1864, he returned with his brigade to the Petersburg lines in February 1865. On March 25, at Hare's Hill, Terry received a flesh wound from a projectile that killed his horse. Disabled by his wounds, when he heard the news of the surrender, he mounted another horse and started out to join the troops in North Carolina. After he returned home from the war, he resumed his law practice and entered politics. Terry drowned on September 5, 1888, while trying to ford a creek near Wytheville, Virginia. He was buried in the City Cemetery in that town.[1]

DEATH CERTIFICATE: RNA

1. CSR; *OR*, vol. 12, pt. 2:657; vol. 21:678, 681; vol. 36, pt. 2:1016, pt. 3:813; vol. 46, pt. 1:382; James I. Robertson, Jr., *4th Virginia Infantry*, 22, 29, 32; idem, *A. P. Hill*, 225, 233, 237–38, 245; *CMH* 3:673; Tyler, *Encyclopedia of Virginia* 3:91.

WILLIAM RICHARD TERRY • *Born March 12, 1827,* at Liberty, Virginia. Terry left his business behind in Virginia and was elected captain of a cavalry company in April 1861. He was made colonel of the 24th Virginia Infantry in September 1861. On May 5, 1862, while leading his regiment during the Battle of Williamsburg, he was wounded in the face. He took part in the battles of August 29 and 30 and took over command when Montgomery Dent Corse was wounded. Terry was supposedly wounded at Gettysburg during the charge on July 3, 1863. However, he was listed as in command at the end of the month and in August. In the fall he assumed command of James L. Kemper's brigade. His promotion as brigadier general ranked from May 1864. On March 31, 1865, near Dinwiddie Court-House, his horse was killed by a shell, and Terry's leg was broken. He was reportedly wounded seven times during the war. Terry returned to Virginia and entered politics. He also served as superintendent of the Confederate Soldiers' Home in Richmond and superintendent of the penitentiary. Ten years before his death, he had a stroke and never recovered. He died March 28, 1897, at Chesterfield Court House, Virginia, and was buried in Hollywood Cemetery at Richmond.[1] Cause of death: Paralysis.[2]

1. *OR,* vol. 11, pt. 1:567, 604, 609; vol. 12, pt. 2:626–27; vol. 27, pt. 3:1058; vol. 29, pt. 2:682; vol. 46, pt. 1:1264, 1268; *Battles and Leaders* 3:434–39; *CMH* 3:674; *SHSP* 22:116, 35:359, 37:193; *CV* 5:179.

2. Burial Register, Hollywood Cemetery, Richmond, Va.

ALLEN THOMAS • *Born December 14, 1830,* in Howard County, Maryland. Thomas was a Louisiana planter when the war started, and he was elected major of an infantry battalion that had been organized for state service. Other companies were added to his battalion, and he was made colonel of the 29th Louisiana Infantry in May 1862. His promotion as brigadier general ranked from February 1864. Following the war he returned to his plantation in Louisiana. He died from malaria on December 3, 1907, at Waveland, Mississippi. Thomas was buried in an unmarked vault at Donaldsonville, Louisiana, in the Bringier Tomb at the Ascension Catholic Church Cemetery.[1]

DEATH CERTIFICATE: NAD

1. *New Orleans Daily Picayune,* Dec. 4, 1907.

BRYAN MOREL THOMAS • *Born May 8, 1836,* near Milledgeville, Georgia. Graduated from USMA in 1858. After Georgia left the Union, he resigned from the U.S. Army in April 1861 and was appointed a lieutenant in the Confederate service. He was absent on sick leave in December 1862, and reported back to the field on January 2 during the Stones River campaign.[1] Having passed through grades, he was promoted to brigadier ranking from August 1864. Thomas returned to Georgia after the war and is best remembered for his work with the Dalton public schools. He died July 16, 1905, in that city and was buried there in the West Hill Cemetery.

DEATH CERTIFICATE: NAD

1. CSR; *OR,* vol. 20, pt. 1:758.

EDWARD LLOYD THOMAS • *Born on March 23, 1825,* in Clarke County, Georgia. After serving in the Mexican War he returned to his plantation in Georgia; in October 1861 he was made colonel of the 35th Georgia Infantry. He was wounded June 26, 1862, at Mechanicsville during the Seven Days' battles; however, he remained in the saddle and fought throughout the entire series of battles. On August 9 he took part in the fight at Cedar Mountain. His promotion as brigadier general ranked from November 1862. He was given a sick leave for thirty days starting January 2, 1863. He settled on his plantation in Georgia after the war until he was appointed to a position in the Land Bureau. Later he was transferred to the Indian Bureau and was an agent in Indian Territory. Thomas was ill for some time before his death at South McAlester, Indian Territory, on March 8, 1898. He was buried at Kiowa, Oklahoma.[1]

DEATH CERTIFICATE: NAD

1. CSR; *OR,* vol. 11, pt. 2:836, 839, 878; vol. 12, pt. 2:219; vol. 25, pt. 1:912; *CMH* 6:444; *CV* 6:181; Biographical Information, Edward Lloyd Thomas Papers, Library, Emory University, Atlanta, Ga.

LLOYD TILGHMAN • *Born on January 18, 1816,* near Claiborne, Maryland. Graduated from USMA in 1836 and resigned from the U.S. Army afterward. Served in the Mexican War as a volunteer. Tilghman was employed as construction engineer on various railroads until the start of the Civil War, when he was given command of the 3rd Kentucky Regiment. He was not well the last half of 1861. On October 30, 1861, while at Hopkinsville, Kentucky, he was too sick to even write. His promotion as brigadier ranked from that month. On November 17, he was ordered to turn over his command at Hopkinsville and to assume command of Forts Donelson and Henry. During the evening of May 16, 1863, Tilghman was killed on the field at Champion's Hill. In front of the Confederate battery were some cabins being used by Federal sharpshooters, and Tilghman dismounted to direct the gunfire against them. After sighting one of the guns, he went to a nearby knoll and was standing erect using his field glasses when a Federal solid shot or fragment went through his body. He died almost instantly. He was buried in Woodlawn Cemetery in New York City.[1]

1. *OR,* vol. 4:490, 560; vol. 7:144; vol. 24, pt. 1:218, 265; vol. 25, pt. 2:77, 80; *CMH* 2:163, Md.; *CV* 1:296.

ROBERT AUGUSTUS TOOMBS • *Born July 2, 1810,* in Wilkes County, Georgia. A wealthy prewar attorney and politician, Toombs was appointed brigadier general in the Confederate Army in July 1861. On August 1, 1861, he was charging around the Richmond fairgrounds on his horse when he was thrown. He retained the bridle but his foot was still in the stirrup. Dragged about, he was bruised but not seriously hurt. During March 1862, Toombs had a bad sore throat and cough, which had been bothering him for months. Early in April he had a severe choking episode, but by the middle of the month his health had improved. Toombs was severely wounded on September 18, 1862, by a ball through his hand after the engagement at Sharpsburg. He had drawn in his pickets too soon, and Federal cavalry had ridden into his lines. Toombs was still absent in late October. His chronic sore throat was less painful and his cough had decreased by January 1863. His hand had improved so that he could use it, but he could not close it well enough to hold anything. He resigned from the army on March 4. The chronic throat inflammation and nighttime cough bothered him again during the first part of 1864. In the summer of 1866, Toombs took sulfur baths for his throat condition. It improved, but he was not certain if it was the result of the water or because his cold was better. He left the country after the war and returned to Georgia in 1867, where he again took an active part in politics. He died December 15, 1885, at Washington, Georgia, and was buried there in Rest Haven Cemetery.[1]

DEATH CERTIFICATE: NAD

1. *OR*, vol. 12, pt. 2:566–67; vol. 19, pt. 1:841, pt. 2:683; Jeremy F. Gilmer to wife, Oct. 4, 1862, in J. F. Gilmer Papers, SHC; Robert A. Toombs to Julia, Mar. 26, 28, Apr. 3, 16, 1862, Jan. 16, 1863, Jan. 20, Apr. 21, June 24, 1864, and Robert A. Toombs to D. M. Dubose, July 11, 1866, all in Robert A. Toombs Papers, UG; Chesnut, *Diary from Dixie*, 99.

THOMAS FENTRESS TOON • *Born June 10, 1840,* in Columbus County, North Carolina. He left his studies at Wake Forest College in May 1861 and enlisted in the Columbus Guards. After this company became a part of the 20th North Carolina, he was elected lieutenant. At Seven Pines on May 31, 1862, a ball that had passed through another man slightly wounded Toon. He was wounded again at Cold Harbor but returned to his unit in July. In February 1863 he was elected colonel of his regiment. Toon was wounded on May 3, 1863, during the Chancellorsville campaign. Early in the morning he received one wound, and before ten o'clock he had received two more, which forced him to leave the field and give up his command. He returned and was at Gettysburg in July. A shot that went through another man's coat sleeve hit him in the leg on May 12, 1864, at Spotsylvania, but the injury only disabled him for a few days. His promotion as brigadier ranked from May 1864. Toon was admitted to Richmond's general hospital no. 24 on December 9 and returned to duty December 28. At Hare's Hill on March 25, 1865, he was desperately wounded while standing on the breastworks rallying his troops. Dr. Schofield of Petersburg took him into his own home, and he was there at the time of the surrender. Following the war he returned to North Carolina. In late November of 1901, Toon caught a cold while in Washington, which developed into pneumonia. For weeks after he returned to his home in Raleigh, he lingered between life and death. By February 1902, he had recovered enough to walk about the house and go up and down stairs. On February 19, 1902, the day he died, he had gotten up and eaten breakfast. He complained of acute indigestion, and his physician came and soon provided him with some relief. Exhausted, he was going to bed to rest for a short time. He had no sooner put his head on the pillow when he turned purple and died. The attending physician reported his death was due to heart failure. He was buried in Oakwood Cemetery at Raleigh.[1]

DEATH CERTIFICATE: NAD

1. *OR*, vol. 25, pt. 1:947; vol. 27, pt. 3:1059; Thomas F. Toon Papers, 1840–1902 (P.C. 998), NCSA; Clark, *Histories of Several Regiments* 2:112, 114, 118–19, 121, 124, 126; newspaper clippings, n.d, n.t., Ms. Ann Little, Raleigh, N.C.

EDWARD DORR TRACY • *Born on November 5, 1833,* at Macon, Georgia. Tracy was practicing law in Alabama when he raised a militia company, which was mustered into the 4th Alabama in May 1861. He was absent sick from late July through August 1861. In October 1861 he was appointed lieutenant colonel of the 19th Alabama Infantry Regiment, and his promotion as brigadier general ranked from August 1862. At Port Gibson, Mississippi, on May 1, 1863, he was hit in the chest by a minié ball and died instantly. He was buried at Rose Hill Cemetery in Macon.[1]

1. CSR; *OR*, vol. 24, pt. 1:258, 659, 661; *CMH* 12:477, Ala.

JAMES HEYWARD TRAPIER • *Born on November 24, 1815,* near Georgetown, South Carolina. Graduated from USMA in 1838. He was ill while serving in Mexico during March 1847. He resigned from the U.S. Army in 1848 and settled on his plantation in South Carolina. Trapier was active in local militia affairs and aided in the erection of batteries in Charleston harbor. At the beginning of the war, he was first a captain and then a major in the Confederate Army and served with P. G. T. Beauregard as an engineer. He was promoted to brigadier general from October 1861. Soon after reaching Tupelo in June 1862, his health failed and, at his own request, he was relieved from field duty. He returned to South Carolina and in October reported for duty at Charleston. During June and July 1864, he was on sick leave with anasarca, or dropsy of the skin. He survived only a few months after the war and died near Georgetown, South Carolina. According to family papers, he died on December 22, 1865. He was buried in the yard of the Church of St. George, Winyah, at Georgetown.[1]

DEATH CERTIFICATE: NAD

1. CSR; *OR*, vol. 35, pt. 2:593, 598; "Sketch of Life by Wife," Mar. 16, 1847, W. W. Mackall Papers, SHC; Trapier Family Papers, SCL; Manigault, *Carolinian Goes to War*, 21.

ISAAC RIDGEWAY TRIMBLE • *Born on May 15, 1802,* in Culpeper County, Virginia. Graduated from USMA in 1822. After resigning from the U.S. Army in 1832, he was an engineer for a number of railroads. At the outbreak of hostilities, he went to Virginia and was appointed colonel of engineers in the state services. He was commissioned a brigadier general in the Confederate service in August 1861. On August 29, 1862, at the battle of Second Manassas, Trimble was wounded in the left leg by a sharpshooter. He had ridden to the top of a hill to observe the Federal advance when he was hit. In great pain, he rode his horse back and then had to be carried from the field. Dr. Hunter McGuire examined him and stated he had been hit by an explosive shell. William C. Oates also reported that explosive balls were used in this battle. The ball had entered the leg about three inches above the ankle, burst in the tibia, and badly lacerated the structures. There were three distinct openings made by the exit of the fragments. Dr. McGuire recommended that he not have an amputation. Unable to go with the army, Trimble went instead to Mr. Foote's near Haymarket and shared the facilities with William N. Pendleton, who was also recuperating. He then went to private quarters in Front Royal. Trimble's spirits were good in spite of his severe injury. He wrote Robert E. Lee that his fighting qualities were "knocked up" for a week or two by a bad but not dangerous wound, and he was about to ask Lee to delay entering Maryland again until he got well enough to go. In the middle of October he went to a private family home in Staunton. Trimble had expected to return to the army by November, but he developed camp erysipelas and probably osteomyelitis. Boils developed around his ankle in mid-November so that he was unable to use his crutches to walk and thus restore the circulation of the leg. The boils were his chief problem during this period, and lancing them was almost more painful than an amputation would have been. In December 1862, the inflammation of the lower leg alternately increased and abated, and he could not walk without crutches. On the thirteenth of the month, a small piece of bone was removed from above the fracture. The doctor recommended laudanum and lead water as a wash for his leg, which had become very inflamed from the calf to the instep. In January 1863 Trimble could sit up all day and write, read, and converse. He was promoted to major general to rank from January 1863, left Charlottesville for the army on January 28, and assumed command on February 1. On the twelfth, he mounted his mare for the first time in more than five months and rode five miles without pain. He developed a cold in April after getting wet and had a relapse with almost fatal erysipelas. By early May, Trimble had almost recovered and was out riding daily. He had one episode of vomiting undigested food and nighttime fever, which he attributed to having stopped taking iron and quinine. However, improvement continued, and he was able to return in June 1863. On horseback at Gettysburg on July 3, 1863, he was again severely wounded in the left leg and was taken first to the house of David Whistler and then to the Samuel A. Cobean farm. Because of his previous good experience with Dr. McGuire, he called for him. This time the ball had struck the external malleolus, passed through the joint, and came out a little in front of the inner malleolus. A primary amputation of the lower third of the leg was performed by McGuire in the parlor of the Cobean farmhouse. The surgeons said that he had a high risk of developing erysipelas if moved in an ambulance, so Trimble elected to stay and be taken prisoner. Initially he was in the home of Robert McCurdy in Gettysburg, where he was captured by the Federal troops. Two weeks after he had been wounded, he was ordered to be transferred to the Lutheran Theological Seminary Hospital, where he found James L. Kemper. Trimble left for a Federal hospital in Baltimore on August 20 and had a miserable trip lying on the straw in a lime car. He withstood the trip well, and the hospital was clean and comfortable. On September 3 he was measured for an artificial leg. Finally, he was transferred to Johnson's Island in late September. In the winter of 1863–64, he started using his artificial leg but continued with his crutches because his stump had not hardened completely. He was exchanged in February 1865 and was prevented from going back to the army because of the Confederate surrender.[1] Following the war he made his home in Maryland and died January 2, 1888, in Baltimore. He was buried in Green Mount Cemetery in that city.

DEATH CERTIFICATE: Cause of death, primary, bronchitis; immediate, pneumonia of three weeks' duration.

1. CSR; *OR*, vol. 12, pt. 2:704, 712; vol. 19, pt. 2:683; vol. 25, pt. 2:801–2, 812; vol. 27, pt. 1:80, pt. 2:321, 362, 608, 660, pt. 3:867, 923; Trimble, "Civil War Diary of General Isaac Ridgeway Trimble," 1–20; McGuire, "Clinical Reports on Gun-shot Wounds of Joints," 147–50; W. N. Pendleton to wife, Aug. 31, 1862, and J. R. Trimble to R. E. Lee, Sept. 3, 1862, in W. N. Pendleton Papers, SHC; *CV* 4:27; Freeman, *Lee's Lieutenants* 2:274, 414–15, 700; *SHSP* 8:309, 26:118; *MSHW*, vol. 2, pt. 3:501; Coco, *Sea of Misery*, 7, 36, 126, 135.

WILLIAM FEIMSTER TUCKER · *Born May 9, 1827*, in Iredell County, North Carolina. He was elected probate judge in 1855; after studying the law he was admitted to the bar. When the war started in 1861, he was in practice and entered Confederate service as a captain in the 11th Mississippi Infantry. The unit was transferred to the West and became part of the 41st Mississippi, of which he was appointed colonel in May 1862. A severe wound of his right arm on October 8, 1862, during the Battle of Perryville, left him with a stiff extremity that was of little use. He returned to duty, however, and was ordered to assume brigade command in February 1863. He was promoted to brigadier general as of March 1864. At Resaca on May 14, 1864, while the brigade was in reserve and Tucker was observing the Federal movements, he was wounded in the left arm by artillery fire. On the same day, he had an excision of three inches of the humerus to within three quarters of an inch from the anatomical neck. Healing was prompt without bony union, and the limb was shortened three inches. Later Tucker could use his forearm and hand when it rested on a table or was supported, and he said it was "preferable to no arm." He never recovered full use of the left arm; with an already bad right arm, he was forced to retire from duty in the field. Following the close of the war, he returned to his law profession and politics. On September 14, 1881, he was killed in bed by a shot that came through an open window. He died in Okolona, Mississippi, and was buried there in the City Cemetery.[1]

DEATH CERTIFICATE: NAD

1. CSR; *OR*, vol. 23, pt. 2:623; vol. 38, pt. 3:761, 798; *MSHW*, vol. 2, pt. 2:694, Case no. 49; CSR of J. H. Sharp; "Biographical Sketch by Son," William F. Tucker subject file, MDAH; Manigault, *Carolinian Goes to War*, 181.

DAVID EMANUEL TWIGGS · *Born in 1790* in Richmond County, Georgia. Served in the Florida and Mexican wars. Twiggs participated in the War of 1812 and received a brevet of major general for his actions during the Mexican War. On January 15, 1861, he asked to be relieved of his command of the Department of Texas because all he had was in the South and his health would not allow him to take an active part in the action. However, before Twiggs could be relieved, he was forced to surrender his command at San Antonio in February 1861 by

Ben McCulloch and a force of Texas volunteers. Twiggs was dismissed in March from the United States Army because of his actions. When Jefferson Davis sent Twiggs his Confederate commission on May 25, 1861, directing him to take charge of the defenses in New Orleans, he was not sure if Twiggs's health would allow him to perform the service. On September 15, 1861, Twiggs's infirmities confined him to an armchair. Authorities at New Orleans wanted a more competent officer, since Twiggs was not only old—the oldest officer of the U.S. Army to join the Confederacy—but also physically unable to command. In October 1861, Twiggs's health still would not permit him to take the field, and he wanted an officer to relieve him. He died July 15, 1862, near Augusta, Georgia, and was buried west of Augusta in the Twiggs Family Cemetery on the property where he was born.[1]

1. CSR; OR, vol. 1:581; vol. 53:690, 739, 742, 744, 748; J. T. Winnemore to Earl Van Dorn, July 15, 1862, in Earl Van Dorn Papers, ADAH.

ROBERT CHARLES TYLER · Records concerning his birth are lacking, but he was probably born in 1833 in Baltimore. Little to nothing is known about Tyler before the war, and there is even some question about his name. He entered Confederate service as a member of the Fifteenth Regiment of the Tennessee Infantry and had risen to lieutenant colonel by 1861. On April 6, 1862, at Shiloh, Tyler was wounded while advancing into heavy fire and had to leave the field. He was listed as being in command in August; in October he was ordered to procure supplies for the army. On the morning of September 20, 1863, while at the Battle of Chickamauga, Tyler was slightly wounded and had to leave the field; however, he soon came back and took command. He was urged to go to the rear because he was disabled. He finally left the field at about 5:30 P.M. but was back the next day. His left leg was badly injured at Missionary Ridge on November 25, 1863, and had to be amputated, after which he was hospitalized at Marietta. His promotion as brigadier general ranked from February 1864. He spent most of his time on leave recuperating; then, in January 1865, he was placed in command of the post at West Point, Georgia, as he was unfit for field service. His general health was good in February; although he could get around on crutches, his limb was very painful. On April 16, 1865, a week after the surrender at Appomattox, Tyler was killed by a sharpshooter during the Federal attack on Fort Tyler, a small earthwork near West Point, Georgia. The sharpshooter was in one of the houses in front of the fort; earlier Tyler had refused to have the houses burned because he thought the people could not stand the loss. The first shot, which was mortal, was followed by a second, which cut his crutch in two and caused him to fall to the ground. He was taken to the foot of the flagstaff, where he died an hour later. Tyler was buried in the Fort Tyler Cemetery at West Point, Georgia.[1]

1. CSR; OR, vol. 10, pt. 1:442–43, 445; vol. 16, pt. 2:764, 968; vol. 30, pt. 2:385, 387, 398–99; vol. 31, pt. 2:742; vol. 49, pt. 1:364, 387, 429; Ezra J. Warner, "Who Was General Tyler?," CWTI 9:15–19; CV 4:381–82, 13:225, 18:28.

V

Robert Brank Vance • *Born April 24, 1828,* in Buncombe County, North Carolina. A court clerk during the years before the Civil War, he was elected captain of a militia company in 1861. The unit was made part of the 29th North Carolina Infantry in October 1861, and he was promoted to colonel. In January 1863 he became seriously ill with typhoid. In May he was at Shelbyville, Tennessee. While he was sick, his regiment was ordered to Jackson, Mississippi, and Vance never was in command of it again. He was promoted to brigadier general from March 1863. He returned to duty and was assigned to service in western North Carolina. Vance was captured in January 1864 and was not released for exchange until March 1865.[1] After the war he served in Congress and as a member of the North Carolina state house of representatives. He died November 28, 1899, near Asheville, North Carolina, and was buried in Riverside Cemetery in that city. Cause of death: Uremic poisoning.[2]

1. *OR,* vol. 29, pt. 2:860; *CMH* 4:351; Clark, *Histories of Several Regiments* 2:491, 711.
2. Register of deaths in the city of Asheville, Buncombe County Courthouse, Asheville, N.C.

Earl Van Dorn • *Born on September 17, 1820,* near Port Gibson, Mississippi. Graduated from USMA in 1842. Served in Florida and Mexican wars. He was wounded on the foot by a musket ball on September 13, 1847, upon entering the Belen Gate of Mexico City. Commanding an expedition against the Comanche Indians, he was wounded four times in a fight near the Wichita Village, Indian Territory, on October 1, 1858. Two of the wounds were inflicted by arrows and were quite serious. The first arrow entered the left arm just above the wrist, passed between the ulna and the radius, and stopped near the elbow. The second arrow entered the right side of his body at the level of the ninth rib and passed out on the left side between the sixth and seventh ribs. He fell from his horse and would have been killed had his troops not arrived in time. Lying on the ground wounded, he killed one of his attackers, then pulled the arrows out of himself. He, along with other members of the expedition, had to wait at the Wichita Village for five days before Van Dorn could travel. He was placed on a litter suspended between two horses and taken back to Camp Radziminski. He recovered quickly and took a five-week leave at home in Mississippi. He returned to command in November, although he was unable to ride for a number of months. He resigned from the United States Army in January 1861 and was commissioned colonel of cavalry in the Confederate service in March. During the summer of 1861, while at San Antonio, he had chills, fever, and trouble with his eyes. In June he was promoted to brigadier general, and in September 1861 he was commissioned major general. When he took command of the Trans-Mississippi Department in February 1862, he was recovering from a fall and immersion in a cold stream. The wet clothing and bad weather brought on attacks of chills and fever. In early March, his ill health compelled him to travel in a ambulance. At the Battle of Elkhorn Tavern on March 7, he was in the saddle although weak and feverish. On the morning of May 7, 1863, Van Dorn was working at his desk at his Spring Hill, Tennessee, headquarters when a local citizen entered and killed him with a pistol. The pistol ball entered the middle of the back of his head and came to rest under the forehead, causing the right eye to become swollen and dark. He was buried in Winter Green Cemetery at Port Gibson, Mississippi.[1]

1. CSR; "Military History of Earl Van Dorn, Hdq. of the Army, Adjutant General's Office," Aug. 4, 1880, Earl Van Dorn Papers, ADAH; Robert George Hartje, "Major General Earl Van Dorn" (diss.), 16–17, 44–46, 68–69, 94–95, 106; Robert G. Hartje, *Van Dorn: The Life and Times of a Confederate General*, 67–70, 124–25, 127, 142, 313, 316; *CMH* 12:273, Miss.; *SHSP* 2:182–83; Monaghan, *Civil War on the Western Border*, 233, 239; Victor M. Rose, *Ross' Texas Brigade*, 99–101.

ALFRED JEFFERSON VAUGHAN, JR. • *Born May 10, 1830*, in Dinwiddie County, Virginia. Vaughan was a farmer in Mississippi when he entered the Civil War as captain of the Dixie Rifles of Moscow, Tennessee. The company was mustered into Confederate service in June 1861 as part of the 13th Tennessee Infantry, and he was elected lieutenant colonel. The following December he was promoted to colonel. On sick leave and confined to his room on January 13, 1862, he could scarcely see to write. A spent ball struck him April 6, 1862, at Shiloh, but apparently did little harm. His promotion as brigadier general ranked from September 1862. At Vining Station, Georgia, on July 4, 1864, Vaughan was about 150 to 200 yards in the rear of his line behind a battery when he was wounded. After he had finished eating, he was lighting his pipe with a sun glass under a small opening in the trees when a Federal shell exploded just as it hit his left foot and the ground. The explosion left a hole big enough to bury him in. In addition to the injury to his foot, he had a wound on his right leg: a laceration below the knee, about four inches long and down to the bone, as if he had been cut with a sharp knife. Although his shock was severe, there was no blood or pain. The surgeon bound the leg, and after giving him whiskey and morphine, sent him in an ambulance to the hospital. On the way, he was stopped by Gen. Benjamin F. Cheatham, who gave him a drink of whiskey because he looked pale. Later, Gen. William J. Hardee stopped him and gave him a drink, followed by Gen. Joseph E. Johnston, who gave him a drink of brandy. Both men also thought that Vaughan looked pale. From this time on Vaughan knew nothing until he awoke on the platform in Atlanta at sunrise the next morning. During the hottest of weather, he was taken in the boxcar of a freight train from Atlanta to Macon, where he was admitted to a hospital. He had a compound fracture of the tarsus and metatarsus of the left foot. An amputation (Syme's) at the ankle was performed using chloroform. Soon afterward, one-third of the edge of the heel flap sloughed off and a few inches of the anterior surface of the tibia was exposed; however, the surgeon thought there was a serviceable stump. Years later, Vaughan wrote that the site selected for the amputation was poor, believing that had it been higher, he would not have had as many days of suffering. Most of his care took place in private quarters by the wife of his division's quartermaster. He was permanently disabled for further field duty. Following the war he engaged in farming in Mississippi. In 1872 he moved to Memphis and was clerk of the county criminal court. After a prolonged confinement at both his home and at St. Joseph's Hospital in Memphis, he was transferred, about a month before he died, to an infirmary in Indianapolis, Indiana, for treatment by cancer specialists. He appeared to improve until late September, when malarial symptoms appeared and aggravated his condition. His weakened state could not endure the strain, and he died on October 1, 1899. He was buried in Elmwood Cemetery at Memphis.[1]

DEATH CERTIFICATE: RNA

1. CSR; *OR*, vol. 38, pt. 5:865; CR, files 754 and 755; Alfred Jefferson Vaughan, *Personal Record of the Thirteenth Regiment Tennessee Infantry*, 19, 34, 85–88; *CMH* 8:133, 337; *Memphis Commercial Appeal*, morning ed., Oct. 2, 1899.

JOHN CRAWFORD VAUGHN • *Born on February 24, 1824*, in Roane County, Tennessee. Served in the Mexican War. A merchant in Tennessee at the start of the Civil War, he recruited a regiment that entered Confederate service as the 3rd Tennessee Infantry. Vaughn was elected colonel in June 1861 and was commissioned brigadier from September 1862. He was wounded near Martinsburg, West Virginia, during Early's march on Washington in July 1864. Vaughn was given leave and returned to Bristol, Tennessee. In September 1864, he took command of the forces in East Tennessee.[1] At the close of the war he returned to Tennessee and served one term in the state senate. Later he moved to Georgia. He died September 10, 1875, near Thomasville, Georgia, and was buried in Laurel Hill Cemetery in that city.

DEATH CERTIFICATE: NAD

1. *OR*, vol. 39, pt. 2:816; vol. 43, pt. 2:866; *CMH* 8:339.

JOHN BORDENAVE VILLEPIGUE • *Born July 2, 1830*, at Camden, South Carolina. Graduated from USMA in 1854. He resigned from the U.S. Army in March 1861 and was appointed a captain of artillery in the Confederate service. During the bombardment of Fort McRee, Pensacola Harbor, on November 22, 1861, he was wounded in the arm by a shell splinter. Despite the wound, he spent the whole night making necessary repairs to the fortifications. Villepigue was promoted to lieutenant colonel in September and was shortly afterward made colonel. In January 1862 he was appointed chief of artillery and engineers on Braxton Bragg's staff. His promotion to brigadier general ranked from March 1862. He died of pneumonia at Port Hudson, Louisiana, on November 9, 1862. At the time of his death, he had had a sick leave since early August, which he had declined to use as long as he was able to serve. The prolonged period with a possible sick leave suggests that he must have had some other underlying disease or that the pneumonia was not routine. He was buried in the Quaker Cemetery at Camden.[1]

1. CSR; *OR*, vol. 6:472, 489, 491, 493, 816; vol. 15:859; vol. 20, pt. 2:423; vol. 52, pt. 2:219; *CMH* 5:422.

W

HENRY HARRISON WALKER • *Born October 15, 1832,* in Sussex County, Virginia. Graduated from USMA in 1853. Walker resigned from the U.S. Army in May 1861 and joined the Confederacy as a captain of infantry. He was appointed lieutenant colonel of the 40th Virginia the following December. He was wounded twice on June 27, 1862, at Cold Harbor. In July 1863 he was promoted to brigadier general and returned to brigade command after having been in charge of a convalescent camp. On May 10, 1864, during the battle of Spotsylvania Court-House, Walker was wounded, and his shattered left foot was amputated the same day. He was hospitalized in Richmond for the rest of May and June. In August he was in Savannah recuperating. He was ordered to report for general court-martial duty in November. In January and February 1865, Walker was in Richmond and Charlottesville because of the wound.[1] Following the war Walker became an investment broker in New Jersey. He died March 22, 1912, at Morristown, New Jersey, and was buried there in the Evergreen Cemetery.

DEATH CERTIFICATE: Cause of death, primary, senile pneumonia; contributory, general arterial sclerosis.

1. CSR; *OR,* vol. 11, pt. 2:839, 842; vol. 27, pt. 3:998, 1025; vol. 36, pt. 1:1029, pt. 2:983; vol. 42, pt. 3:1204; CR, 178:142, 181:18; *SHSP* 16:268; *CMH* 3:675.

JAMES ALEXANDER WALKER • *Born August 21, 1832,* in Augusta County, Virginia. In 1852, he had difficulties with Thomas J. Jackson and was dismissed from Virginia Military Institute just prior to graduation. It is of interest that later, during the Civil War, the school's board sent him his diploma, supposedly at Jackson's request. Before the war he raised a local militia company and was elected captain. In May 1861 he was assigned as lieutenant colonel of the 13th Virginia Infantry. He was absent sick part of July and August 1861. In April 1862 he was promoted to colonel. At Sharpsburg on September 17, 1862, Walker was wounded by a piece of shell and his horse was killed under him. He remained on the field until his wound became very stiff and painful. In March 1863 he was admitted to the hospital with a urethral stricture; he took sick leave in April and May. During May 1863 he was promoted to brigadier general. That same month, on the nineteenth, Walker was ordered to report for assignment to brigade command. On May 12, 1864, at Spotsylvania Court-House, he was hit by a ball that fractured his left elbow. Carried to the rear, he was examined by Dr. Hunter McGuire, whom he urged not to allow an amputation. It appears that surgery could not be avoided, however, and Dr. Galt of Baltimore later performed the operation. Using chloroform and cold water for a disinfectant, the doctor removed some six to eight inches of bone and applied wooden splints. Four days later, Walker was delirious and had a fever. He went by ambulance to his father's house, where his wife joined him, but because of a Federal raid, they had to leave in a buggy to a safer location. His weight decreased while he had the fever and his wound suppurated for weeks. Each morning a tub of ice was brought from the icehouse and used to fill a piggin every hour or so. He would sit with his burning elbow buried in the ice while he read or played with children. In July 1864, with his arm still in a sling and his health poor, Walker was called back into service and assigned to the defense of the Richmond and Danville railroads. When he rejoined his unit, his arm still needed daily dressings. In January 1865, his arm was out of the sling and he participated in the fighting. He was in temporary command of a division in February 1865, although the arm continued to mend slowly. After the war he returned to his law practice and politics in Virginia. In 1893, Walker had a courtroom argument with a young lawyer that ended in a fight. Walker was bent backward over the bar rail and was hit repeatedly in the left side. He defended himself the best he could with his one good arm. In August 1893 he had urinary retention and had to have his bladder catheterized. Initially, there was only old and new blood but, when the catheter was reintroduced, urine was obtained. The surgeon thought small blood vessels about the kidneys had been broken during the fight. On December 26, 1898, Walker was operated on by Dr. McGuire in Richmond. Because Walker had a chronic urethral problem, it is assumed that the operation performed was most likely a suprapubic cystotomy for the formation of an artificial urethra, a procedure McGuire was credited with devising. It took only two minutes to perform and carried a much lower mortality rate than other procedures. Walker was shot during another legal confrontation on August 11, 1899, in Bristol. The opposing lawyer pulled a gun on Walker, who in turn pulled a derringer from his pocket and shot him. The defendant's secretary then shot Walker twice. The first bullet severed an artery in the right breast, just under the collarbone, and the second entered the right shoulder. Walker was initially semicomatose and was in critical condition for two weeks. When he went home on the third week following the shooting, his right arm was paralyzed. Because his left arm was already useless, he had to be helped with everything he did. He started his own vigorous physical therapy program and regained entire use of his right arm after several months. Before his death at Wytheville, Virginia, Walker had diarrhea, which developed into flux. After two weeks, he became comatose and died October 20, 1901. He was buried in the City (East End) Cemetery at Wytheville.[1]

DEATH CERTIFICATE: RNA

1. CSR; *OR,* vol. 19, pt. 1:956, 968, 977–78; vol. 25, pt. 2:809; vol. 36, pt. 1:1030, 1074; vol. 46, pt. 2:1270; Mrs. Manley M. Caldwell–Willie Walker Caldwell, "Life of General James A. Walker," 143–46, 273, 327, typescript, James A. Walker to Will, Aug. 24, 1893, Dec. 24, 1898, Jan. 2, 1899, Operator (telegram) to Mrs. M. M. Caldwell, Aug. 12, 1899, all in James A. Walker Papers, SHC; *CV* 9:510; *CMH* 3:676; Hunter H. McGuire, Jr., M.D., to author, Jan. 10, 1984.

JOHN GEORGE WALKER • *Born on July 22, 1822,* in Cole County, Missouri. Walker was directly commissioned into the United States Army in 1846 during the Mexican War. He was wounded on September 8, 1847, at Molino del Rey. In July 1861 he resigned to enter the Confederacy. He was made major of cavalry in the Confederate Army and was appointed lieutenant colonel of the 8th Texas Cavalry. His promotion as brigadier general was in January 1862. He was disabled by an accident on July 1, 1862, during the Seven Days' battles at Malvern Hill, and turned over his command. His promotion to major general ranked from November 1862. At Pleasant Hill, Louisiana, on April 9, 1864, a bullet produced a contusion in his groin. It was not until he was seen to be fainting from the effects of his wound that he was persuaded to dismount. Despite his suffering, he begged to be carried on a litter to command his men. At the end of the month at Jenkins' Ferry, he arrived back just as the battle commenced, still feeble from his unhealed injury.[1] He fled to Mexico at the close of the war. Later he was United States consul general in Colombia and was special commissioner to the South American republics. He died July 20, 1893, at Washington, D.C., and was buried in Mount Hebron Cemetery at Winchester, Virginia.

DEATH CERTIFICATE: Cause of death, primary, cerebral hemorrhage and apoplexy; immediate, paralysis and coma of four days' duration.

1. *OR*, vol. 11, pt. 2:915; vol. 34, pt. 1:565, 568, 592; *SHSP* 1:411; Taylor, *Destruction and Reconstruction*, 168–69; Blessington, *Walker's Texas Division*, 73, 197.

LEROY POPE WALKER • *Born February 7, 1817*, in Huntsville, Alabama. A lawyer and politician, he was appointed Confederate Secretary of War in February 1861. Throughout his life Walker had frequent colds and illness that precipitated absences from his job for short periods of time. In the summer of 1861, some people criticized his work as secretary of war, saying that it was poorly done because of his bad management and because of his frequent absences due to illness. Others, however, concluded that he was active and efficient; they thought his hard work contributed to his poor health. He did take a rest but suffered a relapse when he returned to his job. He resigned for health reasons in September 1861 and was appointed a brigadier general in Confederate service. Dissatisfied with his lack of field duty, he resigned his commission in March 1862 and served as a judge of a military court until the end of the war. Following the end of hostilities he returned to the practice of law and politics in Alabama. During the presidential campaigns in 1876, Walker gave speeches for his party while sitting down due to a back injury. He died August 22, 1884, six days after developing peritonitis during a trial in Huntsville, and was buried there in the Maple Hill Cemetery.[1]

DEATH CERTIFICATE: NAD

1. William Charles Harris, *Leroy Pope Walker: Confederate Secretary of War*, 101–3, 124–25; Rick Halperin, "Leroy Pope Walker and the Problems of the Confederate War Department" (diss.), 139–46.

LUCIUS MARSHALL WALKER • *Born on October 18, 1829*, at Columbia, Tennessee. Graduated from USMA in 1850. He resigned from the U.S. Army in 1852 and entered into business in Memphis. He joined the Confederate Army as lieutenant colonel of the 40th Tennessee Infantry and was made colonel as of November. Although sick on November 11, 1861, he was on the field by early December. His promotion as brigadier general ranked from March 1862. Walker's report on the evacuation of Island 10 and New Madrid, Missouri, was delayed until April 9, 1862, because of illness. According to a surgeon who examined him in April, he was unfit for duty due to intermittent fever and was extremely debilitated because he had had the disease for several weeks. In May 1862 he was told to report to Daniel Ruggles's division and subsequently took part in the engagement at Farmington on May 9. In November 1862, Walker's physical condition was very poor. The previous summer he had suffered two attacks of dysentery that, together with the very long and severe episode of continued fever from which he had just recovered, had enfeebled his health. He felt his condition was such that he would not be able to endure a vigorous campaign in the winter climate. His surgeon stated that Walker's removal to a warmer climate was necessary. On November 14, 1862, he was given a leave of absence. He reported to Kirby Smith in March 1863 and commanded a cavalry brigade. On September 6, 1863, at Little Rock, Arkansas, during a duel with Gen. John S. Marmaduke, he was mortally wounded. Brought across the river after being shot, he died the next evening. He was buried at Memphis, Tennessee, in Elmwood Cemetery.[1]

1. CSR; *OR*, vol. 4:512; vol. 7:748; vol. 8:131, 170, 807; vol. 10, pt. 1:822; vol. 20, pt. 2:508; vol. 22, pt. 1:525; William M. McPheeters's Civil War Diary—June 1, 1863 to June 20, 1865, Sept. 6, 7, 1863, in William M. McPheeters Papers, MHS; *CMH* 8:341.

REUBEN LINDSAY WALKER • *Born on May 29, 1827,* at Logan, Virginia. Before the Civil War he was a civil engineer and farmer. He entered Confederate service in 1861 and was promoted to major in March 1862. He was absent sick in Richmond through the period of the Seven Days' battles and returned July 2, 1862. Apparently this was the only time that he was ill or absent during the whole war. Walker passed through grades and was promoted to brigadier general from February 1865.[1] Following the war, Walker farmed for a few years and then was involved with the construction of railroads and the Texas state capitol. He died June 7, 1890, in Fluvanna County, Virginia, and was buried in Hollywood Cemetery at Richmond. Cause of death: Bright's disease.[2]

1. *OR*, vol. 11, pt. 2:536, 550, 839; *CMH* 3:680.
2. Burial Register, Hollywood Cemetery, Richmond, Va.

WILLIAM HENRY TALBOT WALKER • *Born November 26, 1816,* in Augusta, Georgia. Graduated from USMA in 1837. Served in Florida and Mexican wars. Walker was severely wounded in the battle at Okeechobee, Florida, on December 25, 1837, against the Seminoles. He was shot through the neck and the shoulder, one arm was broken, and he was wounded in one of his legs. Despite the wounds, he continued to lead his men until he was hit in the region of the heart and fell unconscious to the ground. For several months, Walker lay in Fort Brooke, Florida, suffering from the effects of the climate and his wounds. During 1839, while still disabled, he was ordered to rejoin his company. Feeling he could not go back to duty, he resigned. In August and September 1846, back with the army in Mexico, he was in poor health and said he would have blown his brains out had he been a bachelor. After his arrival at Tampico in February 1847, his health improved. A cannonball knocked him down during a fight in the middle of August, but he was not hurt. At the Battle of Molino Del Rey on September 8, 1847, he was wounded again. A doctor who examined him in November thought he should not have any permanent damage. However, Walker's condition was complicated by attacks of fever, ague, and diarrhea. By December he was suffering more from the debility of his long confinement in bed than anything else. He had been bedridden for nearly a year with his last wound and had to sleep in a chair because of his injuries and asthma. Later he was sent to Fort Ripley but had to leave the post and duty on the frontier because of the effects of the intense cold. His health continued to be poor, although Walker felt he was improving. In 1857 he was unable to sit up, yet he did not want to give up his military position as there was nothing for him in civilian life. Walker resigned his commission in the United States Army in December 1860 and was appointed brigadier general in Confederate service in May 1861. A severe attack of asthma brought on by exposure in July 1861 prevented him from doing any writing. He smoked a quantity of saltpeter and, although not confined to his room, had an indisposition to move about. In August 1861, owing to his poor condition and failing health, it was reported that Walker's stay in the Florida climate was injurious; he was relieved from duty to proceed by easy stages to Richmond. He was symptom free in Richmond, but exposure to the rainy weather at Manassas in September brought back his asthma. He kept ether and laudanum in his tent if he needed them. Walker resigned his commission in October 1861, because of either dissatisfaction or poor health. He commanded Georgia state troops for a short time, but for more than a year he was out of the conflict. He was again appointed brigadier to rank from February 1863 and was placed in command at Savannah. His promotion as major general ranked from May. On June 6, 1863, Walker was in private quarters on leave of absence by direction of the Medical Director's Office. He was killed during the battle near Atlanta on July 22, 1864. Leading his troops around a mill pond, he was shot by a Federal picket and fell dead from his horse. He was buried in the family burial area on the grounds of the Augusta College at Augusta.[1]

1. CSR; *OR*, vol. 1:469; vol. 38, pt. 3:631, 758, pt. 5:900; W. H. T. Walker to Molly (wife), Aug. 28, Sept. 2, 4, 1846, Feb. 19, August (n.d.), Nov. 26, Dec. 8, 1847, (date illegible), 1857, July 5, 1858, July 12, 21, Sept. 4, 14, 1861, and W. H. T. Walker to daughter, July 1861, all in W. H. T. Walker Papers, DU; Stephen A. Davis, "A Georgia Firebrand: Major General W. H. T. Walker, C.S.A.," *Confederate Historical Institute Journal* 2:1–15; *CMH* 6:449; *CV* 7:515.

WILLIAM STEPHEN WALKER • *Born April 13, 1822*, in Pittsburgh, Pennsylvania. Walker was honorably mustered out of the army in 1848 following service in Mexico but was commissioned into the regular army in 1855. Although he resigned his commission in May 1861, his rank as captain in Confederate service ranked from March. He held mainly staff and district commands and was promoted through grades to brigadier general ranking from October 1862. On May 20, 1864, near Petersburg, he accidentally rode into the Federal lines and was fired on when he refused to surrender. His horse was killed, and he sustained bullet wounds of the left leg and left arm and a contusion of his hip. When his troops retreated, Walker was left bleeding on the field until he was captured and taken within the Federal lines. The tibia and fibula were fractured. Near midnight in a Federal hospital, a primary circular amputation in the upper third of the left leg was performed using chloroform and the light from a bonfire. Exchanged in September 1864, Walker was transferred to a hospital in Richmond with his wounds healed, but he was still unfit for duty. On October 29 he was placed in command at Weldon, North Carolina. In late November, his stump was tender and had been aggravated by a recent fall. His left arm was still partially paralyzed from the effect of the bullet wound, which had cut the radial nerve, and his arm was sometimes sensitive to the cold. Unable to use his fingers for anything, and his recovery retarded by two falls which had injured his stump, he was not able to travel fifty miles for a medical examination in February 1865.[1] Following the war he settled in Georgia and died in Atlanta on June 7, 1899. He was buried in Oakland Cemetery in that city.

DEATH CERTIFICATE: Cause of death, uremia.

1. CSR; *OR*, vol. 36, pt. 3:34, 69, 820, 841; *MSHW*, vol. 2, pt. 3:474, Case no. 725; Robertson, *Back Door to Richmond*, 222.

WILLIAM HENRY WALLACE • *Born on March 24, 1827,* in Laurens District, South Carolina. Wallace finished his term as a member of the South Carolina legislature and enlisted as a private in Confederate service. In May 1862 he was elected lieutenant colonel of the 18th South Carolina. He had remittent fever during December 1863 but was listed as in command the following month. He was confirmed as colonel and brigadier general in 1864.[1] At the close of hostilities he returned to his law practice, his plantation, and politics. He died March 21, 1901, at Union, South Carolina, and was buried there in the Presbyterian Cemetery.

DEATH CERTIFICATE: NAD

1. CSR.

EDWARD CARY WALTHALL • *Born April 4, 1831,* in Richmond, Virginia. An attorney before the Civil War, he was elected lieutenant of the Yalobusha Rifles in 1861. The unit was mustered into Confederate service in June as part of the 15th Mississippi, and the following month Walthall was elected lieutenant colonel. In April 1862 he was elected colonel of the 29th Mississippi; his promotion as brigadier ranked from December. On December 27, 1862, he was on sick leave and did not return until about two weeks after the Battle of Murfreesborough. He was in the field in February 1863. On November 25, 1863, following the fight on Missionary Ridge, he remained in his saddle until after his men went into camp in spite of a severely wounded foot. Unable to walk, he had to be lifted from his horse. He was slightly wounded near Resaca in May 1864 but did not mention it in his report. His promotion to major general ranked from that month. Two horses were killed under him and he was severely bruised at Franklin on November 30, 1864, but he was back on the field shortly afterward. He returned to his law practice after the war. He was appointed to the U.S. Senate in 1885 and, reelected, served until 1894, when he resigned because of poor health. He resumed his seat in March 1895. He died April 21, 1898, in Washington, D.C., and was buried in Hillcrest Cemetery in Holly Springs, Mississippi.[1]

DEATH CERTIFICATE: Cause of death, typhoid pneumonia for two weeks.

1. CSR; *OR*, vol. 20, pt. 1:762; vol. 23, pt. 1:59; vol. 38, pt. 3:794; vol. 45, pt. 1:708–9; Edward C. Walthall subject file, MDAH; Confederate States Army Casualties, Roll 1; *CMH* 12:275, 278, Miss.; Manigault, *Carolinian Goes to War*, 54.

RICHARD WATERHOUSE • *Born on January 12, 1832*, in Rhea County, Tennessee. Served in the Mexican War. Engaged in business with his father when the Civil War started, he helped recruit the 19th Texas Infantry. In May 1862 he was appointed colonel of this regiment, and he was commissioned brigadier general to rank from March 1865. He returned to Texas after the war and was engaged in land speculation. Waterhouse was in Waco, Texas, regarding land matters when his business rivals tried to convince a young man to get Waterhouse so drunk that he could not attend to his duties. The young man warned Waterhouse of his rivals' intentions, yet Waterhouse was either drugged or became intoxicated and fell down the hotel stairs. He dislocated his shoulder and was confined to his bed. Within a few days he died, on March 20, 1876, from pneumonia. A grand jury inquest concerning his death was supposedly called but records are no longer available. He was buried in Oakwood Cemetery in Jefferson, Texas.[1]

DEATH CERTIFICATE: NAD

1. *Waco Daily Examiner*, Mar. 21, 22, 1876; *Houston Daily Telegraph*, Mar. 21, 22, 24, 1876.

STAND WATIE • *Born on December 12, 1806*, in the area that is now Rome, Georgia. He became part of the minority faction in the Cherokees when he signed the treaty to move the remaining members of his tribe from Georgia to Indian Territory. During the westward movement of the Indians in March 1837, Watie's health was poor. His face and jaw were swollen, and the doctor prescribed fermentations and cathartics. His condition had worsened by the middle of the month, and the cold, wet weather brought on headaches and a cough. More cathartics were prescribed. When his cough became worse and his condition further deteriorated, a blister was applied to his chest and he was given mucilaginous drinks and expectorants. In a grocery store in May 1842, a man started a fight with Watie and beat him with a whip. Watie stabbed his attacker and then killed him with a pistol shot. The majority of the Cherokees who had not favored the move west joined the Federal forces, whereas the minority under Watie joined the Confederacy. Watie raised a company of Indian troops early in 1861 and later that year was appointed colonel of the First Cherokee Mounted Rifles. During the war in the fall of 1863, he did not feel as well as he had in the past, although no further details are available. His promotion as brigadier general ranked from May 1864. Watie surrendered in June 1865, the last Confederate general to surrender. He later engaged in farming and business in what is now Oklahoma. His health was bad because of the long period of military campaigning, and in December 1867 he had a three-day episode of chills. In October 1870, he had some type of injury and was in poor health. He was stricken acutely by his final illness and died September 9, 1871, in what is now Delaware County, Oklahoma. Watie was buried there in Old Ridge Cemetery, which has since been renamed Poulsen Cemetery.[1]

DEATH CERTIFICATE: NAD

1. Kenny A. Franks, *Stand Watie and the Agony of the Cherokee Nation*, 42, 46–48, 81, 149, 194, 196, 202, 208.

THOMAS NEVILLE WAUL • *Born January 5, 1813*, in Sumter District, South Carolina. Bad health and poor finances forced him to leave South Carolina College before graduating. He studied the law, and after practicing in Mississippi a short time, he moved to Texas. He was elected to the Provisional Congress of the Confederacy and was one of those from Texas who signed the Confederate Constitution. After returning to Texas, he raised Waul's Texas Legion and was made its colonel in May 1862. His promotion as brigadier ranked from September 1863. In the Battle of Jenkins' Ferry on April 30, 1864, Waul was severely wounded and his left arm broken. After the enemy had retired, he left the field weakened by loss of blood. He spent June 1864 convalescing in Texas. In April 1865 he asked for extension of his leave on surgeon's certificate, as the bones in his arm had not yet fully reunited.[1] After the war he farmed and practiced the law in Texas. He died July 28, 1903, in Hunt County, Texas, and was buried in the Oakwood Cemetery at Fort Worth. Cause of death: Tuberculosis.[2]

1. CSR; *OR*, vol. 34, pt. 1:537, 818; *CV* 3:380; Blessington, *Walker's Texas Division*, 271.
2. Death records, no. 24 (1903–17), p. 30, Hunt County, Greenville, Tex.

HENRY CONSTANTINE WAYNE • *Born September 18, 1815*, in Savannah, Georgia. Graduated from USMA in 1838. Served in the Mexican War. He left the U.S. Army in December 1860 and was appointed adjutant and inspector general of Georgia. He held his commission as brigadier general in the Confederate Army from only December 1861 to January 1862, when he resigned and resumed his previous duties in Georgia. In early February 1865, he had an accidental injury to his right hand that prevented him from writing.[1] Following the war he was in business in Savannah, where he died March 15, 1883. He was buried in that city's Laurel Grove Cemetery.

DEATH CERTIFICATE: Cause of death, ascites.

1. *OR*, vol. 53:32.

DAVID ADDISON WEISIGER • *Born December 23, 1818,* in Chesterfield County, Virginia. Served in the Mexican War. He was in command of a militia battalion in 1861 and was made its colonel when the unit was accepted in the Confederate service as the 12th Virginia. On August 30, while at Second Manassas, Weisiger was wounded by a bullet and was disabled until July 1863. He was also wounded in the side by a bullet during the Battle of the Crater on July 30, 1864, just as he reached the entrenchment line. Later in the day he was helped off of the field by his aide-de-camp and was only absent for a few days. His promotion as brigadier ranked from July 1864.[1] Weisiger was a bank clerk and businessman after the war. He died February 23, 1899, in Richmond, Virginia, and was buried in the Blandford Cemetery in Petersburg. Cause of death: La Grippe.[2]

1. CSR; *CV* 3:68–70, 137, 7:362–64; George S. Bernard (speaker), "The Battle of the Crater," copy of an address before the A. P. Hill camp of Confederate Veterans of Petersburg, Va., June 24, 1890, pp. 18, 79, 86 in *CWTI* Coll., USAMHI.

2. Burial Records, Blandford Cemetery, City of Petersburg, Va.

GABRIEL COLVIN WHARTON • *Born July 23, 1824,* in Culpeper County, Virginia. Prior to the Civil War he was a civil engineer and engaged in mining. In July 1861 he was elected major of the 45th Virginia Infantry and the next month was appointed colonel of the 51st Virginia. His promotion as brigadier ranked from July 1863. Following the war he resided in Virginia, served in the state senate, and helped develop mining in the state. He died May 12, 1906, at Radford, Virginia, and was buried there in the family cemetery.

DEATH CERTIFICATE: RNA

JOHN AUSTIN WHARTON • *Born on July 3, 1828,* near Nashville, Tennessee. Wharton was an attorney in Texas at the start of the Civil War and was elected a member of the secession convention. He entered Confederate service as a company captain in Terry's Texas Rangers (8th Texas Cavalry). He was in Nashville from November 7, 1861, through the seventh of January 1862, on sick leave due to measles. After the deaths of the regiment's commanders, Wharton was elected colonel. Although very weak, he was with his troops in February. In March 1862, Wharton was sick at Franklin following an expedition to Charlotte. His right lung was involved by the illness, and on March 3 he turned over command of the 8th Texas Cavalry to Tom Harrison. At Shiloh on April 6, 1862, he was wounded in the right leg during a cavalry charge. By the morning of the eighth, he had been in the saddle for two days, and his wound had become so painful that he again had to turn over his command. He was unable to pay his respects in person to P. G. T. Beauregard in mid-April because of the pain. He was given a leave of absence on April 17 but was back on the field on May 11. In an engagement at Murfreesborough on July 13, 1862, Wharton and his Texas Rangers charged the Federal camp; he was severely wounded in the arm. However, he was able to take the captured Federal prisoners to Knoxville. He planned to remain near Rome, Georgia, during the last of July until his wound healed. He also did not feel he could endure another winter in the cavalry because of the damage to his right lung from the illness of the previous year. On the morning of September 20, 1862, Wharton arrived with his brigade and rejoined Joseph Wheeler. His promotion as brigadier general ranked from November 1862. He accompanied Nathan B. Forrest and Joseph Wheeler in the attack on Fort Donelson on February 3, 1863, where his chest was grazed by a ball. In late May 1863, while going full speed, his horse ran against a tree, injuring Wharton's left leg and foot. He was in bed for almost a week, then had to ride in a carriage and use crutches. By early June, he had almost recovered. He was commissioned major general to rank from November 1863. During January 1864, Wharton was confined to his room because the weather did not agree with him, and he had ruptured a blood vessel, probably in his right lung. In 1864, on account of his impaired health and because of command feuds, he was transferred to the Trans-Mississippi Department. His home leave was terminated when Richard Taylor assigned him to command of the cavalry after Tom Green was killed. On April 6, 1865, in a personal altercation with Col. George Wyeth Baylor at Houston, Wharton was killed by a bullet that entered below his short ribs. He was buried in the Texas State Cemetery in Austin.[1]

1. CSR; *OR*, vol. 10, pt. 1:569, 627, 895; vol. 16, pt. 1:806, 810–11, 894–95; Paul R. Scott, "Eighth Texas Cavalry Regiment," *Houston Tri-Weekly Telegraph*, Feb. 21, Apr. 25, 1862, July 8, 15, 1863, June 13, 1864, and "Testimony Before the Jury of Inquest on the Body of General Wharton," Apr. 10, 1865; Jno. A. Wharton to Wigfall, July 21, 1862, Louis T. Wigfall Family Papers, Letters of Gen. Joseph Eggleston Johnston to Louis T. Wigfall, UTA; *CMH* 11:261, Tex.; *CV* 5:530.

JOSEPH WHEELER · *Born on September 10, 1836*, at Augusta, Georgia. Graduated from USMA in 1859. Wheeler resigned his commission and entered Confederate service in 1861 as a lieutenant of artillery. Supposedly, Wheeler received three slight wounds as well as a painful one during the war, but in spite of all that has been written about him, there is confusion about the dates, and documentation is poor. In September 1861 he was appointed colonel of the 19th Alabama Infantry, and his promotion to brigadier ranked from October 1862. During an engagement outside of Nashville on November 27, 1862, he was wounded when a shell exploded under his horse. However, he stayed on the field. His commission as major general ranked from January 1863. During the fighting between November 23–26, he was struck twice by flying missiles. At Ringgold on November 27, 1863, he was wounded in the foot but again remained on the field. He was captured in Georgia in May 1865 and released the next month. In late August 1865, two former Federal officers broke into his room at the City Hotel in Nashville. While one held a gun on him, the other beat him about the head with a stick, which produced head and facial lacerations. Ill from his recent confinement in Federal prisons and bandaged from the beating, he returned to Augusta. Wheeler later lived in New Orleans until January 1869, when he was obliged to leave because the climate did not agree with him. He moved to Alabama and served eight terms in Congress. Wheeler was commissioned major general of volunteers in May 1898 during the Spanish-American War. He had a fever the last four days of June 1898 and, barely able to remain on the field, temporarily relinquished command. While the charge on San Juan Hill on July 1 was under way, Wheeler was ill in his tent. After the worst of the fighting was over, and in spite of his condition, he went to the front in the afternoon to help fortify the area. On the afternoon of the second, he returned briefly to the rear for a conference. Although his health was still poor, he returned to command. Wheeler next went to the Philippines and from July 1899 through January 1900 participated in the fighting against the insurrection. He retired as a brigadier general of the regular army. Following a brief illness, he died at the home of his sister in Brooklyn, New York, on January 25, 1906. He was buried in the National Cemetery at Arlington.[1]

DEATH CERTIFICATE: RNA

1. Dodson, *Campaigns of Wheeler*, 42, 155, 365, 372; Thompson, *History of the Orphan Brigade*, 969; John P. Dyer, *From Shiloh to San Juan: The Life of "Fightin Joe" Wheeler*, 64, 116, 190–91, 232–36; Jos. Wheeler to Jos. E. Johnston, June 18, 1874, in Jos. E. Johnston Papers, CWM; *CV* 14:154.

JOHN WILKINS WHITFIELD • *Born on March 11, 1818*, in Franklin, Tennessee. Served in the Mexican War. Whitfield was Indian agent in Missouri and Arkansas for a number of years, and when the Kansas Territory was established, he was elected its delegate to Congress. From 1857 until 1861 he was register of a land office in Kansas. He went to Texas and entered Confederate service as major of the Fourth Battalion Texas Cavalry. When the First Texas Legion (later the 27th Texas Cavalry) was organized in April 1862, Whitfield was made its colonel. On September 19, 1862, at the Battle of Iuka, he was wounded twice. The wound in the right shoulder produced a slight fracture of the humerus near its surgical neck. At the close of the year, Whitfield had recovered and was at Yazoo City with his command. He obtained a thirty-day leave on surgeon's certificate in April 1863 to go to Richmond because of rheumatism. His promotion as brigadier general ranked from May. Whitfield reported to Joseph E. Johnston in June and was assigned to the command of a brigade. The following fall, in addition to residual problems with his wounds, he developed diarrhea and rheumatism. In December he went to Texas; it was believed he would not return. Medicine had failed to produce even temporary relief, and a change of climate offered the best method of accomplishing a cure, according to his doctor. Symptoms from his whole muscular and osseous system along with the intermittent chronic diarrhea and the residual difficulties from his wounds added to his problems in October 1864. Following the war he lived in Texas and for a while was a member of the state legislature. He died October 27, 1879, near Hallettsville, Texas, and was buried in the Hallettsville Cemetery.[1]

DEATH CERTIFICATE: NAD

1. CSR; *OR*, vol. 17, pt. 1:123, 128, pt. 2:709; vol. 24, pt. 1:225; Sul Ross to Lizzie Ross, Sept. 24, 1862, Apr. 12, 1863, both in Ross Family Papers, BU; CSR of L. S. Ross; *CMH* 11:263, Tex.

WILLIAM HENRY CHASE WHITING • *Born on March 22, 1824*, in Biloxi, Mississippi. Graduated from USMA in 1845. An excellent student at West Point, he served as an engineer in the U.S. Army until he resigned in February 1861. He entered the Confederate service as a major of engineers and in the summer of 1861 received a battlefield promotion to brigadier general. His commission as major general ranked from February 1863. When called from Wilmington to come to Petersburg in early May 1864, he was ill. Then, during the action on May 15 through May 17, he was physically unfit from the disordered condition of his whole system, body and mind. His poor physical state was further aggravated by exertion and lack of sleep. At his own request, he was ordered on the twentieth to return to Wilmington and resume command of the Third Military District. While leading his men in the defense of Fort Fisher on January 15, 1865, Whiting was wounded by two balls in the right leg. One, which passed through the hip, produced a very severe wound. Initially he was taken to the hospital but then was transferred to Battery Buchanan when the garrison retired. The wounded men were then captured and had to wait for two days and a night before being placed on the steamer that transported them to the northern prisons. Whiting was taken to the military hospital at Fort Columbus, on Governor's Island. At first he seemed to do well, but he developed diarrhea, and the day before his death he did not have the strength to finish or sign a letter. He died March 10, 1865, and was buried in Oakdale Cemetery at Wilmington, North Carolina.[1]

1. OR, vol. 36, pt. 2:259–60, pt. 3:811; vol. 46, pt. 1:435, 438–42, 447; C. B. Denson, An Address containing a Memoir of the Late Major-General William Henry Chase Whiting, of the Confederate Army, 42–50; SHSP 26:165–74; Battles and Leaders 4:651, 654.

WILLIAMS CARTER WICKHAM • *Born on September 21, 1820, at Richmond, Virginia.* An attorney, politician, and presiding justice of a county court before the war, he entered Confederate service as captain of a militia company. In September 1861 he was elected lieutenant colonel of the 4th Virginia Cavalry. In the cavalry charge at Williamsburg on May 4, 1862, he received a severe saber wound in the side but continued in the saddle during the fight. He went to his father's home near Ashland to recover; too ill to be moved, he was captured on the twenty-ninth by Federal troops sent for that purpose. By the end of June he had recovered sufficiently, and he wrote to Confederate officials requesting that they try to get him released from his parole so that he could bear arms. After his exchange, he was promoted to colonel in August. East of Upperville, Virginia, on November 3, 1862, a piece of shell hit him in the neck. Recovering from this wound, he rejoined his command in time to take part in the Battle of Fredericksburg in December 1862. His promotion as brigadier general ranked from September 1863. In October, Wickham was absent from his brigade because of a serious injury sustained by a fall off his horse. In December he was listed as in command of his brigade.[1] He resigned his commission on November 9, 1864, and took his elected seat in the Confederate Congress. After the war he returned to politics and also became president of two railroads. He died in Richmond on July 23, 1888, and was buried in Hickory Hill Cemetery in Hanover County, Virginia.

DEATH CERTIFICATE: Cause of death, angina pectoris.

1. *OR*, vol. 11, pt. 1:443, 445, 572; vol. 19, pt. 2:143; vol. 29, pt. 1:452, 463, pt. 2:143; ser. 3, vol. 4:794–95; *CMH* 3:685; Von Borcke, *Memoirs of the Confederate War* 2:29.

LOUIS TREZEVANT WIGFALL • *Born April 21, 1816,* near Edgefield, South Carolina. He was admitted to the bar in 1839. During October and November 1840, Wigfall fought a series of three duels. In the first, he mortally wounded his opponent; in the second, neither combatant was hit. In the third exchange, Wigfall was shot through both thighs. A murder charge against Wigfall for killing his first opponent was dismissed in March 1841. He had an inflamed eye during July 1841; then, in September, he was on his back with a fever and was unable to work or take a legal case. The next month he was still debilitated and fatigued but slowly improving. Although he had not been out of his room, he had been able to walk around some. A light diet of hominy and boiled milk was started on the seventeenth. His sickness prevented him from making the proper arrangements for his wedding. Wigfall returned to his legal practice in October, a year after the first duel. Because of his vocal Southern stand, he was expelled from the United States Senate in July 1861. He was appointed colonel of the 1st Texas Infantry in August 1861 and promoted to brigadier general the following October. In February 1862 he resigned the commission and served in the Confederate Senate for the rest of the war. Following the war he lived in England until 1872. In late 1870 he developed a severe case of gout. He moved to Texas in January 1874, where he became ill. He died at Galveston on February 18, 1874, and was buried in the Episcopal Cemetery in that city.[1] Cause of death: Apoplexy.[2]

1. James P. Carroll to Hammond, Nov. 1, 7, 1840, June 1841; L. T. Wigfall to John L. Manning, July 22, Oct. 17, 24, 1841; Millege L. Bonham, III, to C. M. Lord, May 18, 29, 1925, all in Louis T. Wigfall Family Papers, UTA; Alvy Leon King, "Louis T. Wigfall: The Stormy Petrel" (diss.), 54–56, 58–59, 370, 374.
2. Internment Record, Galveston Health Department, Galveston, Tex.

CADMUS MARCELLUS WILCOX • *Born on May 29, 1824,* in Wayne County, North Carolina. Graduated from USMA in 1846. Served in the Mexican War. In the summer of 1857, because of poor health, he was sent to Europe on a twelve-month furlough from the United States Army. He left the army and in July 1861 was commissioned colonel of the 9th Alabama. He was promoted to brigadier as of October. He fought at Manassas Plains in August 1862, but afterward was absent because of sickness. In December he participated in the battle at Fredericksburg. During early May 1863, Wilcox was sick for several days with dysentery. His commission as major general ranked from August 1863. He was sick in the winter of 1864 and again in March 1865, but was back to duty by April 1.[1] Following the war he moved to Washington, D.C., and served as chief of the railroad division of the Land Office from 1886 until his death on December 2, 1890. He was buried in Oak Hill Cemetery in Washington.

DEATH CERTIFICATE: Cause of death, cerebral hemorrhage.

1. *OR*, vol. 12, pt. 2:567; vol. 21:610; vol. 29, pt. 2:686; Clark, *Histories of Several Regiments* 4:478; Freeman, *Lee's Lieutenants* 2:619, 3:631; *CMH* 8:342; *SHSP* 18:420–21.

JOHN STUART WILLIAMS • *Born on July 29, 1818,* near Mount Sterling, Kentucky.[1] Served in the Mexican War. A lawyer and politician, he served in the Kentucky legislature for two terms before the Civil War. He joined the Confederate service as colonel of the 5th Kentucky Infantry in November 1861, and his promotion as brigadier general ranked from April 1862. On October 11, 1863, at the time of the fight at Pugh's Hill, Tennessee, Williams was about two and a half miles from Rheatown, reclining on the ground quite sick. He had his unsheathed sword in his hand and, mad as a hornet, was "swearing something awful."[2] After the war he returned to Kentucky where he farmed and served both in the state legislature and in the United States Senate. He died July 17, 1898, at Mount Sterling and was buried in Winchester Cemetery at Winchester, Kentucky.

DEATH CERTIFICATE: NAD

1. Tombstone, Winchester Cemetery, Winchester, Ky.
2. George Dallas Mosgrove, *Kentucky Cavaliers in Dixie: Reminiscences of a Confederate Cavalryman,* 81–82.

CLAUDIUS CHARLES WILSON • *Born on October 1, 1831,* in Effingham County, Georgia. After entering the Georgia bar, Wilson spent most of his years before the Civil War in the practice of his profession. In August 1861 he was made captain of a militia company; the next month he was elected colonel of the 25th Georgia. According to some sources, Wilson died of dysentery in camp near Chattanooga on November 24, 1863. Others say he developed camp fever and died at Ringgold, Georgia, on the twenty-seventh of November.[1] His promotion to brigadier was confirmed by the Confederate Senate on February 17, 1864. He was buried in Bonaventure Cemetery at Savannah, Georgia.

1. CSR; *CMH* 6:453; Warner, *Generals in Gray,* 339.

CHARLES SIDNEY WINDER • *Born on October 18, 1829,* in Talbot County, Maryland. Graduated from USMA in 1850. Prior to the Civil War, Winder was stationed in the Oregon and Washington Territory, but the climate was detrimental to his health, and he had to return back East on sick leave. In April 1861 he was feeling better. There are few details concerning his prior illness, and it is not possible to make a diagnosis. Winder resigned his commission that month and was appointed major of artillery in Confederate service to rank from March. In July 1861 he was made colonel of the 6th South Carolina Infantry and was promoted to brigadier general from March 1862. During the first of August 1862, Winder was sick with a fever. He rested on the seventh and went toward the battle on the eighth. It was very hot, and Winder lay down when he arrived without giving formal notice he was there. Looking very pale and sick, he was urged by the medical director to take no part in the fighting on the ninth at Cedar Mountain. At the suggestion of Dr. Hunter McGuire, Henry Kyd Douglas was sent by Thomas J. Jackson to tell Winder that he had better turn over his command to the next officer and go to the rear until he recovered. Winder, taking this only as a suggestion, did not leave his brigade. While he was directing the artillery battery in his shirtsleeves, he was mortally wounded. A shell fragment passed through his left arm and side, tearing the flesh from the arm above and below the elbow, and lacerated his left side as far back as the spine. Initially, Winder was able to use the arm and recognize those around him. Placed on a stretcher, he was borne off the field and expired in a few hours on August 9, 1862. He was buried at the Wye House near Easton, Maryland.[1]

1. CSR; *OR*, vol. 12, pt. 2:178, 182–83, 191–92; Howard, *Recollections*, 162–64, 170–71; Douglas, *I Rode with Stonewall*, 128–29; Edward A. Moore, *The Story of a Cannoneer Under Stonewall Jackson*, 95.

JOHN HENRY WINDER • *Born on February 21, 1800,* in Somerset County, Maryland. Graduated from USMA in 1820. Served in the Florida and Mexican wars. Except for a four-year period when he was a planter, he served in the U.S. Army from the time of his graduation from West Point to the start of the Civil War. Returning home from duty in Florida in August 1837, he was afflicted with malaria. He was confined to his bed for four or five weeks and did not return to duty until November. In the fight for the Belen causeway in Mexico on September 13, 1847, a projectile hit the head of a nearby soldier and caused his brains to spatter over Winder's face, a piece of bone cutting his cheek. During the occupation of Mexico he was appointed lieutenant governor of Veracruz from December 1847 to July 1848. His health was impaired from an unknown cause, although not fever, while at Indian Key, Florida, in 1857. In May 1860 he became quite ill and returned to Baltimore. Although he was supposedly ill for a year, he left the United States Army and was appointed a major in Confederate service in April 1861. In June 1861 he was appointed brigadier general. Winder was made provost marshal of Richmond, and in 1864 he took on the duties of commissary general of prisoners east of the Mississippi. At one point he had "gangrene" of the face and was forbidden by his surgeon to go inside the stockade at Andersonville. While he was inspecting the prison at Florence, South Carolina, on the evening of February 6, 1865, he had chest pain and apparently died from a heart attack. He was buried in Green Mount Cemetery at Baltimore.[1]

1. CSR; *OR*, vol. 47, pt. 2:1121; *SHSP* 3:205; *CMH* 1:630; Arch Fredric Blakey, *General John H. Winder, C.S.A.*, 5–7, 37, 103, 104–5, 117, 201; Telegram from Henry Louis to Gen. S. Cooper, from Florence, S. C., Feb. 7, 1865, John Henry Winder Papers, Special Collections, DU.

HENRY ALEXANDER WISE • *Born December 3, 1806,* at Drummondtown, Virginia. Wise's health was poor during the early years of his life. While participating in the 1842–43 winter session of Congress, he was sick, partly from a long period of fever. His health remained bad, and finally on February 8, 1844, he resigned his seat in Congress. In May 1855 he was hardly able to talk and suffered from the effects of having drank limestone water. After the signing of the ordinance of secession in April 1861, Wise returned to his farm near Norfolk. His health had been poor for some time, and he was confined to his bed. Although he may be a "dying man," he wrote, he was going to Richmond to seek military service. Leaving his sick bed, he went to Richmond in May and was still an invalid when he left for Charleston in June to raise the Wise Legion. In June 1861 he was appointed brigadier general in Confederate service. When he turned over his command and returned to Richmond on September 30, 1861, Wise was ill from exposure to the mountain country's rainy season and was confined to his bed for several weeks. When his health had improved, he officially reported ready for duty by letter on November 18. On January 22, 1862, he was ordered to take command at Roanoke Island. After visiting the troops on the island on January 31, he returned to Nag's Head. The next day he had the sudden onset of acute pleurisy, developed a high fever, and spat up blood. He was in bed issuing orders until late on the evening of February 8, when, still prostrated, he was placed in a wagon and taken to Gallop's Ferry. Wise declined a leave to go home on the eleventh because his condition and strength were improving and he planned to stay in the field with his men. Finally, able to sit on a horse, he reached Great Bridge on February 16 after marching for three days in a steady rain with a few of his troops. Soon afterward he went home on furlough to improve his health. By March he was in Richmond. Later in the year, Wise was given command of the district between Mattapony and the James. In January 1864, at Adam's Run, South Carolina, he had a cough, catarrh, and influenza. Once during the war when he was critically ill with pneumonia, Wise awoke at midnight and had his servant get him a large cabbage, which he ate. In spite of what his physician predicted, it did not kill him. Following the war he practiced law in Richmond. His health was poor in 1875, and he was frequently ill. In January 1876, his chronic cough produced more distress from an enlarged hernia. Worsening of his health confined him to his house in Richmond from April until his death on September 12, 1876. Shortly before his death his cough became worse, his sputum was offensive, and ulcerations appeared on his mouth and tongue. He was buried in Hollywood Cemetery at Richmond.[1]

DEATH CERTIFICATE: Cause of death, consumption.

1. CSR; *OR*, vol. 5:150–51; vol. 9:112, 121–22, 139, 145, 150, 152–53, 158, 164–65, 428; vol. 51, pt. 2:32, 106, 519–23, 535; ser. 4, vol. 1:1016; Barton H. Wise, *The Life of Henry A. Wise of Virginia, 1806–1876*, 40–41, 102–5, 282, 303–5, 309–17, 418, 421–22; *CMH* 3:689; CSR of Beverly H. Robertson; Craig M. Simpson, *A Good Southerner: The Life of Henry A. Wise of Virginia*, 8, 15, 48, 113, 150, 313.

JONES MITCHELL WITHERS • *Born on January 12, 1814,* in Madison County, Alabama. Graduated from USMA in 1835. He resigned from the army the year he graduated and became an attorney. Following his service in the Mexican War he was a merchant and politician. Withers entered Confederate service in 1861 as a colonel of the 3rd Alabama Infantry, was promoted to brigadier general July 1861 and to major general from April 1862. Ill in early May 1862, he relinquished his command and went to the rear. In June, Braxton Bragg requested that Withers be assigned to some local duty for a few months to avoid the exposure of camp life; otherwise he would not be fit for field duty. He was relieved from command of his division on October 12, 1862, and was told to report to the commanding general for instructions. Withers took command again on November 10. He was on sick leave in late December 1862 and had not resumed command of his division by March. During the summer of 1863, he was relieved of command at his own request because of failing health and his inability to withstand conditions in the field. In February 1864 he commanded the District of North Alabama. Following the war Withers returned to his business in Mobile, where he also was editor of a newspaper, city mayor, and city treasurer. He was in failing health for two years before his death on March 13, 1890, but his final illness was only of a month's duration. He was buried in Magnolia Cemetery at Mobile.[1]

DEATH CERTIFICATE: Cause of death, mitral insufficiency. Duration of illness—years.[2]

1. CSR; OR, vol. 16, pt. 2:938; vol. 20, pt. 1:685, pt. 2:418; vol. 23, pt. 2:720; Manigault, Carolinian Goes to War, 16, 53, 78; Mobile Daily Register, Mar. 15, 1890.

2. Health Department of the City of Mobile, Ala.

WILLIAM TATUM WOFFORD · Born June 28, 1824, in Habersham County, Georgia. Served in the Mexican War. Prior to the Civil War, Wofford was an attorney, farmer, and politician. In April 1861 he was commissioned colonel of the 1st Georgia State Troops, which was redesignated the 18th Georgia Volunteers. His promotion as brigadier general ranked from January 1863. He was absent sick November to December 1864, and returned in January 1865.[1] After the war he participated in politics in Georgia. He died May 22, 1884, near Cass Station, Georgia, and was buried in Cassville City Cemetery, Cassville, Georgia.

DEATH CERTIFICATE: NAD

1. CSR.

STERLING ALEXANDER MARTIN WOOD · Born on March 17, 1823, at Florence, Alabama. He studied law in 1841 and was an attorney and politician prior to the war. Wood entered the military as captain of the Florence Guards in January 1861. In the middle of April 1861, he developed dysentery, occasional fever, and piles. On April 28, after being sick for more than a week with only slight improvement, and not having dressed or been out of bed, he requested a leave to stay in private quarters. There was also no physician present in whom he had confidence. When his unit was incorporated into the 7th Alabama Infantry in May 1861, he was elected colonel. Severe diarrhea, which even prevented him from sitting up, recurred in late October. Wood felt that if he continued to be sick all the time, he would quit the army by Christmas. However, by the nineteenth of December his health had improved; his promotion as brigadier general ranked from January 1862. At Shiloh, on April 6, 1862, his horse was wounded and became unmanageable. Wood was thrown and dragged among the tents. He was disabled for about three hours and then returned to his command. He was absent the next morning to obtain treatment for his injuries. In June 1862 he again questioned if his health would allow him to continue. Diarrhea, which he presumed was due to the water, confined him to his bed in the middle of September. Having recovered in private quarters from his sickness and complicating piles, he stated he would be ready to return to duty by October. At Perryville on October 8, 1862, while leaning against a tree, Wood was hit on the head by a shell fragment. The wound was dressed on the field, and he was sent to the hospital. He took a leave and returned by late December. His health was good during May and June 1863, and there was no recurrence of the illness he had had the previous summer. However, in September he was sick almost all of the time while on the march. He resigned his commission in October 1863 and did not serve for the rest of the war. Wood returned to civilian life where he engaged in politics and practiced law. He died January 26, 1891, at Tuscaloosa, Alabama, and was buried there in the Evergreen Cemetery.[1]

DEATH CERTIFICATE: NAD

1. *OR*, vol. 10, pt. 1:568, 570, 592, 599; vol. 16, pt. 1:1087, 1121; S. A. M. Wood to wife, Apr. 29, Oct. 31, Dec. 19, 1861, June 9, Sept. 14, Oct. 23, 1862, May 23, June 17, Sept. 12, 14, 1863, Surgeon's Certificate by Wm. C. Cross, Brigadier Surgeon, Apr. 28, 1862, S. A. M. Wood to Capt. T. B. Roy, Apr. 28, 1862, Daniel Coleman to ---, May 21, 1862, and Undersigned officers to ---, May 21, 1862, A. L. Hamilton, et al. to S. A. M. Wood, Apr. 14, 1863, Special Order no. 21, Oct. 27, 1862, and S. A. M. Wood to Hardee, Dec. 26, 1862, all in S. A. M. Wood Papers, ADAH.

AMBROSE RANSOM WRIGHT • *Born on April 26, 1826*, at Louisville, Georgia. Active in politics before the war, he was appointed colonel of the 3rd Georgia Infantry in May 1861 and was promoted to brigadier in June 1862. Badly wounded twice at Sharpsburg on September 17, he had to be carried from the field. He recovered in time to lead his brigade in the Battle of Fredericksburg in December. Six miles from Gettysburg on July 2, 1863, he became sick and had to leave his command. He returned at seven o'clock the next morning and was in command throughout the rest of the battle. Wright was absent on sick leave for thirty days in July 1864. On August 12, 1864, John B. Hood wrote that Wright was not able to take the field. Because he was unfit for field service, he was placed in command at Augusta in September. His promotion as major general ranked from November 1864. Following the war he returned to politics; he died on December 21, 1872, at Augusta, Georgia, and was buried there in the Magnolia (City) Cemetery.[1] Cause of death: Brain inflammation.[2]

1. *OR*, vol. 19, pt. 1:150, pt. 2:683–84; vol. 21:617–18; vol. 27, pt. 2:622–25; vol. 38, pt. 5:957; vol. 39, pt. 2:862; *CMH* 6:456; CSR of V. J. Girardey.

2. Burial Records, Magnolia Cemetery, Augusta, Ga.

MARCUS JOSEPH WRIGHT • *Born June 5, 1831*, at Purdy, Tennessee. Prior to the Civil War, Wright was lieutenant colonel of a local Tennessee militia regiment. He entered Confederate service with this regiment, which was designated the 154th Senior Tennessee Infantry. For a few months he acted as military governor of Columbus, Kentucky. At Shiloh on April 6, 1862, he was struck on the leg by a minié ball; although in much pain, he continued in command. He did not mention the wound in his report on the battle, written on the fourteenth from Camp Blythe near Corinth. He was promoted to brigadier general from December 1862. His health was poor at the Battle of Missionary Ridge, and in November 1863, he turned over command of his brigade. He was assigned to command of the post at Atlanta, Georgia, in February 1864. In June 1864, Generals William J. Hardee and Benjamin F. Cheatham thought Wright was physically disqualified for command. He was assigned to West Tennessee on December 14, 1864.[1] Wright returned to his law practice after the war but was best known for collecting Confederate records for official publications. He died December 27, 1922, in Washington, D.C., and was buried in the National Cemetery at Arlington.

DEATH CERTIFICATE: Cause of death, primary, arteriosclerosis and senility; contributory, embolism.

1. *OR*, vol. 10, pt. 1:449–51; vol. 32, pt. 3:581; vol. 38, pt. 4:788; vol. 45, pt. 2:690; Head, *Sixteenth Regiment, Tennessee Volunteers*, 209, 211, 253.

Y

ZEBULON YORK • *Born on October 10, 1819*, in Avon, Maine. Following graduation from law school, he practiced in Louisiana, where he and his partner accumulated large landholdings. He organized a militia company, which became part of the 14th Louisiana Infantry, and was elected major. In February 1862 he was promoted to lieutenant colonel. On May 5, 1862, he was wounded at Williamsburg, Virginia. In early August he was commissioned as colonel. York was wounded in the neck during the battle of Second Manassas on August 29, 1862. Along with other officers, he was sent to Louisiana in December 1862 as a drill officer, but as his services were not required, he was returned to his regiment in Virginia. His promotion to brigadier general ranked from May 1864. He was severely wounded at the Battle of Winchester on September 19, 1864, and his left arm was amputated. Incapacitated for further service in the field, he was assigned to recruiting. Economically ruined by the war, he later ran the York House in Natchez, Mississippi. He died on August 5, 1900, in Natchez and was buried there in the City Cemetery.[1] He died with paralysis.[2]

DEATH CERTIFICATE: NAD

1. CSR; *OR*, vol. 15:920–21; Terry L. Jones, *Lee's Tigers*, 61; *SHSP* 10:260; *CMH* 10:320, La.; *Battles and Leaders* 4:523.
2. Widow's application for pension (no. 8822), Catahoula Parish, La.

PIERCE MANNING BUTLER YOUNG • *Born on November 15, 1836*, at Spartanburg, South Carolina. He resigned from West Point on the secession of Georgia, and in March 1861 was appointed a lieutenant of artillery in the Confederate service. In the middle of November 1861, he had a high fever, chills, and delirium. Sent on leave, he was taken care of in private quarters; his father, a physician, came to see him. Young's condition was severe enough that he was unable to travel, and he did not arrive home until mid-December. His mother and family nursed him back to health. After trying to raise troops and buy horses, he returned to his men in April 1862. On September 13, 1862, near Crampton's Gap while on patrol toward Burkettsville, Young was wounded in the calf, but no bones were broken. He was taken into Virginia in a carriage, where his recovery in private quarters was helped by the presence of a number of pretty girls. He returned to the field in November. On August 1, 1863, he received a pistol ball in the chest during the fight near Brandy Station. The ball went through the flesh and passed out without entering the chest cavity; however, the wound was deeper than first thought. After hospitalization for ten days, he went home on leave and returned in early September. He was promoted to brigadier general that month. Near Hanover Court-House, Virginia, on May 31, 1864, he was wounded in the chest again, but this wound was more severe and was considered to be mortal. By late June, he went to private quarters in Richmond; although able to walk, his right arm was paralyzed. He went home in July and returned to duty in August with a stiff arm. His promotion as temporary major general ranked from December 1864. On May 3, 1865, he was home on sick leave. Following the war he was active in politics and served in Congress from 1868 to 1875. Young was ill in Washington, D.C., in the fall of 1876. He was consul general to St. Petersburg, Russia, for two years, and in 1893 he was appointed United States minister to Guatemala and Honduras. He had gout in January and February 1895, while in Guatemala. Continuing to have poor health, he took home leave to the United States in June and did not return to his position until October. His feet bothered him all the time, and he became tired when he walked. Because of his health, he started home in May 1896 and was hospitalized in New York City the next month. He had dropsy and orthopnea. Following a sudden sinking spell, he died July 6, 1896. He was buried in Oak Hill Cemetery at Cartersville, Georgia.[1] DEATH CERTIFICATE: Cause of death, primary, cirrhosis of the liver; contributory, nephritis and endocarditis.

1. CSR; *OR*, vol. 19, pt. 1:817–18, 824; vol. 27, pt. 2:312; vol. 47, pt. 3:870; Lynwood M. Holland, *Pierce M. B. Young: The Warwick of the South*, 49, 59–60, 67–69, 74–75, 83–88, 173, 232–39; *SHSP* 25:148–49.

WILLIAM HUGH YOUNG • *Born on January 1, 1838*, in Booneville, Missouri. Young left the University of Virginia in September 1861 and returned to Texas. He recruited and was elected captain of a militia company that became part of the 9th Texas Infantry. Following the Battle of Shiloh in April 1862, he was elected colonel of the regiment. At the Battle of Murfreesborough, on December 31, 1862, Young was wounded in the right shoulder by a minié ball; two horses were killed under him. On January 6, he reported on the operations of his regiment in the battle. At Jackson, on July 13, 1863, he received a flesh wound of the upper third of the right thigh and was disabled from duty for thirty days. In the Battle of Chickamauga in September 1863, he was shot through the left chest. In February 1864, he was listed as in command. During the Atlanta campaign at Kenesaw in June 1864, he was wounded in the neck and in the jaw. He took command of

Matthew Duncan Ector's brigade in late July. His commission as brigadier general ranked from August 1864. Young was wounded in the left leg in the engagement at Allatoona on October 5, 1864. Placed in an ambulance, he was taken to the rear, and when the vehicle took a wrong road, he was captured by Federal cavalry at New Hope Church. After many days without medical attention, he finally reached a hospital. The wound had apparently become infected, so Young was strapped to a stretcher and treated without benefit of an anaesthetic; nitric acid was poured into the infected area "until smoke reached the ceiling." He had a compound fracture of the lower third of the left fibula. The ball had entered the lateral aspect of the left leg about one and a half inches above the ankle joint, passed transversely across the fibula, and emerged from the posterior aspect of the leg. He was operated on December 24, 1864, through a three-inch lateral incision, and had a 1½-inch portion of the lower third of the shaft of the fibula resected. No arterial ligations were necessary. For four months he was in Federal hospitals at Marietta, Atlanta, Chattanooga, and Nashville. After the close of the war he returned to Texas and was a real estate operator and attorney. Years later, Young was on a train going east from Denver when it stopped, having come upon thousands of buffalo on the plains. Young got out to shoot one; when he fired, his rifle burst. Pieces of the steel gashed his forehead and knocked him unconscious. The engineer, seeing him lying on the track, picked him up and put him back on the train. Later, Young and his son were swimming when the son noticed a large depression, the result of a wound, in his father's leg. This was not the only evidence of his war experiences, as there were also scars below his collarbone and in the areas of his shoulder blade, thigh, arm, neck, and scalp. He died November 28, 1901, at San Antonio, Texas, and was buried there in the Confederate Cemetery.[1]

DEATH CERTIFICATE: Cause of death, pulmonary congestion, cardiac degeneration. Length of illness—few hours.[2]

1. CSR; *OR*, vol. 20, pt. 1:749; vol. 32, pt. 1:333; vol. 38, pt. 3:909; vol. 39, pt. 1:725, 727, 818; Confederate States Army Casualties, Roll 4; *CMH* 11:266, Tex.; Hugh H. Young, "Two Texas Patriots," *Southwestern Historical Quarterly* 44:16–32.

2. San Antonio, Tex., Metro Health District, File 113 for 1901, Ledger p. 121.

Z

FELIX KIRK ZOLLICOFFER • *Born on May 19, 1812*, in Maury County, Tennessee. Served in the Florida wars. After fighting the Seminoles in 1837, he returned and edited a newspaper until his health gave way. In 1840, he spent several months on a farm recuperating from an illness that caused the loss of a lung. He regained his health and in 1842 became editor of a paper in Nashville. Although very ill during Col. William B. Campbell's campaign for governor, he conducted the editorial portion of the campaign in his newspaper with great skill, and Campbell won the election. An argument with the editor of another paper led to a duel on August 20, 1852. His opponent fired and missed, and Zollicoffer's gun misfired. He was struck in the right hand when the other duelist fired a second time. Ignoring his wound, Zollicoffer supported his pistol on his left arm and shot the other man below the eye. He was appointed brigadier general in July 1861. On January 19, 1862, near Fishing Creek, with the smoke and rain causing poor visibility, Zollicoffer became confused in his directions. Attired in a conspicuous white rubber raincoat, he mistook Federal troops for his own. When he was recognized as being a Confederate, they fired a volley, and he fell dead from his horse. He died with his head resting on the root of an oak tree. Zollicoffer was hit by a number of bullets, but their exact number and locations vary even between those who supposedly examined the body. One surgeon who examined him reported that he was hit by several pistol balls from the rear and by a minié ball that passed clear through him from side to side. Another surgeon reported that he had been hit by four minié balls, one in the thigh, one through the heart, and two in the head, all from the front. He was buried in the City Cemetery at Nashville.[1]

1. OR, vol. 7:81, 86, 107, 565, 844–45; Battles and Leaders 1:392; CV 18:161–63; SHSP 31:167, 171; Susan Merle Dotson, comp., Who's Who of the Confederacy, 332–37; Head, Sixteenth Regiment, Tennessee Volunteers, 296–98, 309; Raymond E. Myers, The Zollie Tree, 21, 24–25, 96, 120–25.

A Sequence of Medical Incidents during the Civil War

KEY:

Accident (A)
Bruise (B)
Concussion (C)
Died (D)

Grazed (G)
Killed in action (KIA)
Killed in duel (KID)

Mortal wound (MW)
Suicide (S)
Wounded (W)

DATE	PLACE	NAME
1861		
May 31/June 1	Fairfax Courthouse, Va.	Ewell, R. S. (W)
June 10	Big Bethel, Va.	Hill, D. H. (C)
June 26	Kelly's Island, Potomac River	Ashby, T. (W)
July 11	Rich Mountain, W.Va.	de Lagnel, J. A. (W) Pegram, J. (A)
July 13	Corrick's Ford, Cheat River, W.Va.	Garnett, R. S. (KIA)
July 18	Blackburn's Ford, Va.	Moore, P. T. (W)
July 21	First Manassas, Va.	Bee, B. E. (MW) Gardner, W. M. (W) Gist, S. R. (W) Hampton, W. (W) Imboden, J. D. (C) Jackson, T. J. (W) Kennedy, J. D. (W) Law, E. M. (W) Paxton, E. F. (B) Pendleton, W. N. (G) Smith, E. K. (W) Stevens, C. H. (W)
July 22	Near battlefield, Manassas, Va.	Bee, B. E. (D)

DATE	PLACE	NAME
July 25 (1861)	Raleigh, N.C.	Ramseur, S. D. (A)
August 1	Richmond, Va.	Toombs, R. A. (A)
August 10	Wilson's Creek, Mo.	Clark, J. B., Jr. (W) McIntosh, J. M. (W) Price, S. (W) Slack, W. Y. (W)
August 25	Near Piggot's Mill, W.Va.	Jenkins, A. G. (A)
September 10	Carnifix Ferry, W.Va.	Floyd, J. B. (W)
October 8/9	Santa Rosa Island, Fla.	Anderson, Richard H. (W)
October 21	Tallahassee, Fla.	Grayson, J. B. (D)
November 7	Belmont, Mo. Ft. Beauregard, S.C.	Jackson, W. H. (W) Elliott, S., Jr. (W)
November 11	Columbus, Ky.	Polk, L. (A)
November 22	Ft. McRee, Pensacola Harbor, Fla.	Villepigue, J. B. (W)
December 13	Alleghany Mountain, W.Va.	Deshler, J. (W)
December 20	Dranesville, Va.	Forney, J. H. (W) Forney, W. H. (W)
December 26	Pohatan County, Va.	Cocke, P. S. G. (S)
December 28	Sacramento, Ky.	Forrest, N. B. (A)

1862

DATE	PLACE	NAME
January 19	Fishing Creek, Ky.	Zollicoffer, F. K. (KIA)
February 13	Ft. Donelson, Tenn.	Gholson, S. J. (W)
February 15	Ft. Donelson, Tenn.	Forrest, N. B. (C)
March 7	Elkhorn, Ark.	Hebert, L. (W) McCulloch, B. (KIA) McIntosh, J. McQ (KIA) Price, S. (W) Slack, W. Y. (MW)
March 21	Moore's Mill, Ark.	Slack, W. Y. (D)
March 23	Battle of Kernstown, Va.	Echols, J. (W)
March 28	Glorieta, N.M.	Scurry, W. R. (G)
April 6	Shiloh, Tenn.	Adams, D. W. (W) Allen, H. W. (W) Bate, W. B. (W)

DATE	PLACE	NAME
April 6 (1862)	Shiloh, Tenn.	Bell, T. H. (A) Bowen, J. S. (W) Campbell, A. W. (W) Clark, C. (W) Duke, B. W. (W) Gladden, A. H. (MW) Hindman, T. C. (A) Holtzclaw, J. T. (W) Johnson, B. R. (C) Johnston, A. S. (KIA) Lowry, R. (W) Tyler, R. C. (W) Vaughan, A. J., Jr. (G) Wharton, J. A. (W) Wood, S. A. M. (A) Wright, M. J. (W)
April 7	Shiloh, Tenn.	Breckenridge, J. C. (W) Cheatham, B. F. (W) Deas, Z. C. (W) Gilmer, J. F. (W) Hardee, W. J. (W) Marmaduke, J. S. (W) Mouton, J. J. A. A. (W) Smith, P. (W)
April 8	Shiloh, Tenn.	Forrest, N. B. (W)
April 12	Near Corinth, Miss.	Gladden, A. H. (D)
April 17	Near Rude's Hill, Va.	Ashby, T. (G)
May 4	Williamsburg, Va.	Wickham, W. C. (W)
May 5	Williamsburg, Va.	Early, J. A. (W) Forney, W. H. (W) Garland, S., Jr. (W) Harris, N. H. (W) Payne, W. H. F. (W) Terry, W. R. (W) York, Z. (W)
May 8	McDowell, Va.	Johnson, E. (W)
May 16	Near Corinth, Miss.	Hogg, J. L. (D)
May 23	Mechanicsville, Va.	Rosser, T. L. (W)
May 25	Winchester, Va.	Kirkland, W. W. (W) Nicholls, F. R. T. (W)
May 31	Seven Pines, Va.	Battle, C. A. (W) Bratton, J. (W) Fry, B. D. (W) Grimes, B. (A)

DATE	PLACE	NAME
May 31 (1862)	Seven Pines, Va.	Hampton, W. (W)
		Hatton, R. H. (KIA)
		Jenkins, M. (W)
		Johnston, J. E. (W)
		Johnston, R. D. (W)
		O'Neal, E. A. (W)
		Pettigrew, J. J. (W)
		Rodes, R. E. (W)
		Smith, W. (W)
		Toon, T. F. (W)
June 6	South of Harrisonburg, Va.	Ashby, T. (KIA)
June 8	Cross Key, Va.	Elzey, A. (W)
		Posey, C. (W)
		Steuart, G. H. (W)
June 9	Port Republic, Va.	Hays, H. T. (W)
June 26	Mechanicsville, Va.	Conner, J. (W)
		Hoke, R. F. (W)
		Starke, W. E. (W)
		Thomas, E. L. (W)
June 27	Cold Harbor, Va.	Elzey, A. (W)
		Evans, C. A. (W)
		Ewell, R. S. (W)
		Iverson, A., Jr. (W)
		Lane, J. H. (W)
		Logan, T. M. (W)
		McComb, W. (W)
		McGowan, S. (B)
		Pender, W. D. (W)
		Pickett, G. E. (W)
		Robertson, J. B. (W)
		Walker, H. H. (W)
June 28	Cold Harbor, Va.	Toon, T. F. (W)
June 29	Savage's Station, Va.	Griffith, R. (MW, died in Richmond, Va.)
June 30	Frayser's Farm, Va.	Anderson, J. R. (C)
		Barry, J. D. (W)
		Featherston, W. S. (W)
		Harris, N. H. (W)
		Jenkins, M. (W)
		Lane, J. H. (W)
		Perry, E. A. (W)
		Sanders, J. C. C. (W)
	Near Malvern Hill, Va.	Daniel, J. (C)

DATE	PLACE	NAME
July 1 (1862)	Malvern Hill, Va.	Anderson, G. B. (W) Brandon, W. L. (W) Cook, P. (W) Cumming, A. (W) Doles, G. P. (W) Jones, J. R. (W) Ramseur, S. D. (W) Ransom, M. W. (W) Walker, J. G. (A)
July 13	Murfreesborough, Tenn.	Wharton, J. A. (W)
July 15	Augusta, Ga.	Twiggs, D. E. (D)
August 2	Orange Court-House, Va.	Jones, W. E. (W)
August 5	Baton Rouge, La.	Allen, H. W. (W) Clark, C. (W) Helm, B. H. (A)
August 9	Cedar Mountain, Va.	Winder, C. S. (KIA)
August 28	Groveton, Va.	Ewell, R. S. (W) Taliaferro, W. B. (W) Terry, W. (W)
August 29	Second Manassas, Va.	Field, C. W. (W) McGowan, S. (W) Pender, W. D. (W) Trimble, I. R. (W) York, Z. (W)
August 30	Second Manassas, Va. Richmond, Ky.	Corse, M. D. (W) Jenkins, M. (W) Mahone, W. (W) Robertson, J. B. (W) Weisiger, D. A. (W) Cleburne, P. R. (W) Hill, B. J. (W) Polk, L. E. (W)
August 31	Stewart's farm, Va.	Lee, R. E. (A)
September 5	Crossing the Potomac	Grimes, B. (A)
September 6	Outside Frederick, Md.	Jackson, T. J. (A)
September 13	Road to Burkitsville, Md.	Young, P. M. B. (W)
September 14	South Mountain, Md.	Corse, M. D. (W) Garland, S., Jr. (KIA) O'Neal, E. A. (W)
September 15	Boonsboro, Md.	Lee, W. H. F. (A)
September 17	Sharpsburg, Md.	Anderson, G. B. (MW)

DATE	PLACE	NAME
September 17 (1862)	Sharpsburg, Md.	Anderson, Richard H. (W)
		Armistead, L. A. (W)
		Battle, C. A. (W)
		Branch, L. O. (KIA)
		Cooke, J. R. (W)
		Corse, M. D. (W)
		Cumming, A. (W)
		Fry, B. D. (W)
		Gordon, John Brown (W)
		Gregg, M. (B)
		Jones, J. R. (C)
		Kennedy, J. D. (W)
		Lawton, A. R. (W)
		McComb, W. (W)
		Ripley, R. S. (W)
		Rodes, R. E. (W)
		Sanders, J. C. C. (W)
		Smith, W. (W)
		Sorrel, G. M. (C)
		Stafford, L. A. (C)
		Starke, W. E. (KIA)
		Walker, J. A. (W)
		Wright, A. R. (W)
	Munfordville, Ky.	Forrest, N. B. (A)
September 18	Sharpsburg, Md.	Toombs, R. A. (W)
September 19	Iuka, Miss.	Little, L. H. (KIA)
		Whitfield, J. W. (W)
October 3	Corinth, Miss.	Cabell, W. L. (C)
October 4	Charleston, S.C.	Smith, W. D. (D)
October 5	Hatchie River, Miss.	Cabell, W. L. (A)
October 7	Camp Hope, near Austin, Ark.	Nelson, A. (D)
October 8	Perryville, Ky.	Allen, W. W. (W)
		Brown, J. C. (W)
		Carter, J. C. (W)
		Cleburne, P. R. (W)
		Lowrey, M. P. (W)
		Polk, L. E. (W)
		Tucker, W. F. (W)
		Wood, S. A. M. (W)
October 16	Raleigh, N.C.	Anderson, G. B. (D)
November 3	Upperville, Va.	Wickham, W. C. (W)
		Stuart, J. E. B. (B)
November 9	Port Hudson, La.	Villepigue, J. B. (D)

DATE	PLACE	NAME
November 27 (1862)	Outside Nashville, Tenn.	Wheeler, J. (W)
December 13	Fredericksburg, Va.	Barksdale, W. (W) Cobb, T. R. R. (KIA) Cooke, J. R. (W) Gregg, M. (MW) Pender, W. D. (W)
December 15	Battlefield, Fredericksburg, Va.	Gregg, M. (D)
December 18	Knoxville, Tenn.	Duncan, J. K. (D)
December 29	Rolling Fork, Ky.	Duke, B. W. (W)
December 31	Murfreesborough, Tenn.	Adams, D. W. (W) Allen, W. W. (W) Brantley, W. F. (W) Chalmers, J. R. (W) Clayton, H. D. (W) Gordon, G. W. (W) Johnston, G. (W) Kelly, J. H. (W) Rains, J. E. (KIA) Smith, T. B. (W) Young, W. H. (W)

1863

DATE	PLACE	NAME
January 1	Murfreesborough, Tenn.	Harrison, T. (W)
January 2	Murfreesborough, Tenn.	Hanson, R. W. (MW) Miller, W. (W) Palmer, J. B. (W)
January 4	Near battlefield, Murfreesborough, Tenn.	Hanson, R. W. (D)
January 11	Hartsville, Mo.	Shelby, J. O. (W)
January 19	Richmond, Va.	Jones, D. R. (D)
February 3	Ft. Donaldson, Tenn.	Forrest, N. B. (A) Wharton, J. A. (G)
March 17	Kelly's Ford, Va.	Rosser, T. L. (W)
April 14	On the Teche, La.	Gray, H. (W)
April 17	Montvale Springs, Tenn.	Donelson, D. S. (D)
April 29	Below Hamilton's Crossing, Va.	Battle, C. A. (A)
May 1	Port Gibson, Miss.	Tracy, E. D. (KIA)

DATE	PLACE	NAME
May 1 (1863)	Above Fredricksburg, Va.	Battle, C. A. (A)
May 2	Chancellorsville, Va.	Cook, P. (W) Fry, B. D. (W) Hill, A. P. (G) Jackson, T. J. (MW) Nicholls, F. R. T. (W)
May 3	Chancellorsville, Va.	Cox, W. R. (W) Evans, C. A. (W) Forney, W. H. (W) Grimes, B. (C) Heth, H. (W) Iverson, A., Jr. (C) McComb, W. (W) McGowan, S. (W) O'Neal, E. A. (W) Paxton, E. F. (KIA) Ramseur, S. D. (W) Scales, A. M. (W) Toon, T. F. (W)
May 4	Chancellorsville, Va. Fredericksburg, Va.	Pender, W. D. (W) Godwin, A. C. (W) Hoke, R. F. (W)
May 7	Spring Hill, Tenn.	Van Dorn, E. (Assassinated)
May 10	Chandler House, Guinea's Station, Va.	Jackson, T. J. (D)
May 14	Near Jackson, Miss.	Capers, E. (W)
May 16	Champion Hill, Miss.	Baker, A. (W) Lee, S. D. (W) Tilghman, L. (KIA)
May 18	Near Tennessee River Vicksburg, Miss.	Dibrell, G. G. (A) Cockrell, F. M. (B)
May 22	Vicksburg, Miss.	Baldwin, W. E. (W)
June 9	Brandy Station, Va.	Barringer, R. (W) Butler, M. C. (W) Lee, W. H. F. (W)
June 13	Columbia, Tenn.	Forrest, N. B. (W)
June 14	Millwood Road, Va.	Ewell, R. S. (B)
June 17	Vicksburg, Miss.	Garrott, I. W. (KIA)
June 20	Middleburg, Va.	Beale, R. L. T. (W)
June 24	Hoover's Gap, Tenn.	Bate, W. B. (W)

DATE	PLACE	NAME
June 25 (1863)	Vicksburg, Miss.	Green, M. E. (W)
June 27	Vicksburg, Miss.	Green, M. E. (KIA)
June 28	Donaldsonville, La.	Major, J. P. (W)
June 30	Hanover, Pa.	Payne, W. H. F. (W)
July 1	Vicksburg, Miss.	Cockrell, F. M. (C)
	Gettysburg, Pa.	Archer, J. J. (W)
		Evans, C. A. (W)
		Heth, H. (W)
		Johnston, R. D. (W)
		Leventhorpe, C. (W)
		Scales, A. M. (W)
July 2	Gettysburg, Pa.	Alexander, E. P. (G)
		Anderson, G. T. (W)
		Barksdale, W. (MW)
		Forney, W. H. (W)
		Hampton, W. (W)
		Hood, J. B. (W)
		Jenkins, A. G. (W)
		Jones, J. M. (W)
		Kennedy, J. D. (W)
		Pender, W. D. (MW)
		Perry, W. F. (C)
		Robertson, J. B. (W)
		Sanders, J. C. C. (W)
		Semmes, P. J. (MW)
		Sorrel, G. M. (W)
July 3	Gettysburg, Pa.	Armistead, L. A. (MW)
		Davis, J. R. (W)
		Fry, B. D. (W)
		Garnett, R. B. (KIA)
		Hunton, E. (W)
		Johnson, E. (W)
		Kemper, J. L. (W)
		Lane, J. H. (A)
		Pettigrew, J. J. (W)
		Terry, W. R. (W)
		Trimble, I. R. (W)
	Federal Field Hospital	Barksdale, W. (D)
July 4	Helena, Ark.	Shelby, J. O. (W)
July 5	Federal Field Hospital	Armistead, L. A. (D)
July 9	Martinsburg, W.Va.	Semmes, P. J. (D)
July 13	Near Raymond, Miss.	Bowen, J. S. (D)
	Jackson, Miss.	Young, W. H. (W)

DATE	PLACE	NAME
July 14 (1863)	Falling Waters, Md.	Pettigrew, J. J. (MW)
July 17	Bunker Hill, Va.	Pettigrew, J. J. (D)
July 18	Staunton, Va.	Pender, W. D. (D)
August 1	Brandy Station, Va.	Baker, L. S. (W) Young, P. M. B. (W)
August 26	Near Abingdon, Va.	Floyd, J. B. (D)
September 6	Little Rock, Ark.	Walker, L. M. (MW— Duel)
September 7	Little Rock, Ark.	Walker, L. M. (D)
September 11	Tunnel Hill, Ga.	Forrest, N. B. (A)
September 13	East of Brandy Station, Va.	Beale, R. L. T. (W)
September 19	Chickamauga, Ga.	DuBose, D. McI. (W) Granbury, H. B. (W) Gregg, J. (W) Holtzclaw, J. T. (A) Palmer, J. B. (W) Smith, P. (KIA) Smith, T. B. (W)
September 20	Chickamauga, Ga.	Adams, D. W. (W) Brown, J. C. (W) Capers, E. (W) Clayton, H. D. (W) Deshler, J. (KIA) Helm, B. H. (MW) Hindman, T. C. (W) Hood, J. B. (W) McNair, E. (W) Stevens, C. H. (W) Tyler, R. C. (W)
	Federal Hospital	Helm, B. H. (D)
October 7	Near Farmington, Tenn.	Humes, W. Y. C. (W)
October 11	Collierville, Tenn.	Chalmers, J. R. (B)
October 12	Near Fleetwood, Va.	Rosser, T. L. (W)
October 14	Bristoe Station, Va.	Barringer, R. (W) Cooke, J. R. (W) Kirkland, W. W. (W) Posey, C. (MW)
	Near Warrenton Road, Va.	Gordon, James B. (W)
November 7	Near Kelly's Ford and Wheatly, Va.	Cox, W. R. (W)

DATE	PLACE	NAME
November 13 (1863)	Charlottesville, Va.	Posey, C. (D)
November 18	Knoxville, Tenn.	Kennedy, J. D. (W)
November 25	Missionary Ridge, Tenn.	Smith, J. A. (W) Tyler, R. C. (W) Walthall, E. C. (W)
November 26	Near Ringgold, Ga.	Maney, G. E. (W)
November 27	Payne's Farm, Va.	Jones, J. M. (W) Steuart, G. H. (W) Terry, W. (W)
	Ringgold, Ga.	Wheeler, J. (W) Wilson, C. C. (D)
November 29	Fort Loudon, Tenn.	Simms, J. P. (W)
December 11	Ft. Sumter, S.C.	Elliott, S., Jr. (W)
December 14	Bean's Station, Tenn.	Gracie, A., Jr. (W)
December 21	Clinch River, Tenn.	Dibrell, G. G. (W)

1864

February 1	Near New Bern, N.C.	Clingman, T. L. (B)
February 19	Near Dog River Factory, Ala.	Baldwin, W. E. (D—Accident)
February 24	Near Pearl River, Miss.	Ferguson, S. W. (W)
April 8	Mansfield, La.	Lane, W. P. (W) Mouton, J. J. A. A. (KIA)
April 9	Pleasant Hill, La.	Bee, H. P. (W) Scurry, W. R. (W) Walker, J. G. (W)
April 12	Blair's Landing, La. Ft. Pillow, Tenn.	Green, T. (KIA) Forrest, N. B. (A)
April 14	Moscow and Camden Road, Ark.	Gano, R. M. (W)
April 30	Jenkins' Ferry, Ark.	Clark, J. B., Jr. (W) Scurry, W. R. (KIA) Waul, T. N. (W)
May 5	Wilderness, Va.	Jones, J. M. (KIA) Pegram, J. (W) Stafford, L. A. (MW)
May 6	Wilderness, Va.	Benning, H. L. (W) Field, C. W. (W) Jenkins, M. (KIA)

DATE	PLACE	NAME
May 6 (1864)	Wilderness, Va.	Kennedy, J. D. (W) Longstreet, J. (W) Perry, E. A. (W)
May 8	Richmond, Va.	Stafford, L. A. (D)
May 9	South of James River Cloyd's Mountain, Va. Spotsylvania Court- House, Va.	Battle, C. A. (A) Jenkins, A. G. (MW) Hays, H. T. (W)
May 10	Spotsylvania Court- House, Va.	Walker, H. H. (W)
May 11	Yellow Tavern, Va.	Stuart, J. E. B. (MW)
May 12	Spotsylvania Court- House, Va.	Daniel, J. (MW) Johnston, R. D. (W) McGowan, S. (W) Perrin, A. M. (KIA) Ramseur, S. D. (W) Terry, W. (W) Toon, T. F. (W) Walker, J. A. (W)
	Meadow Bridge, Va. Richmond, Va.	Gordon, James B. (MW) Stuart, J. E. B. (D)
May 13	Near Spotsylvania Court- House, Va.	Daniel, J. (D)
May 14	Resaca, Ga. Wooldridge Hill, Va.	Finley, J. J. (W) Manigault, A. M. (W) Tucker, W. F. (W) Ransom, M. W. (W)
May 16	Drewry's Bluff, Va.	Moody, Y. M. (W) Corse, M. D. (G)
May 18	Richmond, Va.	Gordon, James B. (D)
May 20	Ware Bottom Church, Va.	Walker, W. S. (W)
May 21	Federal Hospital	Jenkins, A. G. (D)
May 27	New Hope Church, Ga.	Reynolds, A. W. (W)
May 28	Near James River, Va.	Dunovant, J. (W)
May 30	Bethesda Church, Va.	Terrill, J. B. (KIA)
May 31	Near Hanover Court- House, Va. Cold Harbor, Va.	Young, P. M. B. (W) Clingman, T. L. (W)
June 2	Near New Hope Church, Ga.	Ector, M. D. (W)

DATE	PLACE	NAME
June 2 (1864)	Cold Harbor, Va.	Doles, G. P. (KIA) Kirkland, W. W. (W) Lane, J. H. (W)
June 3	Cold Harbor, Va.	Breckenridge, J. C. (A) Law, E. McI. (W) Roberts, W. P. (W)
June 5	Piedmont, Va.	Jones, W. E. (KIA)
June 11	Trevilian Station, Va.	Rosser, T. L. (W)
June 13	Riddell's Shop, Va.	Logan, T. M. (W)
June 14	Pine Mountain, Ga.	Polk, L. (KIA)
June 16	East of Mud Creek, Ga.	Polk, L. E. (W)
June 19	Kennesaw Mountain, Ga.	Cockrell, F. M. (W)
June 30	Petersburg Trenches, Va.	Alexander, E. P. (W)
July 3	Atlanta campaign, Ga.	Hindman, T. C. (W)
July 4	Vining Station, Ga.	Vaughan, A. J., Jr. (W)
July 7	Jackson, Miss.	Gholson, S. J. (W)
July 9	Monocacy, Md.	Evans, C. A. (W)
July 15	Tupelo, Miss.	Forrest, N. B. (W)
July 20	Stephenson's Depot, Va. Near Winchester, Va. Peach-Tree Creek, Ga.	Lewis, W. G. (W) Lilley, R. D. (W) Stevens, C. H. (MW)
July 22	Atlanta campaign, Ga.	Benton, S. (MW) Gist, S. R. (W) Smith, J. A. (W) Strahl, O. F. (W) Walker, W. H. T. (KIA)
July 25	Atlanta, Ga.	Stevens, C. H. (D)
July 27	Atlanta campaign, Ga. First Deep Bottom, Va.	Ector, M. D. (W) Barry, J. D. (W)
July 28	Griffin, Ga. Ezra Church, Ga. Lickskillet Road, Ga.	Benton, S. (D) Baker, A. (W) Brown, J. C. (W) Johnston, G. D. (W) Stewart, A. P. (W) Loring, W. W. (W) Quarles, W. A. (W)
July 30	Newnan, Ga. Crater, Petersburg Trenches, Va.	Anderson, Robert H. (W) Elliott, S., Jr. (W) Weisiger, D. A. (W)

DATE	PLACE	NAME
August 3 (1864)	Near Atlanta, Ga.	Bullock, R. (W)
August 10	Near Atlanta, Ga.	Bate, W. B. (W)
August 16	Second Deep Bottoms, Va.	Chambliss, J. R., Jr. (KIA) Girardey, V. J. B. (KIA)
August 19	Weldon Railroad, Va.	Clingman, T. L. (W)
August 21	Weldon Railroad, Va. Grubb's Crossroads, Ky.	Sanders, J. C. C. (KIA) Johnson, A. R. (W)
August 25	Near Shepherdstown, W.Va.	Gordon, John B. (W)
August 31	Jonesborough, Ga.	Anderson, J. P. (W) Cumming, A. (W) Finley, J. J. (W) Lewis, J. H. (B) Palmer, J. B. (W)
September 2	Franklin, Tenn.	Kelly, J. H. (MW)
September 3	Near Berryville, Va.	Humphreys, B. G. (W)
September 4	Near battlefield, Franklin, Tenn. Greeneville, Tenn.	Kelly, J. H. (D) Morgan, J. H. (KIA)
September 19	Winchester, Va. Cabin Creek, Indian Territory	Godwin, A. C. (KIA) Lee, F. (W) Peck, W. R. (W) Rodes, R. E. (KIA) Terry, W. (W) York, Z. (W) Gano, R. M. (W)
September 22	Strasburg, Va.	Grimes, B. (A)
September 27	Pulaski, Tenn.	Bell, T. H. (W)
October 1	Vaughan Road, Va.	Dunovant, J. (KIA)
October 5	Allatoona, Ga.	Young, W. H. (W)
October 7	Near New Market Road, Va. Charles City Road, Va.	Bratton, J. (W) Gregg, J. (KIA)
October 13	Near Cedar Creek, Va.	Conner, J. (W)
October 19	Cedar Creek, Va.	Battle, C. A. (W) Grimes, B. (W) Ramseur, S. D. (MW)
October 20	"Belle Grove," near Meadow Mills, Va.	Ramseur, S. D. (D)

DATE	PLACE	NAME
October 24 (1864)	Richmond, Va.	Archer, J. J. (D)
November 28	Waynesboro, Ga.	Allen, W. W. (W)
	Buck Head Creek, Ga.	Robertson, F. H. (W)
November 30	Franklin, Tenn.	Adams, J. (KIA)
		Brown, J. C. (W)
		Capers, E. (W)
		Carter, J. C. (MW)
		Cleburne, P. R. (KIA)
		Cockrell, F. M. (W)
		Deas, Z. C. (W)
		Gist, S. R. (KIA)
		Gordon, G. W. (W)
		Granbury, H. B. (KIA)
		Manigault, A. M. (W)
		Quarles, W. A. (W)
		Reynolds, D. H. (W)
		Scott, T. M. (C)
		Strahl, O. F. (KIA)
		Walthall, E. C. (B)
December 2	Petersburg Trenches, Va.	Gracie, A., Jr. (KIA)
December 4	Near Murfreesborough, Tenn.	Bullock, R. (W)
December 9	Coosawatchie, S.C.	Gartrell, L. J. (W)
December 10	Near battlefield, Franklin, Tenn.	Carter, J. C. (D)
December 15	Nashville, Tenn.	Sears, C. W. (W)
December 16	Outside Nashville, Tenn.	Govan, D. C. (W)
	Shy's Hill, Tenn.	Smith, T. B. (W)
December 17	Franklin, Tenn.	Buford, A. (W)
		Holtzclaw, J. T. (C)
	Spring Hill, Tenn.	Lee, S. D. (W)
December 24	Richland Creek, Tenn.	Buford, A. (W)
December 28	Egypt, Miss.	Gholson, S. J. (W)

1865

January 15	Fort Fisher, N.C.	Whiting, W. H. C. (MW)
February 6	West of Hatcher's Run, Va.	Pegram, J. (KIA)
February 7	Hatcher's Run, Va.	Sorrel, G. M. (W)
	Florence, S.C.	Winder, J. H. (D)

DATE	PLACE	NAME
March 10 (1865)	Near Fayetteville, N.C.	Harrison, T. (W)
		Humes, W. Y. C. (W)
	Ft. Columbus, New York Harbor	Whiting, W. H. C. (D)
March 11	Near Fayetteville, N.C.	Anderson, Robert H. (W)
March 19	Bentonville, N.C.	Elliott, S., Jr. (W)
		Palmer, J. B. (W)
		Pettus, E. W. (W)
		Reynolds, D. H. (W)
March 25	Bluff Springs, Fla.	Clanton, J. H. (W)
	Hare's Hill (Ft. Stedman), Va.	Cook, P. (W)
		Gordon, John B. (W)
		Johnston, R. D. (A)
		Terry, W. (W)
		Toon, T. F. (W)
March 30	Near Five Forks, Va.	Payne, W. H. F. (W)
March 31	Near Dinwiddie Courthouse, Va.	Rosser, T. L. (W)
		Terry, W. R. (W)
April 1	Ebenezer Church, Ala.	Forrest, N. B. (W)
April 2	Petersburg Line, Va.	Hill, A. P. (KIA)
April 5	Near Pineville, Va.	Dearing, J. (W)
April 6	High Bridge, Va.	Dearing, J. (MW)
		Rosser, T. L. (W)
	Houston, Tex.	Wharton, J. A. (D—Duel)
April 7	Farmville, Va.	Lewis, W. G. (W)
April 9	Near Appomattox, Va.	Beale, R. L. T. (W)
April 16	Fort Tyler, Ga.	Tyler, R. C. (KIA)
April 22	Lynchburg, Va.	Dearing, J. (D)

Glossary

THE WORDS IN this glossary were selected from the text to provide definitions of medical terms that may not be familiar to the reader. The glossary is organized to allow comparison of the meanings of some of the medical words used in the mid-1800s with their present usage. If the meaning of the word has not changed essentially, or if it is used to describe the same complex of signs and symptoms, only the recent usage is presented.

Scientific discoveries implicating a specific microorganism as the cause of a disease did not occur until after the Civil War. Some of the diagnoses of the 1800s were so all-encompassing that there is confusion as to what was actually meant. The older definition, enclosed in brackets and following today's meaning is, in many cases, more of a discussion of the theories about the possible causes of the condition, with the aim of providing the reader with some insight into the medical thinking of the time. Dr. J. J. Chisolm's *Manual of Military Surgery, for the use of Surgeons of the Confederate States Army* (3rd edition) and Joseph Janvier Woodward's *Outlines of the Chief Camp Diseases of the United States Armies* provide the clearest concepts in many instances and are recommended to the interested reader.

ABSCESS A cavity formed by the breakdown of tissue containing a collection of pus. [The causes of an acute abscess were thought to be: an injury, such as a blow, pressure, irritation of a foreign body, or of a poison introduced from without; or in connection with blood poisoning.]

ACROMION PROCESS OF SCAPULA The lateral extension of the spine of the scapula (shoulder bone), which constitutes the highest point of the shoulder.

ADHESION A fibrous strand or connection that abnormally adheres parts.

AFFECTION A diseased state.

AGUE Fever, or any other recurrent symptom resulting from malaria or a chill. [A popular synonym for intermittent fever.]

AMPUTATION The removal of a limb or other appendage of the body. CIRCULAR AMPUTATION: Performed by using a single flap and by making a circular cut at a ninety-degree angle to the long axis of the limb. PRIMARY AMPUTATION:

The surgery is conducted following the period of shock and before the development of inflammation. [It was believed that when an amputation was required, there was no period as favorable for the surgery as the first twenty-four hours, before reaction set in, and while the patient had his sensibilities depressed by shock.] SECONDARY AMPUTATION: [Performed after the onset of suppuration or to improve a previous circular amputation with open flaps.] SYME'S AMPUTATION: Amputation of the foot at the ankle joint with removal of both malleoli.

ANAL FISSURE A linear ulcer at the edge of the anus.

ANAL FISTULA An abnormal opening of the skin near the anus, which may or may not communicate with the rectum. [This was a common affection, particularly in the cavalry, caused by an abscess in the vicinity of the rectum, which, after discharging its purulent contents either into the rectum or externally, did not heal. Chisolm thought the only treatment was surgical. His recommendation was to convert the incomplete fistula into a complete one by dividing the sphincter muscle at the site using a probe that had been placed through the fistula. A tent of greased lint was then put into the incision each day and, in his experience, the patients would subsequently regain control of their bowels.]

ANASARCA Generalized accumulation of large amounts of body fluid. [Passage of fluid into the subcutaneous connective tissues, not limited to a particular locality, but becoming more or less diffused. See DROPSY.]

ANEMIA A decrease below normal limits in the number of red blood cells per volume of blood, or in the amount of hemoglobin, when the balance between bleeding or destruction and blood production is abnormal. [Deficiency of blood in quantity, either general or local; also, deficiency of the most important constituents of blood, particularly albuminous substances and red corpuscles. From the clinical point of view, anemia was a condition of the system in which impoverishment of the blood, whether from want or from waste, was associated with symptoms of imperfect discharge of the vital functions.]

ANGINA Chest pain that almost always refers to angina pectoris. [A condition in which difficulty in breathing and swallowing existed, caused by disease situated between the mouth and the lungs, or between the mouth and stomach.] ANGINA PECTORIS: Paroxysmal pain characterized by a severe crushing or constrictive sensation in the chest caused by lack of oxygen to the heart muscles. The pain frequently radiates to the neck or to the left shoulder and down the arm. [An affection of the chest, characterized by severe pain, faintness, and anxiety, occurring in paroxysms: connected with disorders of the pneumogastric and sympathetic nerves and their branches; and frequently associated with organic disease of the heart.]

ANTERIOR SUPERIOR SPINOUS PROCESS The boney projection from the anterior portion of a spinal vertebrae.

ANTIMONY A crystalline metallic element. [Tartar emetic was a tartrate of antimony and potassium. In small doses (gr. $\frac{1}{60}$–$\frac{1}{40}$) it was used in acute inflammatory affections of the respiratory tract such as pneumonia, acute edema of the lungs, catarrhal colds, laryngitis, and tonsillitis. Antimony oxide was used for its ability to promote mild perspiration.]

APHASIA Impairment or loss of expression by speech, writing or signs, or of understanding spoken or written language, due to brain damage.

APOPLEXY 1. A stroke; sudden neurologic impairment due to an intracranial hemorrhage or to cerebrovascular occlusion. 2. Extravasation of blood within any organ. [It was customary to include among the forms of apoplexy only that sudden loss of consciousness that was due to cerebral congestion, and to consider as apoplectic states only those that resulted from distinct toxemia. The apoplectic conditions were considered due to: (a) the influence on the brain of a poison circulating in the blood; (b) a sudden cerebral lesion, such as hemorrhage or vascular obstruction; or (c) a sudden shock or other impression arresting the cerebral functions, but causing no visible alteration in the brain.]

ARTERIOSCLEROSIS A group of diseases involving the arterial walls and characterized by thickening and loss of elasticity.

ARTERY A vessel that carries blood away from the heart. BRACHIAL ARTERY: Major artery of the arm that divides into two branches, the radial and ulnar, at the elbow. FEMORAL ARTERY: The main artery going to the leg. POPLITEAL ARTERY: Continuation of the femoral artery in the posterior portion of the knee. TIBIAL ARTERY: Originates from the popliteal artery, and its branches supply the leg below the knee.

ARTICULATION The junction between two or more bones of the skeleton.

ASCITES The accumulation of fluid in the abdominal cavity. [It was considered a consequence of certain preexisting organic diseases, such as direct mechanical obstruction affecting the portal circulation, cardiac or pulmonary diseases obstructing the general venous circulation, disease of the kidneys, and morbid conditions of the peritoneum.]

ASSIMILATION The change of food into living tissue after digestion and absorption.

ASTHENIA Weakness. Lack or loss of energy.

ATROPHY A wasting away or a decrease in size.

AUDITORY PROCESS The projection of the mastoid bone behind the ear.

BILIOUS ATTACK The term is applied to a group of symptoms consisting of nausea, abdominal distress, headache, and constipation. [The term was used when the patient presented a sallow or more or less yellowish tint of the skin, but especially if distinctly jaundiced. Bilious diarrhea signified the discharge of a quantity of bile mixed with loose stools. Certain febrile diseases, attended with yellowing of the skin, were sometimes designated bilious fever. One of the most frequent applications of the term was to certain so-called bilious attacks, which were commonly attacks of acute dyspepsia or migraine.]

BITTER WINE OF IRON [Combination of wine and iron with a bitter taste. Used for supportive therapy or a tonic.]

BLACK VOMIT Vomiting of black material that obtains its color from the action of gastric juice on blood in the stomach. May be present in yellow fever and other conditions in which blood collects in the stomach.

BLEEDING Incision of a vein, as for the letting of blood. (See DEPLETION.)

BLUE MASS Mercury mass. [Also known as the "blue pill." It contained 33 parts mercury, 5 liquorice, 25 althaea, 3 glycerine, and 34 of honey of rose. Used for a number of conditions without much rationale.]

BRIGHT'S DISEASE A general descriptive term used for kidney disease and associated with protein in the urine. [Generic term that included at least three different diseases of the kidney: (a) inflammatory affection caused by exposure to cold, scarlatina, diphtheria, erysipelas, typhus, ague, acute rheumatism, and pneumonia; (b) waxy or amyloid affection—from constitutional syphilis, tuberculosis, prolonged suppuration, caries, or necrosis of bone; (c) cirrhotic or gouty affection—most common cause was considered the abuse of alcohol, particularly in the form of ardent spirits, then gout, lead-poisoning, and unknown causes.]

BRONCHITIS Inflammation of one or more of the larger air passages of the lungs. [Two causes: (a) predisposing-age (youngest and oldest), breathing air when many people were present, heated rooms, cold, dampness, and other diseases were all thought to play a role; (b) exciting causes: transition from cold to heated atmosphere, and irritants, such as particles of cotton or pollen.]

BUBO SIMPLEX An enlarged, inflamed lymph node found in such infections as plague, syphilis, gonorrhea, lymphogranuloma venereum, and tuberculosis. [BUBO SYMPATHETIC: Simple bubo, due to inflammation of a gland through ordinary irritation from an inflamed surface.]

CALOMEL Mercurous chloride. (See BLUE MASS.)

CAMP STATE [A term that included various symptoms such as fever or diarrhea that occurred in troops crowded together in camp for a long period. In some instances, it was used specifically for the continued fevers, including yellow fever, malarial remittent fever, and typho-malarial fever.]

CAMPHOR A ketone obtained from the wood of *Cinnamomum camphora*, an evergreen tree, with a distinctive odor and an aromatic taste. It is applied topically to the skin as an antipruritic and anti-infective. [It was prepared as camphor-water, spirit of camphor, and as a liniment. Taken orally, it supposedly had a useful effect in cholera, diarrhea, vomiting, stomach pains, cardiac depression, nervousness, bronchitis, catarrhal colds, typhoid, and eruptive fevers. Locally, it was used as a counterirritant or to relieve pain when needed for conditions such as myalgia, lumbago, toothache, or gangrene.]

CANNULA A hollow tube that is placed into a cavity or duct for purposes of drainage or flushing.

CARBOLIC ACID Phenol. [Added to cold water, it was used as wet dressings for its supposed disinfectant qualities, primarily for postsurgery wound care.]

CARBUNCLE An infection of the skin and subcutaneous tissue that usually produces localized destruction of tissue and forms a group of boils, due to *Staphylococcus aureus*. [It was considered a constitutional affection, dependent on conditions of general debility or plethora, and often associated with gouty or diabetic tendencies.]

CARDIORENAL Pertaining to the heart and the kidney.

CATARACT An opacity of the crystalline lens of the eye.

CATARRH Inflammation of the mucous membranes of the air passages of the head and throat, which is accompanied by a discharge. [Used to describe any fluid discharge.]

CATHARTIC An agent that causes evacuation of the bowels by increasing bulk, stimulating peristaltic action, or increasing secretion of fluid into the intestine.

CAUTERY The application of a caustic material, a hot object, or other agent to destroy tissue.

CAYENNE PEPPER The dried fruit of various species of Capsium, which is used as an irritant or to relieve flatulence or pain. [Cayenne pepper was prepared as an alcoholic fluid extract and as a plaster for topical preparation. The oral preparation was purportedly an excellent stomach tonic, and it was also used in low fevers and cholera as a stimulant. In chronic nephritis it supposedly checked the loss of albumin, and helped in infections of the prostate.]

CEREBRAL HEMORRHAGE Bleeding into the main portion of the brain occupying the upper part of the cranial cavity.

CEREBROVASCULAR ACCIDENT A condition with sudden onset caused by acute vascular lesions of the brain, such as hemorrhage, embolism, clot, or a ruptured aneurysm. May result in paralysis, vertigo, numbness, aphasia, and difficulty with speech. It is often followed by permanent neurologic damage.

CHLOROFORM A volatile liquid used as an inhalation anesthetic and analgesic. [Most Confederate surgeons thought chloroform should be given to every patient requiring a serious or painful operation. Noisy breathing was considered a sign that the anesthetic effect had been produced and that inhalation should be suspended and the operation commenced. Only when the operation was very prolonged was inhalation repeated. Personally, Chisolm had known of only two deaths attributed to this agent. As a liniment, chloroform was applied as a rubefacient and to reduce pain in pruritus and rheumatic and neuralgic pains. Internally, it was administered in cholera, hepatic colic, colic, vomiting, and similar pains of internal and spasmodic character.]

CHOLERA An acute infectious disease caused by *Vibrio cholerae* and characterized by severe diarrhea with extreme fluid and electrolyte depletion, producing prostration. The resulting severe dehydration may lead to shock, kidney failure, and death. [Caused by decomposing animal or vegetable substances. Climatic and meteorological influences were thought to materially affect the susceptibility of the human subject to the disease. The malady was apt to prevail as an epidemic in moist or wet seasons of the year. It occurred especially among people whose bodies were predisposed to pass into a diseased condition because they had habitually breathed impure air and consumed unwholesome food and water, or became debilitated from other causes.]

CIRRHOSIS OF THE LIVER A group of chronic diseases of the liver that is characterized by loss of normal liver structure, formation of fibrosis, and by the destruction of liver cells and their regeneration to form nodules. The disease has a lengthy latent period, followed by the sudden appearance of fluid retention, vomiting of blood, or jaundice. [It was usually considered to be caused by the abuse of spirituous liquors, but also resulted from syphilis and the immoderate use of certain foods such as curry or coffee.]

CLAVICLE The curved collar bone that joins the sternum and the scapula to form the front of the shoulder.

COCAINE [Was available as a fluid extract, a crystalline form, and as a hydrochloride salt. The hydrochlorate form was used as a local anesthetic. The leaves were smoked to provide relief from asthma and irritable throat affections.]

COLIC Acute intermittent abdominal pain that increases and decreases in severity in association with smooth muscle contractions.

CONCUSSION A severe blow or shock, or the condition that results from such an injury. Usually refers to this type of injury to the brain.

CONGESTION An increase in the accumulation of blood. PASSIVE CONGESTION OF BRAIN: Results from a decrease or blockage of blood flow from the organ. Also is called venous congestion. CONGESTION OF LUNG: Excessive or abnormal accumulation of blood in the lung.

CONJUNCTIVA The membrane that lines the eyelids and covers the exposed surface of the sclera.

CONSUMPTION A wasting away of the body. [This was a term for any wasting disease, but it was generally applied to pulmonary phthisis (tuberculosis). Phthisis was used to designate a disease characterized by progressive wasting of the body, persistent cough, and expectoration of opaque matter or sometimes blood. There was loss of color and strength, shortness of breath, fever, night sweats, and diarrhea. General causes were considered family predisposition, fevers and exanthemata, syphilis, insufficient food, alcohol, bad ventilation, climatic influences, dampness of soil, and infection.]

CONTAGION The passage of disease from a sick person to a well individual. [The property and process by which, in certain sorts of disease, the affected body or part caused a disease like its own to occur in other bodies or other parts. It implied transmission by contact. Contagium denoted the specific material, shown or presumed, in which the infective power ultimately resided.]

CONTUSION A bruise or injury of a part without a break in the skin.

CORONARY ARTERY DISEASE Pathologic changes in the arteries that supply the heart muscle.

COUNTER-IRRITANTS [Any irritation artificially established with a view to diminish, counteract, or remove certain morbid processes that may be present in a more or less remote part of the system. The substances employed in establishing this state were called counter-irritants and were classified as follows: (1) Rubefacients: Those remedies, applied to the skin, which produced local warmth and redness from increased flow of blood in the cutaneous vessels. Examples were mustard plasters, oils of turpentine, and mustard foot baths. (2) Blistering agents: A blister acted primarily as a rubefacient and powerful stimulant to the cutaneous vessels. Examples were Spanish fly, glacial acetic acid, liquor ammonia on a piece of lint, or application of a heated piece of metal. (3) Pustulants: These agents produced a pus-containing eruption. An example was a strong solution of nitrate of silver.]

COURTSPLASTER An adhesive plaster, in particular one made of silk, that is coated with isinglass and glycerin.

CUPPING [Dry cupping was performed by heating a glass or metal cup that was then applied to the skin over the affected part. On cooling, there was contraction of the air contained in the cup and the skin was forcibly sucked up into the cup. (See DEPLETION.)]

CYSTOTOMY Surgical production of an opening into the urinary bladder.

DEBILITY Lack or loss of strength. [The body or any of its organs were considered to be in a state of debility when their vital functions were discharged with less than the normal vigor, being reduced in the amount of activity that they displayed and of work that they could accomplish.]

DENGUE An infectious, febrile disease that produces severe pains in the head, eyes, and extremities and is accompanied by catarrhal symptoms and sometimes a cutaneous eruption. It is caused by a virus and is transmitted by the bite of a mosquito. [Thought to be infectious because of the many cases in which the disease was supposedly conveyed from person to person.]

DEPLETION The act or process of emptying or the removal of a fluid. [This was the method for the unloading, or rendering less full, of that which was considered overburdened or overfull, for example, portions of the turgid vascular system. The methods used for depletion were as follows: (1) General Bloodletting: Performed by cutting a vein or artery. Indications were engorgement of the right heart and venous system, visceral congestion and arterial turgescence. (2) Local Bleeding: Bleeding by means of leeches, scarifications, or cupping. (3) Purgation: For general depleting purposes, a watery purge was said to be the most efficacious and safe agent. This was thought to be particularly good for brain, cardiac, and hepatic congestions, when it was required to give relief to turgid vessels without removing blood. (4) Vomiting: Depletion primarily from the stomach. (5) Sweating: A less effective method of depletion that was occasionally combined with purging. (6) Abstinence: General depletion could be produced by abstinence from food and drink.]

DEVITALIZE To deprive of vitality or life.

DIARRHEA An increase in fecal frequency and liquidity. [A point of differentiation from dysentery was that diarrhea was not accompanied by painful straining at stool. It was supposed to be caused by food in excess or of improper quality; diseased, decomposed, or imperfectly masticated food; impure water; excessive bile; retained feces; parasites; defective hygiene and living in dwellings that were damp, cold, dark, and unventilated; foul emanations from decaying animal matter; chills; climatic variations; and nervous disturbances.]

DILATATION The stretching of an orifice or tubular structure beyond its previous size.

DIPHTHERIA An acute infectious disease that is produced by the toxin-producing bacteria *Corynebacterium diphtheriae*, affecting primarily the membranes of the nose, throat, or larynx, and is characterized by the presence of a gray white pseudomembrane. [The disease was considered contagious and due to poverty; its concomitants were tuberculous, scarlatina, measles, and whooping-cough.]

DROPSY Increase in the accumulation of fluid in tissue or body cavities. [The term included edema, anasarca, or ascites. It was recognized that the accumulation of fluid in the tissues, or in a serous cavity, depended on more fluid exuding from the blood vessels than could pass back into the vessel. The fluid retention was considered to result from obstruction of venous and lymphatic vessels or by dilatation of arteries. Fluid retention with scurvy was believed to be due to a blood-vascular disorder. Alterations in the composition of the blood resulting from anemia or albuminuria were also thought to be causative factors without vascular changes.]

DYSENTERY This includes a number of conditions in conjunction with inflammation of the intestines and particularly involving the colon. There is painful, colicky abdominal pain, straining at stool, and frequent bowel movements containing blood and mucus. The causative agent may be chemical irritants, bacteria, or parasites. [Regarded as a specific febrile disease, characterized by considerable nervous prostration and inflammation of the glands of the large intestine. It could sometimes resolve, but frequently terminated in, intestinal ulceration. It appeared to exist in direct proportion to the presence of malarious fevers. The belief was that paroxysmal fevers interferred materially with the nutrition and functions of the digestive organs. Dysentery was considered to be secondary to portal congestion, unwholesome drinking water, bad and unwholesome food, impure air, bile, indigestible articles of diet, and sudden changes in temperature.] DYSENTERY, BILIOUS: Stools have a green, bilious appearance. [This was considered by many as being more severe than other forms of dysentery.]

DYSPEPSIA A decrease in digestion of food. The term is often used to describe epigastic discomfort following meals.

EFFUSION Passage of fluid into an area.

EMBOLISM   The sudden blocking of an artery by a clot or foreign material that is carried there by the bloodstream.

EMPYEMA   Accumulation of pus in a cavity of the body. Usually it refers to thoracic empyema.

ENDOCARDITIS   Inflammation of the lining membranes of the cavities of the heart and the connective tissues around it. It is characterized by the presence of bacterial growths on the surface of the lining of the heart or in the heart muscle itself, and usually involves a heart valve.

ENGORGED LIVER   The liver is distended, swollen, or congested with fluid.

ENSIFORM CARTILAGE (XIPHOID)   The pointed process of cartilage that is supported by a core of bone and is connected with the lower end of the body of the sternum (breastbone).

ERYSIPELAS   A contagious disease of skin and subcutaneous tissue due to infection with *Streptococcus pyogenes*, marked by redness and swelling of affected areas and with constitutional symptoms. [The features common to all inflammations usually spoken of as erysipelas were fever and an inflammation that tended to spread indefinitely by means of the lymph spaces and lymphatic vessels of the affected part. Chisolm said that idiopathic erysipelas, which was often seen in isolated cases, was usually found attacking persons without wounds. Patients with gunshot wounds who were debilitated by the many depressing influences of camp life were peculiarly prone to attacks of erysipelas. Overcrowding, bad ventilation, and a dirty environment could all contribute by producing a poisoned atmosphere. However, it could not always be traced to the depressing effect of bad food or a vitiated atmosphere, as cases occurred in private quarters where ventilation was good. The disease was believed to be contagious as well as infectious. It was recognized that sponges, bandages, and other objects required by such a patient should be restricted exclusively to that individual. A strong recommendation was that all the windows be left open for thorough ventilation, even at the risk of catarrhal affections, which were trivial when compared to the serious character of erysipelas.]

ESOPHAGITIS   Inflammation of the lining of the esophagus that is caused by reflux of acid gastric content into the esophagus.

ETHER   A very volatile liquid, with a characteristic odor, and highly inflammable: it is inhaled as a general anesthetic.

EUSTACHIAN TUBE   Auditory tube. The channel that establishes communication between the cavity behind the eardrum and nasopharynx and serves to adjust the pressure of air in the cavity to the external pressure.

EXCISION   Removal by cutting. [Some surgeons removed by excision a segment of bone and left the two remaining ends in place, instead of performing an amputation.]

EXCORIATION   Any superficial loss of substance, such as that which is produced on the skin by scratching. (See DEPLETION.)

EXPECTORANTS Medications that cause the passage of mucus or exudate from the lungs, bronchi, and trachea.

FATTY DEGENERATION OF THE HEART Deposition of fat globules in the heart tissue.

FEBRIS COMMINICUS [A fever that could be communicated from one individual to another.]

FEMUR The bone that extends from the pelvis to the knee, also called the thigh bone.

FEVER Elevation of body temperature above normal. [Derangement of function was attributed to the febrile condition itself and was considered, in part, independent of the initial cause. It was thought that the fever itself was the chief antagonist with which the physician or surgeon had to contend.] ACCLIMATING FEVER: [A fever that supposedly occurred as one became accustomed to a new environment.] BILIOUS FEVER: Fever that is accompanied by the vomiting of bile or with yellowing of the skin. CAMP FEVER: [A group of conditions that included typhus, typhoid, typhomalaria, common continued fever, remittent fever, and intermittent fever.] CONTINUED FEVER: Persistently elevated body temperature, showing little or no variation and never falling to normal during any twenty-four-hour period. [Three types were recognized: typhus, enteric, and relapsing. They resulted from the introduction into the body of a poison from without; this poison was thought to reproduce in the system. It was noted that the continued fevers rarely affected the same individual twice, and they had a more or less definite duration.] INTERMITTENT FEVER: Recurring paroxysms of temperature elevations separated by intervals during which the temperature is normal. Usually malarial in origin. [Three forms of ague were recognized, namely, the quotidian, which recurred in twenty-four hours; the tertian in forty-eight hours; and quartan in seventy-two hours.] RECURRENT FEVER: Relapsing. REMITTENT FEVER: A fever that varies two degrees Fahrenheit or more each day, but in which the temperature never reaches a normal level. [Typhoid fever.] ROMAN FEVER: [A virulent type of malaria that prevailed in the low plain surrounding the city of Rome.] TYPHOID FEVER: Infection by *Salmonella typhosa* involving primarily the lymphoid tissue of the distal small intestine. The disease may start suddenly with chills and fever, transient rose spots on the skin, abdominal distension, and an enlarged spleen. [In common with other continuous fevers, typhoid fever was considered to be due to the introduction from without of a specific poison into a system more or less predisposed to the disease. There were two views as to the origin of the poison: First, that it was specific in nature and derived only from some preexisting case of the disease. Second, that it could be generated anew by the decomposition of sewage, and perhaps of other forms of animal filth. The most common vehicle of the poison was drinking water.] SWAMP FEVER: Leptospiral disease or malaria. YELLOW FEVER: An acute, infectious, viral disease that mosquitoes transmit to man. The patient manifests fever, jaundice, and protein in the urine. [A contagious fever of a continuous and special type that was noted to have two well-defined stages. The first extended from 36 to 150 hours, depending on its severity, and was marked by rapid circulation and elevated temperature. The second was characterized by depression of the nervous and muscular powers, and of the circulation, with slow and often intermittent pulse, jaundice, suppression of urine, protein in the urine, passive bleeding from the mucous surfaces, black vomit, convulsions, delirium, and coma. A certain degree of density of population appeared to be essential to the production of yellow fever, and it was a disease of crowded cities located on the shores of the ocean or large rivers as well as of ships. It was also the disease of strangers in the warm, moist climates of the islands and tropical parts of America.]

FIBULA   The outer and smaller of the two bones in the lower leg.

FLUX   An excessive flow or discharge. [An increased discharge from a mucous surface through any of the natural passages, of serum, blood, mucus, pus, or the various secretions.]

FOMENTATION   The application of hot, moist substances to the body to ease pain or the material so applied.

FRACTURE   The breaking of a part, especially of a bone. COMMINUTED FRACTURE: The bone is splintered or crushed. COMPOUND FRACTURE: An open fracture.

GANGRENE   Death of tissue, which is usually associated with loss of vascular supply to the area and is followed by bacterial infection and putrefaction. GANGRENE, HOSPITAL: [This disease was seldom seen, except when large numbers of wounded soldiers were kept in foul hospitals near a battlefield. It was characterized by rapid tissue destruction; the microorganisms causing it are uncertain to this time. The cause was thought to be a blood poisoning, which depended on a foul, infected atmosphere, operating on an enfeebled constitution. The presence of a wound ensured an attack. Surgeons recognized its contagious as well as infectious character and the facility of transmitting it by sponges or dressings used in common by the patients of a ward. The air of a ward or a hospital was also thought to become impregnated with the poison from the breath of those suffering from the disease.]

GASTRODUODENITIS   An inflammation of the lining of the stomach and the first portion of the small intestine.

GOUT   A hereditary form of arthritis that is associated with an increase of uric acid in the blood, and by recurrent attacks of acute arthritis, usually of a single peripheral joint, which is then followed by complete remission.

GRANULATION   Formation in wounds of small, rounded masses of tissue composed mainly of capillaries and connective tissue, usually with inflammatory cells.

HEMORRHAGE, SECONDARY   [Any bleeding after forty-eight hours was considered secondary by most surgeons. All injuries to large arteries or any wound that remained unhealed for a long time could produce secondary hemorrhage. Suppuration was usually established about the fifth or sixth day following a wound. When the walls of blood vessels were involved and the precaution of rest and absolute quiet had not been enforced, secondary hemorrhage occurred.]

HEMOTHORAX   A collection of blood in the chest cavity.

HEMICRANIA   A pain or discomfort in one side of the head.

HEMATEMESIS   The vomiting of blood.

HEPATITIS   Inflammation of the liver.

HUMERUS   The bone that extends from the shoulder to the elbow. ANATOMICAL NECK OF THE HUMERUS: The slightly narrowed area of the humerus just distal to the head of the bone.

HUMOR   A fluid or semifluid material. [Humoral was chiefly used as a term for a pathological doctrine that associated all diseases with morbid states of the fluids of the body.]

HYPERTROPHY   An enlargement or overgrowth of an organ or part due to an increase in the size of its cells.

INANITION   A condition usually brought about by weeks to months of very inadequate nutrition. There is extreme weight loss and considerable weakness.

INDIGESTION   Usually refers to vague, nonspecific abdominal discomfort following meals.

INFERIOR MAXILLA   The bone of the lower jaw.

INFARCTION   An area of tissue death due to a local decreased blood flow, which results from obstruction or loss of the circulation to the area.

INFECTION   Invasion and growth of microorganisms in tissues. [A disease that was capable of transmission from one animal to another of a different class, or from one individual to another of the same species, and could be transmitted by contact or through the air.]

INFLUENZA (GRIPPE)   An acute viral infection of the respiratory tract. There is inflammation of the mucous membranes of the nasal passages, pharynx, and conjunctiva. Generalized muscle pain, headache, fever, chills, and prostration are usual. [This disease was not regarded as simply an unusually prevalent common catarrh but was considered as a specific affection, which appeared occasionally over wide districts, simultaneously or at about the same time. It was characterized by marked febrile symptoms, often attended by serious complications, and caused great and prolonged prostration of strength.]

INTENTION   A manner of restoring integrity of injured tissue. HEALING BY first intention: Healing in which union or restoration of continuity occurs directly without the intervention of granulation.

IRITIS   Inflammation of the circular pigmented membrane of the eye that lies behind the cornea and is perforated by the pupil. The condition is usually marked by pain, sensitivity to light, contraction of the pupil, and discoloration of the iris. [It was classified according to its actual or supposed causes, as rheumatic or syphilitic; or according to the nature of the morbid process, as plastic, serous, or suppurative.]

IRON [Various iron compounds were taken internally to build blood and support the body. Mineral acid salts of iron were used locally for their astringent and coagulating action, especially to stop bleeding.]

JAUNDICE A condition manifest by a yellow color of the skin, mucous membranes, and sclera because of increased bile.

LA GRIPPE Influenza.

LANGUOR A lack of vigor and a feeling of weakness, listlessness, or indifference.

LAUDANUM Opium tincture containing about 10 percent opium and some morphine. [It was often used for "nervousness" or sedation, or to prepare liniments for superficial pain.]

LEECHES Blood-sucking annelids used for depletion. (See DEPLETION.) [An average leech abstracted nearly half an ounce of blood. Useful, since fairly definite amounts of blood could be withdrawn from the affected or adjacent parts, or from more distal parts. Care was taken not to apply leeches to parts over which sufficient compression could not be made to control the bleeding. When they did not bite readily, the area was wetted by a little milk and sugar, or a slight needle prick sufficient to draw a speck of blood was used.]

LICHEN PLANUS An often chronic inflammatory skin disease with violet-colored, itchy, polygonal flat papules having a shiny surface and occurring in circumscribed patches.

LINT An absorbent surgical-dressing material that is made by taking apart old woven linen.

LITHEMIA An excess of lithic or uric acid and urates in the blood. An old term for uremia.

LUMBAGO Pain in the back between the thorax and the pelvis.

MALADY Any disease or illness.

MALARIA An infectious disease that is caused by the protozoa of the genus *Plasmodium* that is parasitic in the red blood cells and is transmitted by infected mosquitoes of the genus *Anopheles*. The attacks of chills, fever, and sweating occur at intervals that are determined by the time needed for development of a new generation of parasites. Following recovery from the acute attack, there is a tendency for the disease to become chronic with occasional relapses. [MARSH MIASM: By many, this was considered to be due to an earth-born poison generated in soils, the energies of which were not expended in the growth and sustenance of healthy vegetation. This poison was supposed to be the cause of all the types of intermittent and remittent fevers, and of the degeneration of the blood and tissues resulting from long residence in places where this poison was generated.]

MALLEOLUS The rounded projection on either side of the ankle joint.

MASTOID PORTION TEMPORAL BONE The rounded protrusion behind the ear.

MAXILLA, INFERIOR The bone of the lower jaw.

MEASLES A highly contagious viral infection involving primarily the respiratory tract. [A specific infectious eruptive fever. The contagium of measles, except in the catarrhal stage, was not thought to be diffusible very far in the air, but would cling to surfaces, and could be carried from place to place.]

MENTAL COMPRESS A compress that is applied to the chin.

MERCURY A metallic element. [Its salts were employed therapeutically as purgatives to restore normal function in chronic inflammations, and as antisyphilitics, intestinal antiseptics, disinfectants, and astringents. (See BLUE MASS.)]

METACARPALS The part of the hand between the wrist and fingers, made up of five bones.

MIASMATIC Pertaining to or caused by miasma. MIASMA: A supposed noxious material that is derived from the soil or earth. [The unknown atmospheric influences could arise either from sources such as vegetable decomposition or from those produced by the decomposition of matters derived from the human body. MIASMATIC DISEASES In its broadest sense this included a number of conditions, such as typhoid fever, yellow fever, remittent fever, intermittent fever, diarrhea, dysentery, erysipelas, hospital gangrene, pyaemia, smallpox, measles, mumps, and epidemic catarrh. In its narrowest sense, only intermittent and remittent fevers and other malarial diseases were included.]

MIGRAINE Periodic attacks of unilateral, temporal vascular headaches. Nausea, vomiting, diarrhea, or constipation are often concomitant symptoms. [The chief predisposing causes of attacks of migraine were considered to be a hereditary tendency, anemia, a general want of tone of the system, and a nervous temperament. Among the exciting causes were included those of a depressing or exhausting nature, whether physical or mental, such as prolonged mental work, mental excitement, grief, anxiety, bodily fatigue, late hours, sexual excesses, breathing impure air of a crowded room, and improper food.]

MITRAL INSUFFICIENCY A diseased mitral valve in the heart that allows blood to flow back from the left ventricle into the left atrium.

MUCILLAGINOUS DRINKS A viscous drink made of gum or dextrin that is used either as a vehicle for some medication or to soothe irritated surfaces. [A drink made of barley-water, flaxseed tea, toast-water, gum, or dextrin.]

MYOCARDITIS Inflammation of the muscular walls of the heart.

NEPHRITIS A general term for inflammation of the kidney.

NERVE, RADIAL The posterior nerve of the brachial plexus descending in the back of the arm and forearm. NERVES, SUPRAORBITAL: Nerves above the eye.

NEURALGIA, FACIAL Paroxysmal pain that extends along the course of one or more nerves of the face. [Applied to a condition marked by paroxysmal pain, which was for the most part unilateral, and in the course of nerves. Causes were thought to be premature aging, malaria, anemia, malnutrition, sexual excesses and perhaps, likewise, a state of celibacy. The most frequent exciting causes were cold, especially damp cold; injury to the nerve by violence; and the presence of lead or mercury in the system.]

NITRO-MURIATIC ACID (NITROHYDROCHLORIC) It is prepared by mixing 1 volume of nitric acid and 4 volumes of hydrochloric acid. DILUTE: A solution of 22 cc. of nitrohydrochloric acid that is diluted with water to 100 cc. [Used to increase the flow of bile and to slow diarrhea.]

NUX VOMICA The dried ripe seed of *Strychnos nux-vomica* that contains alkaloids, mainly strychnine and brucine. [It was used as a bitter tonic and central nervous system stimulant. In five-drop doses it was thought to be useful in atonic dyspepsia and gastric catarrh, whereas in ten-drop doses it appeared to increase peristalsis in constipation due to atony of the bowels. Its supposed action on the pneumogastric and nervous system made it useful for all types of coughs, asthma, and irregular heart action.]

OBSTRUCTIVE SLEEP APNEA Transient failure of automatic respiratory control, resulting in decreased exchange of air by the lungs, which becomes more pronounced during sleep.

OPERATION, FLAP Any operation involving the raising of a flap of tissue.

OPHTHALMIA Severe inflammation of the eye.

OPIUM An exudate that is obtained by incising the unripe capsules of *Papaver somniferum*. Various principles and derivatives of opium are used for their narcotic and analgesic effects.

ORBIT PROCEP The bony cavity of the skull that contains the eye and its associated structures.

ORGANIC AFFECTION OF HEART A general term meaning a diseased state of the heart.

OS CALCIS The irregular quadrangular bone at the back of the area of articulation between the foot and the leg.

OS FRONTIS Pertaining to the forehead.

OSTEOMYELITIS Inflammation of bone that is caused by a pus-producing micro-organism. It may remain localized or may spread throughout the various parts of the bone.

PAPULES Small, solid elevations of the skin that are circumscribed.

PAREGORIC A medication containing powdered opium, benzoic acid, anise oil, camphor, glycerin, and diluted alcohol. One teaspoon full yields about 1.5 to 2 mg. of anhydrous morphine. It is used orally in the treatment of diarrhea.

PATELLA The kneecap.

PECTORAL MUSCLES Muscles of the breast or chest.

PELVIS, ORIFICES The pelvis is made up of the sacrum and coccyx posteriorly and by the two hip bones laterally and anteriorly. It has an orifice on top, the inlet, and one at the bottom, the outlet.

PEPPERMINT Peppermint oil, a mixture of oils derived from *Mentha piperita*, is used as a carminative for gastrointestinal symptoms. The major individual constituent of the oil is menthol. [Preparations included peppermint water (2 parts peppermint oil in 1,000 parts distilled water) and essence of peppermint (an alcoholic solution containing 10 percent of the oil and 1 percent of the powdered herb). It was given orally for the relief of nausea and colic and to expel flatus. In combination with purgatives, it prevented griping and covered the taste of many nauseous substances.]

PERICARDIAL EFFUSION Fluid in the sac that surrounds the heart and roots of the great vessels. [Dropsy of the pericardium. It was thought to result from venous congestion due to disease of the heart or of the lungs, or cirrhosis, or from increased blood volume produced by chronic organic diseases of the spleen, liver, or kidneys, or by tubercular diseases.]

PERICARDITIS Inflammation of the sac that surrounds the heart. [Although occasionally idiopathic, more often it was considered to be secondary in its character. Secondary forms could result from wounds, blows, and contusions to the region of the heart, an abscess perforating from the lungs or the liver, or from enteric fever, variola, scarlatina, and pyaemia in all forms, and local spread. Perhaps due to rheumatism or the chronic forms of Bright's disease. By far the larger proportion of cases occurred in connection with the last two named diseases. In rheumatism, pericarditis was thought to occur early and occasionally preceded the joint-affection; although no period of the disease was regarded as free from the tendency to this complication, it usually affected within the first week of the rheumatic onset.]

PERITONITIS Inflammation of the internal serous membrane lining the abdominal and pelvic walls.

PHYSIC A medicine, especially a cathartic.

PILES Hemorrhoids.

PLASTER A pastelike mixture that can be spread over the skin and which is adhesive at body temperature. Plasters protect or may be counterirritant, or may be used to hold a medication to the area. MUSTARD PLASTER: A uniform mixture of powdered black mustard and a solution of suitable adhesive, spread on an appropriate backing material, and used as a local irritant. ISINGLASS PLASTER: A form of gelatin that is prepared from the swimming bladders of the Russian sturgeon.

PLEURA The membrane surrounding the lungs and covering the thoracic cavity that encloses a potential space known as the pleural cavity. The right and left pleurae are separate from each other.

PLEURISY Inflammation of the pleura, with exudation into its cavity and on its surface. It may be primary or secondary to disease of a surrounding structure, such as the lung, and is associated with pain during breathing. [An inflammation of the pleura of whatever nature and extent was considered the most common of the serous inflammations. Chief local causes were wounds or bruises of the chest wall; fracture of the ribs; infections of the spine; escape of irritating matter into the pleural cavity, from the costal side or from the pulmonary side; from disease of the bronchial glands; or from the side of the abdomen. Some thought there were grounds for suspecting that a chill alone was a cause of acute pleurisy. It also occurred as a part or as a complication of other diseases.]

PNEUMONIA Inflammation of the lungs with the air spaces being filled with exudate. [Caused by atmospheric influences—coldness and dampness, sudden changes of temperature and winds from the north.] PLEURAL PNEUMONIA: Secondary to pleural disease or trauma. HYPOSTATIC PNEUMONIA (Formerly also called hydrostatic): Pneumonia due to remaining in one position with shallow breathing, such as in the weak or aged. [A class of consolidations of the lung very common in those who were subjects of other diseases, which were, for the most part, noninflammatory in nature. These consolidations were found at the bases and more dependent portions of the lungs in the course of both chronic and acute diseases, and also in the aged and cachectic. They were the result of weak inspiratory power, feeble circulation, and gravitation. The consolidation thus mechanically induced was increased by more or less exudation of fluid and blood corpuscles into the alveoli.] SENILE PNEUMONIA: Same as hypostatic. TYPHOID PNEUMONIA: Pneumonia associated with typhoid.

POTT'S DISEASE Tuberculosis of the spine.

PRECORDIAL PAIN Pain in the chest occurring in the area in front of the heart.

PROSTRATION Extreme exhaustion.

PULMONARY EDEMA The presence of large amounts of fluid in the intercellular tissue spaces of the lungs.

PULMONARY CONTUSION A bruise or injury of the lung.

PURGATIVE A medication causing evacuation of the bowels.

PYELITIS Infection of the collecting area of the kidney that is drained by the ureter.

PYEMIA A general disease with the presence and persistence of pathogenic microorganisms or their toxins in the blood, with secondary areas of suppuration and formation of multiple abscesses.

QUININE An alkaloid of *Cinchona*. [Its principal action was in the malarial diseases, where it was considered a specific. It was used as a prophylactic for malaria. To control fever, it was used in typhus, typhoid, variola, pneumonia, and acute rheumatism. Neuralgias of malarial origin and neuralgia of the ophthalmic division of the fifth nerve were treated with quinine.]

RADIUS The bone on the outer or thumb side of the forearm.

RESECTION Excision. [The term was used by some surgeons for the removal of one end of a bone when the remaining portion was left in place. It was recommended instead of amputation for certain fractures.]

RHEUMATISM A number of conditions characterized by inflammation, degeneration, or metabolic derangement of the connective tissue structures of the body, especially the joints and related structures, including muscles, bursae, tendons, and fibrous tissue. INFLAMMATORY RHEUMATISM: Rheumatic fever. A febrile disease occurring as a delayed sequel of infections with group A *hemolytic streptococci*. [The disease was considered as having an intimate etiological relation to weather, season, and climate. It was characterized by pyrexia, sweats, and acute shifting inflammation of the joints and other structures. An occasional attack was referred to derangement of digestion and the functions of the liver, or after an injury to a joint. A fatal termination was due to congestion or inflammation of the lungs, and inflammation of the heart and pericardium. The causes of chronic rheumatism were considered to be the same as those of the acute disease.]

RISIN   A boil.

SALTPETER   Potassium nitrate.

SCIATICA   Pain that radiates from the back to the buttock and down into the lower extremity along its posterior or lateral aspect.

SCURVY   A condition due to a deficiency of vitamin C in the diet that is manifest by weakness, anemia, soft gums, and a tendency to bleed into the skin and mucous membranes. [Flagrant scurvy was rare, but what was considered the scorbutic taint was common. This was characterized by general debility, poor appetite, lack of energy, mental apathy, neuralgia, and a tendency for diarrhea. It occurred in men who had a deficient diet or who had been exposed to overexertion of any kind.]

SETON   A thread that is passed through a sinus, fistula, or open tract to keep the passage open or to act as a guide for later dilatation.

SLOUGHING BONE   Necrotic bone that separates from the viable portions.

SPLINTS   An appliance used to immobilize or fix in place a displaced or fractured part. SPLINTS OF COAPTATION: Small splints that are adjusted about a fractured limb for the purpose of approximating the edges of the wound or the ends of a fractured bone. INTERDENTAL SPLINT: An appliance fastened to the teeth that provides lugs for applying mandibular and/or maxillofacial traction or fixation.

STIMULANTS   Medications or chemicals to increase functional activity.

STROKE   A condition with sudden onset. The term is most commonly used to describe an acute vascular lesion of the brain, such as hemorrhage, thrombosis, or ruptured aneurysm. [Was a common synonym for an attack of apoplexy or sudden paralysis.]

STRYCHNINE   An extremely poisonous alkaloid that causes excitation of all portions of the central nervous system. [It was used as a bitter tonic, circulatory stimulant, and with cathartic drugs.]

SUBMAXILLARY GLANDS   One of the three chief paired salivary glands situated beneath the jaw.

SUPPURATE   The act of discharging pus.

SUPRAORBITAL NERVES   Nerves above the eye.

SYNCOPE   A temporary suspension of consciousness due to a generalized decrease in blood to the brain. [A state of suspended animation due to sudden failure of the action of the heart.]

TENESMUS   Ineffectual and painful straining at stool.

TENT A conical and expansible piece of soft material, such as lint or gauze, for dilating an opening or for helping to keep a wound open so that it heals from the bottom.

THROMBOSIS The formation or development of a blood clot in a blood vessel.

THORACENTESIS Surgical puncture through the chest wall into the cavity around the lungs so that fluid can be removed.

TIBIA The shin bone.

TINCTURE An alcoholic or hydroalcoholic solution.

TUMEFACTION A swelling.

ULNA The bone of the forearm, which is on the side opposite that of the thumb.

UREMIA The retention of excessive by-products of protein metabolism in the blood, and the subsequent toxic condition. [A group of nervous symptoms, which occasionally occurred in the course of acute or chronic Bright's disease, as well as in other maladies, which prevented the secretion or the discharge of urine. Evidence at the time seemed to point to the probability of the process being due to retention of some material or materials normally excreted.]

URETHRA The membranous canal that carries urine from the bladder to the exterior of the body.

VERTIGO A feeling of movement, although the subject is stationary. [The consciousness of disordered equilibrium. It appeared in more than one form: ocular, auditory, gastric, nervous, epileptic, migrainous, and with organic brain disease and gout.]

VESICULAR ERUPTION Small saclike bodies or blisters that gradually become visible.

Bibliography

MANUSCRIPT SOURCES

Alabama Department of Archives and History. Montgomery.
   Earl Van Dorn Papers.
   Josiah Gorgas Diaries. July 23, 1863–December 27, 1865. Typed copies.
   William Joseph Hardee Papers.
   Danville Leadbetter Papers.
   Sterling Alexander Martin Wood Papers.
Alamo, Library of the. San Antonio, Tex.
   Walter P. Lane biography file.
Baylor University Library. The Texas Collection. Waco.
   Carter-Harrison Family Papers.
   Ross Family Papers.
Duke University. William R. Perkins Library. Manuscript Department. Durham, N.C.
   Mathew Calbraith Butler Papers, 1851–1920.
   Samuel Wragg Ferguson Papers.
   Elijah T. D. Hawkins Papers.
   Theophilus Hunter Holmes Papers.
   William Henry Talbot Walker Papers.
Emory University. Robert W. Woodruff Library. Special Collections Department. Atlanta, Ga.
   Edward Lloyd Thomas Papers.
The Filson Club. Manuscript Department. Louisville, Ky.
   Johnson Family Papers, 1798–1943.
   Charles Lanman Collection. Autobiographical Sketch. Undated. A.Ms.2p.
   Humphrey Marshall Papers, 1861–1865. 12 pieces. Original MS and typewritten copies.
Georgia, University of. Hargrett Rare Book and Manuscript Library. Athens.
   Carlton-Newton-Mell Collection.
   Alfred H. Colquitt Collection.
   Joseph Henry Lumkin Papers.
   Robert Toombs Papers.
Jones Memorial Library. Lynchburg, Va.
   Diuguid's Burial Records. Roll No. 3. 929.3D. Book no. 7, page 222.

Lloyd House. Alexandria Library. Alexandria, Va.
   Biography of General Montgomery Corse by his son Montgomery D. Corse. Typewritten copy.
   Montgomery Corse Letters.
Louisiana State Museum. New Orleans.
   From the Collection of the Louisiana State Museum Historical Center. Record Group 56. Accession no. 11871.32.
Louisiana State University. Louisiana and Lower Mississippi Valley Collections, LSU Libraries. Baton Rouge.
   P. G. T. Beauregard Civil War Papers.
   Beauregard Miscellany Letters.
   Charles James Johnson Papers.
Mississippi Department of Archives and History. Jackson.
   William Barksdale, subject file.
   Samuel Benton, subject file.
   William L. Brandon, subject file.
   Samuel W. Ferguson Papers.
   Samuel G. French Papers.
   Samuel J. Gholson, subject file.
   Nathaniel H. Harris, subject file.
   Benjamin G. Humphrey, subject file.
   Annie E. Jacobs. "The Master of Doro Plantation." Typescript.
   Stephen D. Lee Letters.
   Mark Perrin Lowrey, subject file.
   Robert Lowry, subject file.
   Claudius W. Sears Diaries.
   William F. Tucker, subject file.
   Edward C. Walthall, subject file.
Missouri Historical Society. St. Louis.
   Dorsey Family Papers.
   Kraines, Oscar. "Incorruptible Cockrell: Presidential Troubleshooter and Senate Watchdog. The Life and Times of Francis Marion Cockrell." Typed copy.
   William M. McPheeters Papers. Civil War Diary, June 1, 1863–June 20, 1865 of William M. McPheeters, Surgeon in the Confederate Army. 204 pages, unbound.
Murray State University. Forrest C. Pogue Library. Special Collections. Murray, Ky.
   H. B. Lyon Letters. Microfilm. 2 rolls.
Museum of the Confederacy. Eleanor S. Brockenbrough Library. Richmond, Va.
   C.S.A. Hospital Department. Surgical notes presented by Dr. H. McGuire to J. W. Powell, Chief Surg. Gen. A. P. Hill's Division.
   E. S. Carrington Book 1863. Richmond. List of sick and wounded allowed to remain in Private Quarters and Furloughed.
   Medical Department. Receiving Hospital, Gordonsville, Va. Register Book. June 1, 1863–May 5, 1864.
   Summary of the sick and wounded of the 21st N.C. Regiment. April 1, 1862–June 30, 1863.

National Archives. Washington, D.C.

Adjutant General's Office. Letters Received. 125A/201A, May 24, 1857, and 201./125.A, July 1857.

Confederate Records. RG 109. Chap. 6. Vols. 145, 178, 181, 754, 755, and 764.

Confederate Records. RG 109. Compiled Service Records of Confederate Generals and Staff Officers, and Nonregimental Enlisted Men. M331. 275 rolls.

Confederate Records. RG 109. Compiled Service Records of Confederate Soldiers Who Served in Organizations from Various States. Organizations from state of Alabama (M311. 508 rolls), Arkansas (M317. 256 rolls), Florida (M251. 104 rolls), Georgia (M266. 607 rolls), Kentucky (M319. 136 rolls), Louisiana (M320. 414 rolls), Maryland (M321. 22 rolls), Mississippi (M269. 427 rolls), Missouri (M322. 193 rolls), North Carolina (M270. 580 rolls), South Carolina (M267. 392 rolls), Tennessee (M268. 359 rolls), Texas (M323. 445 rolls), and Virginia (M324. 1,075 rolls).

Confederate State Army Casualties: Lists and Narrative Reports. 1861–65. M836. Microfilm, 7 rolls.

North Carolina State Archives. Raleigh.

Gen. Lewis A. Armistead Misc.

L. O'B Branch Papers.

W. H. S. Burgwyn Papers.

Bryan Grimes Papers.

Collett Leventhorpe Papers.

Stephen D. Ramseur Papers.

Frederick Tilberg Papers.

Thomas F. Toon Papers, 1840–1902. P.C. 998.

John A. Young Diary, 1861, 4th N.C. Regt. P.C. 629.1.

South Caroliniana Library. Manuscripts Division. University of South Carolina. Columbia.

M. L. Bonham Papers.

John Bratton Papers.

M. C. Butler Papers.

Ellison Capers Papers.

James Conner Papers.

Stephen Elliott, Jr., Papers.

Martin Witherspoon Gary Papers.

States Rights Gist Papers.

Maxcy Gregg Papers.

Joseph Brevard Kershaw Papers.

Trapier Family Papers.

Southern Historical Collection. Library of the University of North Carolina. Chapel Hill.

Jas. Patton Anderson Autobiography.

John Bratton Papers.

J. F. H. Claiborne Papers.

Raleigh E. Colston Papers.

Raleigh E. Colston biographical notes.

Louis Hebert Papers. An Autobiography of Lewis Hebert.

Jeremy F. Gilmer Papers.

Bryan Grimes Papers.

William Gaston Lewis Papers.

Thomas Muldrup Logan Papers.

W. W. Mackall Papers.

William Nelson Pendleton Papers.

Edward Asbury O'Neil Papers.

William Dorsey Pender Letters.

William Dorsey Pender Papers.

Robert Ransom Papers.

James A. Walker Papers.

Gen. James A. Walker, Life of. Typed copies.

Tennessee State Library and Archives. Nashville.

Brown-Ewell Papers 1803–1919. Acc. Number 1358.75-73. Location VIII-G-1-4.

Campbell Brown–Ewell Papers. Acc. Number 5, 647, 649, 1256. Location 1-A-5.

Major Campbell Brown, Military Reminiscences of. 1861–63. Box 2. Folder 4.

Confederate Collection. Casualty list Forrest's Command, 1864. Compiled by J. B. Cowan.

William Hicks Jackson Papers. 1766–1978.

Texas State Library. Archives Division. Austin.

Samuel Bell Maxey Papers.

Texas, University of, at Austin. General Libraries. Barker Texas History Center. Austin.

Bernard E. Bee Papers.

(Ben and Henry Eustace) McCulloch Papers.

Louis T. Wigfall Family Papers.

Tulane University Libraries. Howard-Tilton Memorial Library. Tulane University. New Orleans, La.

Mrs. Mason Barret Collection of Albert Sidney and William Preston Johnston Papers. Box 17. Folder 32.

U.S. Army Military History Institute. Carlisle Barracks, Pa.

Aztec Club Archives Historical Papers. General Information. W. M. Booth Taliaferro. Diary, typed.

Robert L. Brake Collection: The Gettysburg Campaign.

Civil War Miscellaneous Collection.

James Patton Anderson Letters.

Civil War Times Illustrated Collection.

Battle of the Crater.

Daniel Harvey Hill.

Lewis Henry Little. Civil War Diary.

"Mark P. Lowrey autobiography." 1867.

Camille Polignac. Diary of the War between the States.

Charles W. Squires.

R. E. and G. W. C. Lee Papers.

Murray J. Smith Collection.

Smith-Kirby-Webster-Black-Danner Family Papers.

Virginia, University of. Library. Manuscript Division, Special Collections Department. Charlottesville.

Beale Family Papers, no. 7754.

Lawrence O'Bryan Branch Papers, no. 10057.

Benjamin Huger Papers, no. 9942.

Hunter Holmes McGuire Papers, no. 9320.
Rosser Family Papers, no. 1171.
J. E. B. Stuart Collection, no. 7442.
Virginia State Library. Richmond.
Dr. James Richmond Boulware Diary.
Cooke Family Papers.
Dr. Hunter McGuire Collection.
Personal Papers Collection.
Washington and Lee University. The University Library. Lexington, Va.
James Lewis Howe Papers.
G. W. C. Lee Papers.
Robert E. Lee Papers.
William and Mary, College of. Earl Gregg Swem Library. Williamsburg, Va.
Joseph E. Johnston Papers.
William Booth Taliaferro Papers.

UNPUBLISHED MATERIALS

Cemetery Burial and internment records

Alabama
Anniston. Edgemont Cemetery.
Georgia
Augusta. Magnolia Cemetery.
Savannah. Department of Cemeteries, City of Savannah.
Kentucky
Louisville. Cave Hill Cemetery Co., Inc. Warren County, 1877–1913. Vol. 2.
Maryland
Baltimore. Green Mount Cemetery.
Baltimore. New Cathedral Cemetery.
Mississippi
Biloxi. Biloxi Cemetery.
Missouri
Kansas City. Forest Hill Cemetery.
St. Louis. Catholic Cemeteries of the Archdiocese.
New York
Brooklyn. Green-Wood Cemetery.
North Carolina
Winston-Salem. Salem Cemetery Co.
South Carolina
Camden. Quaker Cemetery Association.
Charleston. Magnolia Cemetery Trust.
Tennessee
Memphis. Elmwood Cemetery.
Nashville. Mount Olivet Cemetery.

Texas
 Austin. Oakwood Cemetery.
Virginia
 Petersburg. Blandford Cemetery.
 Richmond. Hollywood Cemetery.

City and County Burial and Death Records

Alabama
 Mobile. Health Department of the City of Mobile.
North Carolina
 Asheville. Register of Deaths in the City of Asheville. Buncombe County Courthouse.
South Carolina
 Charleston. Registers of the Charleston County deaths compiled by the Charleston
  County Health Department. Charleston County Library.
Texas
 Galveston. Galveston Health Department. Internment Records.
 Greenville. Hunt County Death Records.
 Marshall. Register of Deaths and Burials of City of Marshall.
 San Antonio. Metro Health District.
Virginia
 Spring Hill. Diuguid's Burial Records. Roll no. 3, 929.3D Book no. 7, p. 222.

Dissertations

Adams, Grace Rita. "Brigadier-General John Adams, C.S.A.: Biography of a Frontier Amer-
 ican (1825–1864)." Ph.D. diss., Saint Louis University, 1964.
Cummings, Charles Martin. "Seven Ohio Confederate Generals: Case Histories of Defec-
 tion." Ph.D. diss., Ohio State University, 1963.
Hall, Martin Hardwick. "The Army of New Mexico: Sibley's Campaign of 1862." Ph.D. diss.,
 Louisiana State University and Agricultural and Mechanical College, 1957.
Halperin, Rick. "Leroy Pope Walker and the Problems of the Confederate War Department,
 February–September, 1861." Ph.D. diss., Auburn University, 1978.
Hartje, Robert George. "Major General Earl Van Dorn." Ph.D. diss., Vanderbilt University,
 1955.
Hattaway, Herman Morell. "Stephen Dill Lee: A Biography." Ph.D. diss., Louisiana State
 University Agricultural and Mechanical College, 1969.
Jones, Robert Rivers. "Conservative Virginian: The Postwar Career of Governor James
 Lawson Kemper." Ph.D. diss., University of Virginia, 1964.
Kennedy, Larry Wells. "The Fighting Preacher of the Army of Tennessee: General Mark
 Perrin Lowrey." Ph.D. diss., Mississippi State University, 1976.
King, Alvy Leon. "Louis T. Wigfall: The Stormy Petrel." Ph.D. diss., Yale University, 1967.
McKee, James Willette, Jr. "William Barksdale: The Intrepid Mississippian." Ph.D. diss.,
 Mississippi State University, 1966.
Piston, William Garrett. "Lee's Tarnished Lieutenant: James Longstreet and His Image in
 American Society." Ph.D. diss., University of South Carolina, 1982.

Scott, Paul. "Eighth Texas Cavalry Regiment, CSA." Master's thesis, University of Texas, Arlington, 1977.

Settles, Thomas Michael. "The Military Career of John Bankhead Magruder." Ph.D. diss., Texas Christian University, 1972.

Miscellaneous

Florida

Pension application of Evander McIver Law. Filed April 24, 1917. Florida Department of State. Division of Archives, History and Records Management. The Capitol, Tallahassee.

Louisiana

Soldier's application (Louis Hebert) for pension (no. 2663). Filed June 27, 1899. St. Martin Parish.

Widow's application (Mrs. Zebulon York) for pension (no. 8822). Catahoula Parish.

Tennessee

Family Questionnaire (William B. Bate). N.d., marked received October 11, 1922. State of Tennessee. Tennessee Historical Committee. Department of Libraries, Archives and History, Nashville.

PUBLISHED MATERIALS

Alvarez, Eugene. "The Death of the 'Old War Horse' Longstreet." *Georgia Historical Quarterly* 52 (1968): 70–77.

Anderson, Ephraim McD. *First Missouri Confederate Brigade.* Edited by Edwin C. Bearss. 1868. Reprint, Dayton, Ohio: Morningside Press, 1972.

Arceneaux, William. *Acadian General: Alfred Mouton and the Civil War.* 2nd ed. Lafayette: Center for Louisiana Studies, University of Southwestern Louisiana, 1981.

Baird, Nancy Disher. *David Wendel Yandell: Physician of Old Louisville.* Lexington: University Press of Kentucky, 1978.

Baldwin, Helen Pool. Interview. "The Life Story of Brig. General Felix Robertson." *Texana* 8 (1970): 154.

Beale, Richard L. T. *History of the Ninth Virginia Cavalry, in the War Between the States.* Richmond, Va.: B. F. Johnson Publishing, 1899.

Bean, William G. *Stonewall's Man Sandie Pendleton.* Chapel Hill: University of North Carolina Press, 1959.

Benner, Judith Ann. *Sul Ross: Soldier, Statesman, Educator.* College Station: Texas A&M University Press, 1983.

Bevier, Robert S. *History of the First and Second Missouri Confederate Brigades, 1861–1865 and from Wakarusa to Appomattox, a Military Anagraph.* 1879. Reprint, Florissant, Miss.: Inland Printer, 1985.

Blackburn, James K. P. *Terry's Texas Rangers: Reminiscences.* Civil War Series, no. 2. Austin, Tex.: Ranger Press, 1979.

Blakey, Arch Fredric. *General John H. Winder C.S.A.* Gainesville: University of Florida Press, 1990.

Blessington, Joseph P. *The Campaigns of Walker's Texas Division.* New York: Lange, Little, 1875.

Bridges, Leonard Hal. *Lee's Maverick General, David Harvey Hill.* New York: McGraw-Hill, 1961.

Brown, Norman D., ed. *One of Cleburne's Command: The Civil War Reminiscence and Diary of Captain Samuel T. Foster, Granbury's Texas Brigade, C.S.A.* Austin: University of Texas Press, 1980.

Buck, Irving A. *Cleburne and his Command.* Dayton, Ohio: Morningside House, 1985.

Bushong, Millard K. *General Turner Ashby and Stonewall's Valley Campaign.* Verona, Va.: McClure Printing Company, 1980.

————. *Old Jube: A Biography of General Jubal A. Early.* 3rd ed. Shippensburg, Pa.: Beidel Printing House, 1985.

Caldwell, James F. J. *The History of a Brigade of South Carolinians. Known First as "Gregg's" and Subsequently as "McGowan's Brigade."* 1866. Reprint, Dayton, Ohio: Facsimile 16, Press of the Morningside Bookshop, 1974.

Cassidy, Vincent H., and Amos E. Simpson. *Henry Watkins Allen of Louisiana.* Baton Rouge: Louisiana State University Press, 1964.

Casso, Evans J. *Francis T. Nicholls: A Biographical Tribute.* Thibodaux, La.: Nicholls College Foundation, 1987.

Cauthen, Edward, ed. *Family Letters of the Three Wade Hamptons.* Columbia: University of South Carolina Press, 1953.

Chapla, John D. *42nd Virginia Infantry.* Lynchburg, Va.: H. E. Howard, 1983.

Chesnut, Mary Boykin. *A Diary from Dixie.* Edited by Ben Ames Williams. 2nd ed. Cambridge: Harvard University Press, 1982.

Chisolm, J. Julian, M.D. *A Manual of Military Surgery, for the Use of Surgeons in the Confederate States Army.* 3rd ed. 1864. Reprint, Dayton, Ohio: Morningside House, 1983.

Christian, Asbury. *Lynchburg and Its People.* Lynchburg, Va.: J. P. Bell, 1900.

Clark, Walter. "General James Pettigrew, C.S.A." *North Carolina Booklet* 20 (1921): 171–80.

————, ed. *Histories of the Several Regiments and Battalions from North Carolina in the Great War, 1861–1865.* 5 vols. 1901. Reprint, Wendel, N.C.: Broadfoot's Bookmark, 1981.

Coco, Gregory A. *A Vast Sea of Misery.* Gettysburg, Pa.: Thomas Publications, 1988.

Coker, James Lide. *History of Company G, Ninth S. C. Regiment, Infantry, S.C. Army and of Company E, Sixth S.C. Regiment, Infantry, S.C. Army.* Original publication undated. Reprint. Greenwood, S.C.: Attic Press, 1979.

Commager, Henry Steel, ed. *The Blue and the Gray.* 2 vols. 1950. Reprint, New York: American Book-Stratford Press, 1950.

Confederate Veteran Magazine. 40 vols. Nashville: S. A. Cunningham, Founder, 1893–1932; Wendell, N.C.: Broadfoot's Bookmark Reprint, n.d.

Conrad, James L. "From Glory to Contention: The Sad History of 'Shanks' Evans." *Civil War Times Illustrated* 22 (September 1983): 32–38.

Coulter, E. Merton. *William Montague Browne: Versatile Anglo-Irish American, 1823–1883.* Athens: University of Georgia Press, 1967.

Covey, E. N. "The Interdental Splint." *Richmond Medical Journal* 1 (1866): 88–91.

Cowper, Pulaski, comp. *Extracts of letters of Major-General Bryan Grimes to his Wife.* Raleigh, N.C.: Alfred Williams and Co., 1884.

Crenshaw, Ollinger. *General Lee's College: The Rise and Growth of Washington and Lee University*. New York: Random House, 1969.

Cullum, George W. *Biographical Register of the Officers and Graduates of the U.S. Military Academy at West Point, N.Y.: from its establishment, in 1802 to 1890*. 3rd ed. Boston: Houghton Mifflin, 1891.

Cumming, Kate. *Kate: The Journal of a Confederate Nurse*. Edited by Richard Barksdale Harwell. Baton Rouge: Louisiana State University Press, 1959.

Cummings, Charles M. *Yankee Quaker, Confederate General: The Curious Career of Bushrod Rust Johnson*. Rutherford, N.J.: Fairleigh Dickinson University Press, 1971.

Dabney, Robert L. *Life and Campaigns of Lieut. Gen. Thomas J. Jackson (Stonewall Jackson)*. New York: Blelock & Co., 1866.

Davis, Stephen A. "A Georgia Firebrand: Major General W. H. T. Walker, C.S.A." *Confederate Historical Institute Journal* 2 (1981): 1–15.

Davis, William C. *Breckinridge, Statesman, Soldier, Symbol*. Baton Rouge: Louisiana State University Press, 1974.

———. *The Orphan Brigade: The Kentucky Confederates Who Couldn't Go Home*. Garden City, N.Y.: Doubleday, 1980.

Dawson, Francis. *Reminiscences of Confederate Service, 1861–1865*. Edited by Bell I. Wiley. Baton Rouge: Louisiana State University Press, 1980.

Denson, C. B. *An Address containing a Memoir of the Late Major-General William Henry Chase Whiting, of the Confederate Army. Delivered in Raleigh, N.C., on Memorial Day, May 10, 1895*. 1895. Reprint, Wendell, N.C.: Avera Press, n.d.

Dictionary of American Biography. Vols. 1 and 6. New York: Charles Scribner's Sons, 1962.

Dickinson, Jack L. *Jenkins of Greenbottom: A Civil War Saga*. Charleston, W.Va.: Pictorial Histories Publishing Co., 1988.

Diket, A. L. *Wh Hae Wi' (Pender) . . . Bled*. New York: Vantage Press, 1979.

Dinkins, James. *1862–1865, By an Old Johnnie*. Dayton, Ohio: Press of Morningside Bookshop, 1975.

Divine, John E. *8th Virginia Infantry*. Lynchburg, Va.: H. E. Howard, 1983.

Dodson, William Carey. *Campaigns of Wheeler and his Cavalry, 1862–1865*. Atlanta: Hidgins Publishing, 1889.

Donovan, Timothy P., and Willard B. Gatewood, Jr. *The Governors of Arkansas: Essays in Political Biography*. Fayetteville, Ark.: University of Arkansas Press, 1981.

Dotson, Susan Merle, comp. *Who's Who of the Confederacy*. San Antonio, Tex.: Naylor Company, 1966.

Douglas, Henry Kyd. *I Rode with Stonewall*. Covington, Ga.: Mockingbird Books, 1974.

Dufour, Charles L. *Nine Men in Gray*. Garden City, N.Y.: Doubleday, 1963.

Duke, Basil W. *A History of Morgan's Cavalry*. Edited with an introduction and notes by Cecil Fletcher Holland. Civil War Centennial series. Bloomington: Indiana University Press, 1960.

———. *Personal Recollections of Shiloh. Read before the Filson Club, April 6, 1914*. Suffolk, Va.: Robert Hardy Publications, 1986.

———. *Reminiscences of General Basil W. Duke, C.S.A.* Bloomington, Ind.: Indiana University Press, 1960.

Duncan, Robert Lipscomb. *Reluctant General: The Life and Times of Albert Pike*. New York: E. P. Dutton, 1961.

Dyer, John P. *From Shiloh to San Juan: The Life of "Fightin Joe" Wheeler.* Baton Rouge: Louisiana State University Press, 1961.

Eckenrode, Hamilton J., and Bryan Conrad. *James Longstreet: Lee's War Horse.* Chapel Hill: University of North Carolina Press, 1936.

Eckert, Ralph Lowell. *John Brown Gordon: Soldier, Southerner, American.* Baton Rouge: Louisiana State University Press, 1989.

Elliott, Joseph Cantey. *Lieutenant General Richard Heron Anderson: Lee's Noble Soldier.* Dayton, Ohio: Morningside House, 1985.

Evans, Clement A., ed. *Confederate Military History.* 13 vols. N.d. Reprint, New York: Castle Books, 1956.

Flood, Charles Bracelan. *Lee: The Last Years.* Boston: Houghton Mifflin, 1981.

Foote, Shelby. *The Civil War: A Narrative.* 3 vols. New York: Random House, 1958–74.

Franks, Kenny A. *Stand Watie and the Agony of the Cherokee Nation.* Memphis: Memphis State University Press, 1979.

Freeman, Douglas S. *Lee's Lieutenants.* 3 vols. New York: Charles Scribner's Sons, 1942.

———. *R. E. Lee: A Biography.* 4 vols. New York: Charles Scribner's Sons, 1963.

Freemantle, Sir Arthur J. L., and Frank A. Haskell. *Two Views of Gettysburg.* Edited by Richard Harwell. Chicago: Lakeside Press, R. R. Donnelley & Sons, 1964.

French, Samuel G. *Two Wars: An Autobiography of General Samuel G. French.* Nashville: Confederate Veteran, 1901.

Gallagher, Gary W. *Stephen Dodson Ramseur.* Chapel Hill: University of North Carolina Press, 1985.

———, ed. *Extracts of Letters of Major-General Bryan Grimes, to his Wife.* Compiled from original manuscripts by Pulaski Cowper. Wilmington, N.C.: Broadfoot Publishing, 1986.

Garrett, Jill L. *Obituaries from Tennessee Newspapers.* Easley, S.C.: Southern Historical Press, 1980.

Going, Allen J. "A Shooting Affray in Knoxville with Interstate Repercussions: The Killing of James H. Clanton by David M. Nelson, 1871." *East Tennessee Historical Society's Publications* 27 (1955): 39–48.

Gordon, John B. *Reminiscences of the Civil War.* 1903. Reprint, New York: Time-Life Books, 1981.

Govan, Gilbert Eaton, and James W. Livingood. *A Different Valor: The Story of General Joseph E. Johnston, C.S.A.* New York: Bobbs-Merrill, 1956.

Graber, Henry W. *The Life Record of H. W. Graber: A Terry Texas Ranger, 1861–1865.* N.p., 1916.

Green, Wharton J. *Confederate General Robert Ransom. An address before the Ladies Memorial Assoc., May 10, 1899.* Suffolk, Va.: Robert Hardy Publications, 1986.

Hagood, John. *Memoirs of the War of Secession.* 1910. Reprint, Camden, S.C.: J. J. Fox, 1989.

Hale, Virginia Laura, and Stanley S. Phillips. *History of the Forty-Ninth Virginia Infantry, C.S.A. "Extra Billy Smith's Boys."* Lanham, Md.: S. S. Phillips & Associates, 1981.

Hallock, Judith Lee. *Braxton Bragg and the Confederate Defeat. Volume II.* Tuscaloosa: University of Alabama Press, 1991.

Hamlin, Percy Gatling. *The Making of a Soldier: Letters of General R. S. Ewell.* Richmond: Whittet & Shepperson, 1935.

———. *"Old Bald Head" (General R. S. Ewell): The Portrait of a Soldier.* Strasburg, Va.: Shenandoah Publishing House, 1940.

Harris, William Charles. *Leroy Pope Walker: Confederate Secretary of War.* Tuscaloosa, Ala.: Confederate Publishing, 1962.

Harris, Capt. W. N., comp. *Diary of General Nat. H. Harris.* Duncansby, Miss.: Capt. W. N. Harris, Publisher, 1901.

Hartje, Robert G. *Van Dorn: The Life and Times of a Confederate General.* Nashville: Vanderbilt University Press, 1967.

Harvey, Paul J. *Old Tige: General William L. Cabell, C.S.A.* Hillsboro, Tex.: Hill Junior College Press, 1970.

Haskell, John. *The Haskell Memoirs.* Edited by Gilbert E. Govan and James W. Livingood. New York: G. P. Putnam's Sons, 1960.

Hassler, William W. *A. P. Hill: Lee's Forgotten General.* Richmond: Garrett and Massie, 1962.

———. *The General to His Lady: The Civil War Letters of William Dorsey Pender to Fanny Pender.* Chapel Hill: University of North Carolina Press, 1965.

Hattaway, Herman. *General Stephen D. Lee.* Jackson: University Press of Mississippi, 1976.

Head, Thomas A. *Campaigns and Battles of the Sixteenth Regiment, Tennessee Volunteers.* Facsimile rpt. of the 1885 edition. McMinnville, Tenn.: Womack Printing, 1961.

Heitman, Francis B. *Historical Register and Dictionary of the United States Army.* 2 vols. 1903. Reprint. Gaithersburg, Md.: Olde Soldiers Books, 1988.

Henry, Robert Selph. *"First With the Most" Forrest.* Indianapolis: Bobbs-Merrill, 1944.

Hesseltine, Willia B., and Hazel C. Wolf. *The Blue and the Gray on the Nile.* Chicago: University of Chicago Press, 1961.

History of Southern Arkansas. Chicago: Goodspeed Publishing, 1890.

Holland, Lynwood M. *Pierce M. B. Young: The Warwick of the South.* Athens: University of Georgia Press, 1964.

Holtzman, Robert S. *Adapt or Perish: The Life of General Roger A. Pryor, C.S.A.* Hamden, Conn.: Archon Books, 1976.

Hood, John Bell. *Advance and Retreat.* Secaucus, N.J.: Blue and Grey Press, 1985.

Horn, Stanley F. *The Army of Tennessee.* Norman: University of Oklahoma Press, 1952.

Horton, Louis. *Samuel Bell Maxey: A Biography.* Austin: University of Texas Press, 1974.

Howard, McHenry. *Recollections of a Maryland Confederate Soldier and Staff Officer under Johnston, Jackson and Lee.* Edited by James I. Robertson, Jr. 1914. Reprint, Dayton, Ohio: Facsimile 26, Morningside Bookshop, 1975.

Hughes, Nathaniel Cheairs, Jr. *General William J. Hardee: Old Reliable.* Baton Rouge: Louisiana State University Press, 1965.

Hunton, Eppa. *Autobiography of Eppa Hunton.* Richmond: William Byrd Press, 1933.

Johnson, Adam R. *The Partisan Rangers of the Confederate States Army.* Edited by William J. Davis. Louisville, Ky.: George G. Fetter, 1904.

Johnson, Jesse B., and Lowell H. Harrison. "Ogden College: A Brief History." *Register of the Kentucky Historical Society* 67 (1970): 189–220.

Johnson, John Lipscomb. *The University Memorial.* Baltimore, Md.: Turnbull Brothers, 1871.

Johnson, Robert U., and Clarence C. Buel, eds. *Battles and Leaders of the Civil War.* 4 vols. 1884–88. Reprint, New York: Roy F. Nichols, 1956.

Johnston, Joseph E. *Narrative of Military Operation, Directed during the Late War Between the States.* New York: Appleton, 1874.

Johnston, Wm. Preston. *The Life of Gen. Albert Sidney Johnston.* New York: D. Appleton, 1878.

Jones, Terry L. *Lee's Tigers.* Baton Rouge: Louisiana State University Press, 1987.

Jordan, Thomas, and John P. Pryor. *The Campaigns of Lieutenant-General N. B. Forrest, and of Forrest's Cavalry.* Dayton, Ohio: Press of the Morningside Bookshop, 1977.

Klein, Maury. *Edward Porter Alexander.* Athens: University of Georgia Press, 1971.

Krick, Robert K. *30th Virginia Infantry.* Lynchburg, Va.: H. E. Howard, 1983.

Lane, Walter P. *The Adventures and Recollections of General Walter P. Lane.* New York: Pemberton Press, Jenkins Publishing, 1970.

Lawson, Lewis A. *Wheeler's Last Raid.* Greenwood, Fla.: Penkevill Publishing, 1986.

Lee, John F. "John Sappington Marmaduke." *Missouri Historical Society Collections* 6 (1906): 31–40.

Lee, Robert E. *The Wartime Papers of R. E. Lee.* Edited by C. Dowdey and L. H. Manarin. New York: Virginia Civil War Commission, Bramhall House, 1956.

Lee, Susan (Pendleton). *Memoirs of William Nelson Pendleton, D. D.* Philadelphia: J. B. Lippincott, 1893.

Levin, Alexandra Lee. *"This Awful Drama": General Edwin Gray Lee, C.S.A., and His Family.* New York: Vantage Press, 1987.

Lewis, Lloyd. *Sherman, Fighting Prophet.* New York: Harcourt, Brace, 1932.

Liddell, St. John Richardson. *Liddell's Record.* Edited by Nathaniel C. Hughes. Dayton, Ohio: Morningside House, 1985.

Long, Armistead Lindsay. *Memoirs of Robert E. Lee.* Secaucus, N.J.: Blue and Grey Press, 1983.

Lord, Walter, ed. *The Fremantle Diary.* London: Andre Deutsch, and D. R. Hillman & Sons, 1956.

McCaffrey, James M. *This Band of Heroes: Granbury's Texas Brigade, C.S.A.* Austin, Tex.: Eakin Press, 1985.

McCash, William B. *Thomas R. R. Cobb: The Making of a Southern Nationalist.* Macon, Ga.: Mercer University Press, 1983.

McDonald, Archie P., ed. *Make Me a Map of the Valley: The Civil War Journal of Stonewall Jackson's Topographer.* Dallas: Southern Methodist University Press, 1973.

McGuire, Hunter. "Clinical Reports on Gun-Shot Wounds of Joints." *Richmond Medical Journal* 1 (1866): 147–50, 260–65.

———. "Last Wound of the Late Gen. Jackson (Stonewall). The amputation of his arm—His last moments and death." *Richmond Medical Journal* 1 (1866): 402–12.

McKim, Randolph H. *A Soldier's Recollections.* 1910. Reprint, New York: Time-Life Books, 1984.

McMurry, Richard M. *John Bell Hood and the War for Southern Independence.* Lexington: University Press of Kentucky, 1982.

McWhiney, Grady. *Braxton Bragg and Confederate Defeat. Volume 1. Field Command.* New York: Columbia University Press, 1969.

Madison, R. L., and H. T. Barton. "Letter." *Richmond and Louisville Medical Journal* 10 (1870): 516–23.

Manigault, Arthur Middleton. *A Carolinian Goes to War.* Edited by R. Lockwood Tower, and *Mexican War Narrative.* Edited by Warren Ripley and Arthur M. Wilcox. Columbia: Charleston Library Society, University of South Carolina Press, 1983.

Marbaker, Thomas D. *History of the Eleventh New Jersey Volunteers.* Trenton, N.J.: MacCrellish & Quigley, 1889.

Marshall, Park. *A Life of William B. Bate.* Nashville: Cumberland Press, 1908.

Mathis, James L. "The Building of the Wall—Thomas Jonathan Jackson." *Military Medicine* 129 (1964): 449–56.

Maury, Dabney Herndon. *Recollections of a Virginian in the Mexican, Indian, and Civil Wars.* New York: Charles Scribner's Sons, 1894.

Medical and Surgical History of the War of the Rebellion. 2 vols., 3 pts. each. GPO: Washington, D.C., 1870–1883.

Monaghan, Jay. *Civil War on the Western Border, 1854–1865.* New York: Bonanza Books, 1955.

Montgomery, Horace. *Howell Cobb's Confederate Career.* Chicago: Adams Press, 1973.

Moore, Edward A. *The Story of a Cannoneer Under Stonewall Jackson.* 1907. Reprint, New York: Time-Life Books, 1983.

Moore, Robert A., Pvt. *A Life for the Confederacy. As Recorded in the Pocket Diaries of Pvt. Robert A. Moore.* Edited by Bell Irvin Wiley. Jackson, Tenn.: McCowat-Mercer Press, 1959.

Morrison, James L., Jr., ed. *The Memoirs of Henry Heth.* Westport, Conn.: Greenwood Press, 1974.

Mosgrove, George Dallas. *Kentucky Cavaliers in Dixie: Reminiscences of a Confederate Cavalryman.* Edited by Bell Irvin Wiley. Jackson, Tenn.: McCowat-Mercer Press, 1957.

Myers, Frank M. *The Comanches: History of White's Battlion, Virginia Cavalry.* 1871. Reprint. Gaithersburg, Md.: Butternut Press, 1987.

Myers, Raymond E. *The Zollie Tree.* Louisville, Ky.: Filson Club Press, 1964.

Nash, Charles Edward. *Biographical Sketches of General Pat Cleburne and General T. C. Hindman.* Dayton, Ohio: Facsimile 39, Press of the Morningside Bookshop, 1977.

Neff, Robert O. *Tennessee's Battered Brigadier. (The Life of General Joseph B. Palmer).* Nashville: Historic Travellers' Rest, 1988.

Nicholls, Francis T. "Autobiography of Francis T. Nicholls, 1834–1881." Edited by Francis T. Nicholls. *Louisiana Historical Quarterly* 17 (1934): 251–52.

Nichols, G. W. *A Soldier's Story of his Regiment (61st Georgia) and Incidentally of the Lawton-Gordon-Evans Brigade, Army Northern Virginia.* Kennesaw, Ga.: Continental Book Co., 1898.

Nichols, James L. *General Fitzhugh Lee: A Biography.* Lynchburg, Va.: H. E. Howard, 1989.

Nisbet, James Cooper. *Four Years on the Firing Line.* Edited by Bell Irvin Wiley. Wilmington, N.C.: Broadfoot Publishing, 1987.

Noll, Arthur Howard. *General Edmund Kirby Smith.* Sewanee, Tenn.: University Press at the University of the South, 1907.

Nunn, W. C., ed. *Ten More Texans in Gray.* Hillsboro, Tex.: Hill Junior College Press, 1980.

Oates, William C. *The War between the Union and the Confederacy and Its Lost Opportunities.* Dayton, Ohio: Press of the Morningside Bookshop, 1985.

O'Flaherty, Daniel. *General Jo Shelby: Undefeated Rebel.* Chapel Hill: University of North Carolina Press, 1954.

Orr, William C., Richard J. Martin, and C. Dowell Patterson. "When to Suspect Sleep Apnea—the 'Pickwickian Syndrome.'" *Resident and Staff Physician* 25 (1979): 101–4.

Parker, William L. *General James Dearing CSA.* Lynchburg, Va.: H. E. Howard, 1990.

Parks, Joseph Howard. *General Edmund Kirby Smith, C.S.A.* Baton Rouge: Louisiana State University Press, 1954.

———. *General Leonidas Polk, C.S.A.: The Fighting Bishop.* Baton Rouge: Louisiana State University Press, 1962.

Parrish, T. Michael. *Richard Taylor: Soldier Prince of Dixie*. Chapel Hill: University of North Carolina Press, 1992.

Paxton, John Gallatin. *The Civil War Letters of Gen. Frank "Bull" Paxton—A Lieutenant of Lee and Jackson*. Hillsboro, Tex.: Hill Junior College Press, 1978.

Pemberton, John C. *Pemberton: Defender of Vicksburg*. Wilmington, N.C.: Broadfoot Publishing, 1987.

Pfanz, Harry W. *Gettysburg—The Second Day*. Chapel Hill: University of North Carolina Press, 1987.

Pickett, George Edward. *Soldier of the South: General Pickett's War Letters to his Wife*. Edited by Arthur Crew Inman. Boston: Houghton Mifflin, 1928.

Poague, William Thomas. *Gunner with Stonewall: Reminiscences of William Thomas Poague*. Edited by Monroe F. Cockrell. Jackson, Tenn.: McCowat-Mercer Press, 1957.

Pryor, Mrs. Roger. *Reminiscences of Peace and War*. New York: Macmillan, 1904.

Purdue, Howell, and Elizabeth Purdue. *Pat Cleburne, Confederate General*. 2nd ed. Tuscaloosa, Ala.: Portals Press, 1977.

Rhoades, Jeffrey L. *Scapegoat General: The Story of Major General Benjamin Huger, C.S.A.* Hamden, Conn.: Archon Books, Shoe String Press, 1985.

Riley, Harris D., Jr. "General Richard Taylor, C.S.A.: Louisianian, Distinguished Military Commander and Author with Speculations on His Health." *Southern Studies: An Interdisciplinary Journal of the South* 1, n.s. (Spring 1990): 67–86.

———. "Robert E. Lee's Battle with Disease." *Civil War Times Illustrated* 18 (December 1979): 12–22.

Robertson, James I., Jr. *4th Virginia Infantry*. Lynchburg, Va.: H. E. Howard, 1982.

———. *18th Virginia Infantry*. Lynchburg, Va.: H. E. Howard, 1984.

———. *General A. P. Hill: The Story of a Confederate Warrior*. New York: Random House, 1987.

———. *The Stonewall Brigade*. Baton Rouge: Louisiana State University Press, 1981.

Robertson, William Glenn. *Back Door to Richmond: The Bermuda Hundred Campaign, April–June 1864*. Newark: University of Delaware Press, 1987.

Roher, Walter A. "Confederate Generals—The View from Below." *Civil War Times Illustrated* 18 (July 1979): 10–13.

Rose, Victor M. *The Life and Services of Gen. Ben McCulloch*. 1888. Reprint, Austin, Tex.: Steck Company, 1958.

———. *Ross' Texas Brigade*. Louisville, Ky.: Courier-Journal Book and Job Rooms, 1881.

Rowland, Dunbar. *Mississippi*. 1907. Reprint (5 vols.), Atlanta, Ga.: Southern Historical Association, 1916.

Rozear, Marvin P., E. Wayne Massey, Jennifer Horner, Erin Foley, and Joseph C. Greenfield, Jr. "R. E. Lee's Stroke." *The Virginia Magazine of History and Biography* 98 (1990): 291–308.

Rugeley, H. J. H, annotated by. *Batchelor-Turner Letters, 1861–1864. Written by Two of Terry's Texas Rangers*. Austin, Tex.: Steck, 1961.

Sanger, Donald Bridgman, and Thomas Robson Hay. *James Longstreet*. Baton Rouge: Louisiana State University Press, 1952.

Sayre, Lewis A. "The Operation on General John C. Breckinridge—His Remarks, etc. [An Open Letter]." *American Medical Weekly* (Louisville, Ky.) 2 (June 12, 1875): 605–8.

Scharf, J. Thomas. *History of St. Louis City and County*. Philadelphia: Louis H. Everts, 1883.

Schoff, Philip, D.D. "The Gettysburg Week." *Scribner's Magazine* 16 (1894): 21–30.

Shackelford, George Green. *George Wythe Randolph and the Confederate Elite.* Athens: University of Georgia Press, 1988.

Shalhope, Robert E. *Sterling Price: Portrait of a Southerner.* Columbia: University of Missouri Press, 1971.

Shaver, Lewellyn A. *A History of the Sixtieth Alabama Regiment: Gracies Alabama Brigade.* 1867. Reprint, Gaithersburg, Md.: Butternut Press, n.d.

Sheppard, Eric William. *Bedford Forrest: The Confederacy's Greatest Cavalryman.* Dayton, Ohio: Press of Morningside Bookshop, 1981.

Simpson, Craig M. *A Good Southerner: The Life of Henry A. Wise of Virginia.* Chapel Hill: University of North Carolina Press, 1985.

Simpson, Harold B. *Touched With Valor.* Hillsboro, Tex.: Hill Junior College Press, 1964.

Smith, Frank H. "The Forrest-Gould Affair." *Civil War Times Illustrated* 9 (November 1970): 32–37.

Smith, Gustavus. *The Battle of Seven Pines.* Dayton, Ohio: Facsimile 20, Morningside Bookshop, 1974.

Snow, William P. *Lee and his Generals.* 1867. Reprint, New York: Fairfax Press, 1982.

Sommers, Richard J. *Richmond Redeemed: Seige at Petersburg.* Garden City, N.Y.: Doubleday, 1981.

Sorrel, G. Moxley. *Recollection of a Confederate Staff Officer.* 1905. Reprint, Dayton, Ohio: Morningside Bookshop, 1974.

Southern Historical Society Papers. 52 vols. 1876–1959. Reprint, Millwood, N.Y.: Kraus, 1977, 1980.

Southern History of the War. Official reports of battles as published by order of the Confederate Congress at Richmond by Enquirer Book and Job Press, Richmond, Va. 1864. Reprint, New York: Kraus, 1970

Special Staff of Writers. *History of Virginia: Virginia Biography.* 6 vols. Chicago: American Historical Society, 1924.

Steiner, Paul E. *Medical-Military Portraits of Union and Confederate Generals.* Philadelphia: Whitmore Publishing, 1968.

———. "Medical-Military Studies on the Civil War. 1. Lieutenant General Ambrose Powell Hill, C.S.A." *Military Medicine* 130 (1965): 225–28.

———. "Medical-Military Studies on the Civil War. 6. Brigadier General James Johnston Pettigrew, C.S.A." *Military Medicine* 130 (1965): 930–37.

———. "Medical-Military Studies on the Civil War. 7. Major General Stephen D. Ramseur, C.S.A." *Military Medicine* 130 (1965): 1016–22.

———. "Medical-Military Studies on the Civil War. 10. Major General Thomas L. Rosser, C.S.A." *Military Medicine* 131 (1966): 72–80.

———. *Physicians-Generals in the Civil War.* Springfield, Ill.: Charles C. Thomas, 1966.

Stephens, Robert Grier, Jr. *Intrepid Warrior: Clement Anselem Evans.* Dayton, Ohio: Morningside House, 1992.

Stickles, Arndt Mathias. *Simon Bolivar Buckner: Borderland Knight.* Chapel Hill: University of North Carolina Press, 1940.

Tankersley, Allen P. *John B. Gordon: A Study in Gallantry.* Atlanta: Whitehall Press, 1955.

Taylor, Richard. *Destruction and Reconstruction.* 1870. Reprint, New York: Time-Life Books, 1983.

Thomas, Emory M. *Bold Dragoon: The Life of J. E. B. Stuart*. New York: Harper & Row, 1986.

Thomas, John P. *Career and Character of General Micah Jenkins, C.S.A*. Columbia, S.C.: State Co., 1903.

Thompson, Edwin P. *History of the Orphan Brigade*. Louisville, Ky.: L. N. Thompson, 1898.

Thompson, Jerry. *Henry Hopkins Sibley: Confederate General of the West*. Natachitaoches, La.: Northwestern State University Press, 1987.

Trimble, Isaac Ridgeway. "The Civil War Diary of General Isaac Ridgeway Trimble." *Maryland Historical Magazine* 17 (1922): 1–20.

Tucker, Glenn. *Chickamauga: Bloody Battle of the West*. Dayton, Ohio: Press of Morningside Bookshop, 1976.

Tyler, Lyon Gardiner. *Encyclopedia of Virginia*. 5 vols. New York: Lewis Historical Publishing, 1915.

U.S. War Department. *The War of the Rebellion: A Compilation of the Official Records of the Union and Confederate Armies*. 128 vols. GPO: Washington, D.C., 1880–1901.

Vandiver, Frank Everson. *Ploughshares into Swords: Josiah Gorgas and Confederate Ordnance*. Austin: University of Texas Press, 1952.

———, ed. *The Civil War Diary of General Josiah Gorgas*. University: University of Alabama Press, 1947.

Vaughan, Alfred Jefferson. *Personal Record of the Thirteenth Regiment Tennessee Infantry*. Memphis: Press of South Carolina, TOOF & Co., 1897.

Von Borcke, Heros. *Memoirs of the Confederate War for Independence*. 2 vols. Dayton, Ohio: Morningside House, 1985.

Waddell, Jos. A. *Annals of Augusta County, Virginia with Reminiscences*. Richmond, Va.: J. W. Randalph and English, Publishers, 1888.

Walker, Charles D. *Memorial, Virginia Military Institute Biographical Sketches of the Graduates and Eleves of the Virginia Military Institute*. Philadelphia: J. B. Lippincott, 1875.

Warner, Ezra J. *Generals in Gray*. Baton Rouge: Louisiana State University Press, 1975.

———. "Who was General Tyler?" *Civil War Times Illustrated* 9 (October 1970): 15–19.

Watson, William. *Life in the Confederate Army*. 1888. Reprint, New York: Time-Life Books, 1983.

Welch, Spencer Glasgow. *A Confederate Surgeon's Letters to his Wife*. Marietta, Ga.: Continental Book Co., 1954.

Wellman, Manly Wade. *Giant in Gray: A Biography of Wade Hampton of South Carolina*. New York: Charles Scribner's Sons, 1949.

Williams, T. Harry. *P. G. T. Beauregard: Napoleon in Gray*. Baton Rouge: Louisiana State University Press, 1954.

Wills, Brian Steel. *A Battle from the Start*. New York: HarperCollins, 1992.

Wilson, Clyde N. *Carolina Cavalier: The Life and Mind of James Johnston Pettigrew*. Athens: University of Georgia Press, 1990.

Wingfield, Marshall. *General A. P. Stewart: His Life and Letters*. Memphis: West Tennessee Historical Society, 1954.

Wise, Barton H. *The Life of Henry A. Wise of Virginia, 1806–1876*. New York: Macmillan, 1899.

Woodward, Joseph Janvier. *Outlines of the Chief Camp Diseases of the United States Armies*. New York: Hafner Publishing, 1964.

Worshaw, John H. *One of Jackson's Foot Cavalry.* 1912. Reprint, New York: Time-Life Books, 1982.

Wyeth, John Allen. *Life of General N. B. Forrest.* New York: Harper and Brothers, 1899.

Wynne, James. "On the Disease Affecting the Inmates of the National Hotel at Washington, D.C." *American Medical Monthly* (N.Y.) 8 (1857): 347–58.

Young, Hugh H. "Two Texas Patriots." *Southwestern Historical Quarterly* 44 (1940): 16–32.

Newspapers

Alabama
    Anniston. *The Anniston Evening Star,* March 15, 27, April 1–4, 1901.
    Mobile. *Daily Register,* March 15, 1890.
Arkansas
    Little Rock. *Arkansas Gazette,* April 26, 1899.
California
    Oakland. *The Oakland Times,* June 30, 1909.
    San Francisco. *San Francisco Alta,* January 3, 1874; February 1–2, 1875.
Georgia
    Augusta. *Daily Chronicle and Constitutionalist,* April 10, 1881.
    Covington. *The Covington Star,* May 31, 1887.
    Gainesville. *The Gainesville News,* January 6, 1904.
    Milledgeville. *Southern Recorder,* March 6, 1866.
Louisiana
    New Orleans. *Daily Picayune,* February 16, 1870; June 14, 1872; April 22, August 22, 1876; April 13, August 3, 1879; August 30, 1880; June 22, 1891; December 13, 16, 1892; August 31, 1902; December 4, 1907; January 5, 7, 1912.
    Daily Crescent, September 20, 1866.
Maryland
    Baltimore. *Baltimore Sun,* July 4, 1912.
Mississippi
    Holly Springs. *Holly Springs South,* June 3, 1891.
    Vicksburg. *Vicksburg Herald,* May 29, 1908.
New York
    New York. *New York Daily Tribune,* February 10, 1896.
North Carolina
    Greensboro. *Greensboro Patriot,* February 10, 1892.
    Raleigh. *Raleigh News and Observer,* July 4, 1912.
    Shotwell. *Farmer and Mechanic,* August 19, 1880.
    Washington. *North State Press,* August 26, 1880.
    Wilmington. *Daily Journal,* March 26, 1867.
South Carolina
    Charleston. *Charleston Evening Post,* June 12, 1861.
Tennessee
    Columbia. *Maury Democrat,* December 8, 1892; April 6, 1893.
    Knoxville. *Free Press and Herald,* September 29, 1871.
    Memphis. *Commercial Appeal,* October 2, 1899.
        Daily Appeal, September 29, 1871; January 27, September 21, 1872; January 4, 1883.

Memphis Daily, September 14, 1883.
Memphis Press-Scimitar, March 11, 1927.
Public Ledger, January 11, 1870.

Texas
Austin. *Austin Daily Statesman,* January 13, 1885.
Dallas. *Dallas Morning News,* February 23, 1911; March 28, 1913.
Galveston. *Daily News,* February 21, 24, 1871.
News, September 28, 1876.
Houston. *Houston Daily Telegraph,* March 21, 22, 24, 1876.
Tri-Weekly Telegraph, February 21, April 19, 25, August 13, 1862; July 8, 15, 1863; June 13, 1864; April 10, 1865.
San Antonio. *Daily Express,* January 13, 1885.
Waco. *Daily Examiner,* March 21–22, 1976.

Virginia
Alexandria. *Gazette,* December 4, 1876.
Lynchburg. *The News,* April 22, 1865 (Extra Saturday Evening); March 3, 1894.
Richmond. *Times Dispatch,* August 12, 1914.

Washington, D.C.
Washington Post, June 4, 1912.